£80.00

D0267596

Inclusion-body myositis (IBM) is the term used to designate a form of chronic polymyositis in which biopsies show vacuolated muscle fibers containing filamentous inclusions in the cytoplasm and nuclei. The sporadic form is now recognized as the commonest muscle disease to strike those over 50, while the hereditary forms (h-IBMs), which affect younger patients, have many of the same morphologic features but lack mononuclear cell inflammation, hence the term inclusion-body "myopathy," instead of myositis. The possible etiopathological relationships of the different hereditary forms to one another, and to sporadic IBM, are discussed in this book, as are their differences.

This is the first book devoted entirely to the sporadic and hereditary IBMs. The editors and contributors are eminent clinicians and researchers, and experts in various aspects of IBM. The book covers in detail the clinical, pathological, electrophysiological, and therapeutic aspects, and provides a comprehensive review of recent advances in the major fields of IBM research. It aims to clarify the various issues, to gather the newest information to aid physicians in the diagnosis and management of IBM patients, and to help researchers in their efforts to understand the etiology and pathogenesis. It will appeal to clinicians in neurology, rheumatology and physical medicine, and to pathologists, electromyographers, immunologists, and researchers in neuromuscular disease.

INCLUSION-BODY MYOSITIS AND MYOPATHIES

INCLUSION-BODY MYOSITIS AND MYOPATHIES

Edited by

VALERIE ASKANAS, M.D., PH.D.

Neuromuscular Center, Good Samaritan Hospital, University of Southern California School of Medicine, Los Angeles, California

GEORGES SERRATRICE, M.D., F.R.C.P.

Service de Neurologie et des Maladies Neuromusculaires, Centre Hospitalo-Universitaire La Timone, Marseille, France

W. KING ENGEL, M.D.

Neuromuscular Center, Good Samaritan Hospital, University of Southern California School of Medicine, Los Angeles, California

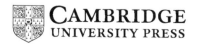
CAMBRIDGE
UNIVERSITY PRESS

PUBLISHED BY THE PRESS SYNDICATE OF THE UNIVERSITY OF CAMBRIDGE
The Pitt Building, Trumpington Street, Cambridge CB2 1RP, United Kingdom

CAMBRIDGE UNIVERSITY PRESS
The Edinburgh Building, Cambridge CB2 2RU, United Kingdom
40 West 20th Street, New York, NY 10011-4211, USA
10 Stamford Road, Oakleigh, Melbourne 3166, Australia

First published 1998

Printed in the United States of America

Typeset in Times Roman

Library of Congress Cataloging-in-Publication Data
Inclusion-body myositis and myopathies / [edited by] Valerie Askanas,
Georges Serratrice, W. King Engel.
p. cm.
Includes index.
ISBN 0-521-57105-7 (hardback)
1. Inclusion body myositis. I. Askanas, Valerie.
II. Serratrice, Georges. III. Engel, W. King.
[DNLM: 1. Myositis, Inclusion Body. WE 544 I37 1997]
RC935.M9I53   1997
616.7′ 43–dc20
DNLM/DLC
for Library of Congress   96-44919

A catalog record for this book is available from the British Library

ISBN 0 521 57105 7 hardback

This book is dedicated to Janine Serratrice, who touched the lives of all of us. We miss you, Janine.

Contents

Contributors

Gabrielle Åhlberg
Department of Neurology, Karolinska Sjukhuset, P.O. Box 130, S-171 76 Stockholm, Sweden

Renate B. Alvarez, M.S.
USC Neuromuscular Center, Department of Neurology, University of Southern California, School of Medicine, Good Samaritan Hospital, 637 South Lucas Avenue, Los Angeles, California 90017-1912, U.S.A.

Maria Anvret
Clinical Genetics, Karolinska Sjukhuset, P.O. Box 130 S-171 76 Stockholm, Sweden

Zohar Argov, M.D.
Hadassah Medical Organization, Service of Neurology, Neuromuscular Diseases, Kyriat Hadassah, Jerusalem 91120, Israel

Valerie Askanas, M.D., Ph.D.
USC Neuromuscular Center, Department of Neurology, University of Southern California, School of Medicine, Good Samaritan Hospital, 637 South Lucas Avenue, Los Angeles, California 90017-1912, U.S.A.

Jean-Phillippe Azulay, M.D.
Service de Neurologie, et des Maladies Neuromusculaires, CHU La Timone, 13385 Marseille cedex 5, France

Alex Baeta-Machado
Laboratoire d'Anatomie Pathologique, CHU La Timone, 13385 Marseille cedex 5, France

Samir Belal
Institut National de Neurologie, La Rabta 1007 Tunis, Tunisia

Christiane Ben Hamida
Institut National de Neurologie, La Rabta 1007 Tunis, Tunisia

Mongi Ben Hamida, M.D.
Institut National de Neurologie, La Rabta 1007 Tunis, Tunisia

Anke Bender
Department of Neuroimmunology, Max-Planck Institute of Psychiatry, Am Klopferspitz 18 A, D-82152 Martinsried, Germany

Françoise Billé-Turc, M.D.
Service de Neurologie, et des Maladies Neuromusculaires, CHU La Timone, 13385 Marseille cedex 5, France

Lori Blechynden
Australian Neuromuscular Research Institute, Queen Elizabeth II Medical Centre, Nedlands, 6009, Western Australia

Kristian Borg, M.D., Ph.D.
Department of Neurology, Karolinska Sjukhuset, P.O. Box 130, S-171 76 Stockholm, Sweden

Stirling Carpenter, M.D.
The Toronto Hospital, University of Toronto, Toronto, Ontario, Canada

Michèle Coquet, M.D.
Laboratoire de Néuropathologie, Hôpital Pellegrin, Place Amélie Raba Leéon, 33000 Bordeaux, France

Olivier Coquet
Laboratoire de Néuropathologie, Hôpital Pellegrin, Place Amélie Raba Léon, 33000 Bordeaux, France

Edward Cupler, M.D.
Neuromuscular Diseases Section, Medical Neurology Branch, National Institute of Neurological Disorders and Stroke, National Institutes of Health, Bethesda, Maryland 20892, U.S.A.

Marinos C. Dalakas, M.D.
National Institutes of Health, National Institute of Neurological Disorders and Stroke, NINCDS Bldg. 10, Room 4N248, 9000 Rockville Pike 10, Bethesda, Maryland 20892, U.S.A.

Claude Desnuelle, M.D.
Service de Neurologie, Laboratoire de Neurobiologie Cellulaire, Hôpital Pasteur, Avenue de la Voie Romaine – BP 69, 06002 Nice, France

Lars Edström, M.D.
Department of Neurology, Karolinska Sjukhuset, Neurologisca Kliniken, P.O. Box 130, S-171 76 Stockholm, Sweden

Andrew G. Engel, M.D.
Department of Neurology and Neuromuscular Research Laboratory, Guggenheim Building G 801, Mayo Clinic, Rochester, Minnesota 55905, U.S.A.

W. King Engel, M.D.
USC Neuromuscular Center, Department of Neurology, University of Southern California, School of Medicine, Good Samaritan Hospital, 637 South Lucas Avenue, Los Angeles, California 90017-1912, U.S.A.

Michel Fardeau, M.D.
INSERM U 153, 17, rue du Fer à Moulin, 75005 Paris, France

Xavier Ferrer
Service de Neurologie, Hôpital Pellegrin, Place Amélie Raba Léon, 33000 Bordeaux, France

Dominique Figarella-Branger, M.D.
Laboratoire d'Anatomie Pathologique, CHU La Timone, 13385 Marseille cedex 5, France

Michael J. Garlepp, Ph.D.
Australian Neuromuscular Research Institute, Queen Elizabeth II Medical Centre, Nedlands, 6009, Western Australia

Robert C. Griggs, M.D.
Department of Neurology, University of Rochester, School of Medicine, 601 Elmwood Avenue, Box 673, Rochester, New York 14642, U.S.A.

Faycal Hentati
Institut National de Neurologie, La Rabta 1007 Tunis, Tunisia

Reinhard Hohlfeld, M.D.
Ludwig-Maximilians-Universität München, Neurologische Klinik, Marchioninistr. 15, 81377 München, Germany

Elisabeth Holme
Göteborg University, Department of Clinical Chemistry, Sahlgrenska University Hospital, S-413 45 Göteborg, Sweden

Isabel Illa, M.D.
Neuromuscular Diseases Section, Medical Neurology Branch, National Institute of Neurological Disorders and Stroke, National Institute of Health, Bethesda, Maryland 10892, U.S.A.

Jean Julien
Service de Neurologie, Hôpital Pellegrin, Place Amélie Raba Léon, 33000 Bordeaux, France

Hannu Kalimo, M.D., Ph.D.
Department of Pathology, University Hospital of Turku, Turku, Finland

George Karpati, M.D., F.R.C.P.
Montreal Neurological Institute and Hospital, 3801 University Street, Montreal, Québec H3A 2B4, Canada

Cassandra Lawson
Australian Neuromuscular Research Institute, Queen Elizabeth II Medical Centre, Nedlands, 6009, Western Australia

Marta Leon-Monzon, Ph.D.
Neuromuscular Diseases Section, Medical Neurology Branch, National Institute of Neurological Disorders and Stroke, National Institutes of Health, Bethesda, Maryland 10892, U.S.A.

Christopher Lindberg, M.D.
Göteborg University, Department of Neurology, Sahlgrenska University Hospital, S-413 45 Göteborg, Sweden

Frank L. Mastaglia, M.D.
Australian Neuromuscular Research Institute, Queen Elizabeth II Medical Centre, Nedlands, 6009, Western Australia

Jerry R. Mendell, M.D.
Department of Neurology, Ohio State University, School of Medicine, 1654 Upham Drive, Room 473, Means Hall, Columbus, Ohio 43210, U.S.A.

Stella Mitrani-Rosenbaum, Ph.D.
Unit for Development for Molecular Biology, and Genetic Engineering, Hadassah University Hospital, Mount Scopus, Jerusalem, Israel

Ali-Reza Moslemi
Göteborg University, Department of Pathology, Sahlgrenska University Hospital, S-413 45 Göteborg, Sweden

Nobuyuki Murakami
National Institute of Neuroscience, National Center of Neurology and Psychiatry, Department of Ultrastructural Research, 4-1-1 Ogawahigashi-cho, Kodaira, Tokyo 187, Japan

Pekka Nokelainen, M.D.
Department of Human Molecular Genetics, National Public Health Institute, Helsinki, Finland

Ikuya Nonaka, M.D.
National Institute of Neuroscience, National Center of Neurology and Psychiatry, Department of Ultrastructural Research, 4-1-1 Ogawahigashi-cho, Kodaira, Tokyo 187, Japan

Anders Oldfors, M.D., Ph.D.
Göteborg University, Department of Pathology, Sahlgrenska University Hospital, S-143 45 Göteborg, Sweden

Véronique Paquis
Laboratoire de Neurobiologie Cellulaire, Hôpital Pasteur, Avenue de la Voie Romaine – BP 69, 06002 Nice, France

Rachel Paul
Laboratoire de Neurobiologie Cellulaire, Hôpital Pasteur, Avenue de la Voie Romaine – BP 69, 06002 Nice, France

Jean François Pellissier, M.D.
Laboratoire d' Anatomie Pathologique, CHU La Timone, 13385 Marseille cedex 5, France

Jean Pouget, M.D.
Service de Neurologie, et des Maladies Neuromuscularies, CHU La Timone, 13385 Marseille cedex 5, France

Giovanni Putzu
Laboratoire d'Anatomie Pathologique, CHU La Timone, 13385 Marseille cedex 5, France

Michael Rose, M.D.
Department of Neurology, University of Rochester, School of Medicine, 601 Elmwood Avenue, Box 673, Rochester, New York 14642, U.S.A.

Menachem Sadeh
Department of Neurology, Sheba Medical Center, and Sackler School of Medicine, Tel Hashomer, Israel

Eijiro Satoyoshi, M.D.
National Institute of Neuroscience, National Center of Neurology and Psychiatry, 4-1-1 Ogawahigashi-cho, Kodaira, Tokyo 187, Japan

Anne Saunières
Service de Neurologie, Hôpital Pasteur, Avenue de la Voie Romaine – BP 69, 06002 Nice, France

Georges Serratrice, M.D., F.R.C.P.
Service de Neurologie, et des Maladies Neuromuscularies, CHU La Timone, 13385 Marseille cedex 5, France

Hannu Somer, M.D., Ph.D.
Department of Neurology, University of Helsinki, Helsinki, Finland

Nobuhiko Sunohara
National Institute of Neuroscience, National Center of Neurology and Psychiatry, 4-1-1 Ogawahigashi-cho, Kodaira, Tokyo 187, Japan

Yume Suzuki
National Institute of Neuroscience, National Center of Neurology and Psychiatry, Department of Ultrastructural Research, 4-1-1 Ogawahigashi-cho, Kodaira, Tokyo 187, Japan

Hyacinth Tabarias
Australian Neuromuscular Research Institute, Queen Elizabeth II Medical Centre, Nedlands, 6009, Western Australia

Fernando Tomé, M.D.
INSERM U 153, 17, rue du Fer à Moulin, 75005 Paris, France

Bjarne Udd, M.D., Ph.D.
Department of Neurology, Vasa Central Hospital, 65130 Vasa, Finland

Frank van Bockxmeer
Department of Biochemistry, Royal Perth Hospital, Perth, Australia

Claude Vital, M.D.
Laboratoire de Néuropathologie, Hôpital Pellegrin, Place Amélie Raba Léon, 33000 Bordeaux, France

Preface

Sporadic inclusion-body myositis (s-IBM) is a great challenge for neurologists, rheumatologists, immunologists, geneticists, gerontologists, internists, pathologists, and electrophysiologists. Previously considered uncommon, s-IBM is now recognized as the most common muscle disease beginning over the age of 50 years. It was first described more than 20 years ago. During the past two decades, increasingly detailed observations have been reported concerning the clinical, pathological and immunological aspects, and various hypotheses have been put forward regarding the etiology and pathogenesis. In spite of the evolving information and concepts, no drug is yet able to provide completely satisfactory treatment of s-IBM, although some forms of treatment can produce slight to moderate benefit.

Hereditary inclusion-body myopathies (h-IBMs) have many of the same morphologic and chemo-morphologic changes in the muscle fiber seen in s-IBM, but the hereditary forms lack mononuclear-cell inflammation. h-IBMs can be inherited in either an autosomal recessive or dominant fashion. h-IBM has been seen especially in certain ethnic groups; however, with greater awareness it is likely that h-IBMs will be identified in various other ethnic groups. Now considered as forms of h-IBMs are conditions that previously have been designated as quadriceps-sparing vacuolar myopathy of Persian Jews, distal myopathy with rimmed vacuoles of the Japanese, Welander distal myopathy among the Swedish, and Finnish distal myopathy (thus, several "distal myopathies" are actually h-IBM). The first genetic linkage for autosomal-recessive h-IBM in the first two groups has recently been found. The possible etio-pathogenic relationship of the different hereditary forms to one another and to s-IBM are discussed here, as are the differences.

This book on sporadic and hereditary IBM arises from the need to clarify various issues and definitions, to gather the newest information to aid physicians in the diagnosis and management of IBM patients, and to help researchers in their efforts to understand the etiology and pathogenesis. The newly developed phenotypic in vitro model of IBM produced by gene transfer is also described. The authors of the chapters in this book are all experts in various aspects of IBM.

Part I is devoted to general considerations and definitions of s-IBM and h-IBM. It also includes a detailed comparison of the chemomorphologic changes in muscle of s-IBM and h-IBM, as well as comparison with Alzheimer brain, with which there are remarkable similarities. There is an updated classification of the various forms of h-IBM. The model of IBM produced by gene transfer is presented.

Part II is devoted to evolving concepts of the IBMs, including an historical perspective.

Part III is devoted to s-IBM. It includes, among other topics, issues related to the natural history of the disease, uncommon clinico-pathologic forms of s-IBM, electrophysiologic findings, and the question of possible genetic predisposition to s-IBM.

Part IV is devoted entirely to the h-IBMs. These different forms occurring in various ethnic groups are described in detail, as is the first genetic linkage in an autosomal-recessive form.

Part V covers special aspects of s-IBM and the h-IBMs. These include inflammation, muscle-fiber nuclear abnormalities, the possible presence of viruses, and mitochondrial abnormalities.

The book concludes in Part VI with consideration of various treatment approaches to s-IBM.

Accordingly, this first book on the IBMs is a comprehensive review of the recent advances in the major fields of IBM research. The volume will be of interest to clinicians in neurology, rheumatology, and physical medicine, and to pathologists, electromyographers, immunologists, and researchers interested in various aspects of neuromuscular diseases.

It is our expectation that this book, containing the latest information presented by eminent clinicians and researchers, not only will serve to disseminate the current knowledge of the IBMs and the diagnosis and management of IBM patients, but will also provide the basis for further clinical and laboratory research studies of sporadic and hereditary IBM.

Valerie Askanas
Georges Serratrice
W. King Engel

Part I

Overview of Pathologic and Pathogenic Comparisions Between Sporadic Inclusion-Body Myositis and Hereditary Inclusion-Body Myopathies

1

Newest Approaches to Diagnosis and Pathogenesis of Sporadic Inclusion-Body Myositis and Hereditary Inclusion-Body Myopathies, including Molecular-Pathologic Similarities to Alzheimer Disease

VALERIE ASKANAS AND W. KING ENGEL

Introduction

The term "inclusion-body myositis" was introduced by Yunis and Samaha (1) in 1971 to designate a subset of chronic polymyositis patients whose biopsies showed, in addition to inflammation, vacuolated muscle fibers containing characteristic filamentous inclusions in the cytoplasm and nuclei. Since that time, *sporadic inclusion-body myositis (s-IBM)* has received considerable attention, and several previous reports have described its unique clinical and pathologic features (2–4).

More recently it has become apparent that there are, in various ethnic groups, hereditary muscle diseases that also have vacuolated muscle fibers containing filamentous inclusions, but do not show inflammation in the biopsy. To emphasize (i) the similarities of these hereditary myopathies to s-IBM, and (ii) their lack of inflammation, we have introduced the term *hereditary inclusion-body myopathy (h-IBM)* (5).

These s-IBM and h-IBM diseases, formerly under-diagnosed and considered to be infrequent, are now being identified more and more often by clinicians and pathologists. Recent interest in s-IBM and the h-IBMs has been generated by the identification, within IBM muscle fibers, of congophilia (6) and other striking pathologic features that had not been thought to occur in diseased human muscle. These features include abnormal accumulation of β-amyloid protein (7), two other epitopes of the β-amyloid precursor protein (8), hyperphosphorylated tau (9), $a_1$antichymotrypsin (10), apolipoprotein E (ApoE) (11), ubiquitin (12), and cellular prion protein (13). Accumulations of these proteins were previously considered strictly neuronal and characteristic of Alzheimer disease and prion brain diseases. In the IBMs, increased accumulation of the β-amyloid precursor protein (βAPP) and prion protein (PrP) results, at least partially, from their increased synthesis (14,15). (Moreover, increased synthesis of cellular PrP has not previously been reported in any human disease.)

In addition, it has become apparent that the "tubulofilamentous" structures, which accumulate in groups that by light microscopy appear as "inclusions" in both s- and h-IBMs, are twisted (9). They actually are *paired-helical filaments (PHFs),* which closely resemble the PHFs of Alzheimer-disease (AD) brain and, like AD-brain PHFs, the IBM PHFs contain hyperphosphorylated tau (9). The demonstration in IBM muscle of several proteins and structures previously considered brain-specific is of great interest and, hypothetically, may suggest that: 1) their accumulation in brain and muscle diseases might result from a cascade of similar pathogenic steps shared by the different cell-types, possibly initiated by different causes; 2) the aberrant expression of those proteins may co-depend on, and be a manifestation of, a specific *aging phenomenon* similar in muscle and brain; and 3) different etiologic factors might up-regulate the same *master-pathogenic gene* whose overexpressed protein is a transcription factor (e.g., for βAPP and for PrP) that, in the IBMs, leads to specific muscle-fiber deterioration. Experimental support for these hypotheses e.g., by βAPP gene-transfer, is presented below.

In this chapter we will concentrate on major new advances that are a) leading to better diagnosis, and b) facilitating the search for the pathogenic mechanisms(s) of s-IBM and the h-IBMs. (When the term "IBMs" is used here, it includes both s-IBM and the h-IBMs.)

I. Diagnostic Approaches to Sporadic Inclusion-Body Myositis and the Hereditary Inclusion-Body Myopathies

1. Sporadic inclusion-body myositis (s-IBM)

a) General clinical features

s-IBM is the most common muscle disease beginning in patients over age 50, and it occurs predominantly in men. The muscle weakness is distal and proximal. There is a characteristic thinning of the forearm muscles associated with weakness of the finger extensors and/or flexors (especially flexor digitorum profundus). Typically, the quadriceps is prominently involved (reviews: 16,17; Chapter 3, this volume). There is also distal lower-limb weakness, which can appear early, and proximal weakness of all limbs. The slowly progressive course usually leads to severe disability and eventually to respiratory-muscle weakness. Dysphagia is fairly common; it can appear during the limb-muscle weakness or sometimes precede it (18). In older patients with dysphagia, s-IBM should be included in the differential diagnosis, and it can be diagnosed on the basis of the characteristic limb-muscle biopsy abnormalities (described below).

Since 1993 we have been following a post-polio patient with a progressive muscle-weakness syndrome consisting of typical IBM pathology in the muscle biopsy (she experienced sustained, moderate improvement on a regimen of 20 mg alternate-day prednisone, and had further improvement with L-carnitine 1 gm/day plus coenzyme Q_{10} 100 mg/day) (W.K. Engel and V. Askanas, unpublished data). Other patients with a post-polio syndrome and IBM pathology have been described (18,20). Not known is whether the previous poliomyelitis virus infection predisposed to development of s-IBM, nor is it known if there is poliovirus genome in those post-polio IBM vacuolated muscle fibers.

An unusual presentation of s-IBM was described in a 70-year-old patient who had weakness of only the paravertebral muscles, and in them the characteristic IBM pathology (21). Two patients were reported with pathologically characteristic IBM along with renal-cell carcinoma (22). Other IBM patients with atypical clinical presentations have recently been described (19).

Recently we had an Iranian patient with s-IBM and blood positive for HTLV-I antibody-immunoblot and antigen-PCR (19a). That patient was referred to us from Iran because h-IBM is very prominent among Iranian Jews (discussed below). However, he came from an HTLV-I-endemic region in Iran, was Muslim not Jewish, and did not have a family history of h-IBM. His muscle biopsy revealed pronounced inflammation and expression of the full spectrum of the s-IBM pathologic phenotype. Monoclonal anti-HTLVI antibody revealed definite sarcolemmal immunoreactivity in some of his muscle fibers (W.K. Engel, K. Haginoya, R.B. Alvarez et al., in press). Whether the HTLV-I retrovirus is causing his s-IBM is not certain, but that possibility is being studied.

There is no completely successful treatment for s-IBM, and none for the h-IBMs. In our experience, most s-IBM patients have some benefit from prednisone (20–60 mg, single-dose on alternate-days) (16,23). The benefit can be modest to moderate, but for some patients there is quite a significant and useful improvement of muscle strength and especially *endurance* (note that clinical quantitation of muscle power usually does not evaluate endurance). Occasional patients have benefited from oral cyclophosphamide (2 mg/kg/day) or total-body irradiation (23). With sustained drug treatment we have found that the benefit can persist for 6 months to 5 years (and sometimes longer), but normal strength is not restored. Similar benefits, although denied by a number of authors, were recently reported by others (24,25). Treatment with in-travenous immunoglobulin (IVIG) was reported to benefit 3 of 4 s-IBM patients (26). That result was not confirmed by another trial in 7 patients (27). In our experience, some s-IBM patients have definite and repro-ducible improvement in muscle function from repeated 5-day courses of IVIG (0.4 gm/kg/day). We have suggested (23) that anti-dysimmune treatment of s-IBM might be benefiting only the inflammatory-myopathy component, not the vacuolar-myopathy or denervation com-ponents (discussed below). Some of our s-IBM patients report increased strength and endurance when given the combination of L-carnitine 1 gm 3–5 times daily, plus coenzyme Q_{10} 100 mg 3–5 times daily; such benefit may relate to the mitochondrial abnormalities present in s-IBM.

b) Light-microscopic histochemistry and ultrastructure of s-IBM muscle biopsies

The light-microscopic pathologic features include: a) degrees of mononu-clear-cell inflammation varying from abundant in the early stages to little or none in the later stages; muscle fibers with one or several irregular, various-sized vacuoles (on a given 10-μm-thick cross-section), which are more common in the middle and later stages of the disease. In the past, s-IBM has often been referred to as a myopathy with "red-rimmed vacu-oles." However, in our recent review of more than 40 s-IBM muscle biopsies stained with the Engel-Gomori trichrome method (28), it was apparent that the majority of the vacuoles were not red-rimmed; some of the vacuoles contained interior reddish or grayish-purple material, and some appeared empty. Only a minority of the vacuoles were truly red-rimmed (Figures 1.1A,B, following page 104).

Small angular muscle fibers that are histochemically dark with the pan-esterase and NADH–tetrazolium reductase reactions are considered indicative of a recent-denervation component; these are also a charac-teristic feature of s-IBM muscle (5) (Figure 1.1C).

The mononuclear inflammatory cells are similar to those in polymyositis, being mainly CD8$^+$ cytotoxic T cells (29). In both diseases, macrophages comprise approximately 20–30% of the mononuclear cells surrounding or invading non-necrotic muscle fibers, while within necrotic fibers macrophages comprise 80% of the invading cells (29). Recently, in 2 patients with long-lasting common variable immunodeficiency and IBM, the inflammatory cells had an increased proportion of natural-killer (NK) CD8$^-$ cells (30). Because the vacuoles can be very small and sometimes are present in only a few muscle fibers, s-IBM, especially in its early stages, can be difficult to distinguish from polymyositis by routine histochemistry. In many countries, s-IBM probably is underdiagnosed; this has recently been emphasized in Great Britain (31).

To help differentiate s-IBM from polymyositis on the basis of light microscopy of fresh-frozen sections, we recommend the following:

1. Engel-Gomori trichrome staining (28) to visualize vacuolated muscle fibers and mononuclear-cell inflammation.
2. Fluorescence-enhanced Congo-red staining (Figures 1.1C–F and 1.2C–F) (32) or nonfluorescent crystal-violet staining for small (or large) foci of amyloid within some of the vacuolated fibers.
3. Alkaline phosphatase reaction to evaluate perimysial connective-tissue staining (typically negative or low in s-IBM, but usually prominent in polymyositis) (Figure 1.2A,B) (23; W.K. Engel and V. Askanas, unpublished data).
4. Immunocytochemical staining for the presence of PHFs, utilizing SMI-31 monoclonal antibody (originally made to react with phosphorylated heavy-chain neurofilament), which recognizes the phosphorylated tau of PHFs in both s-IBM and the h-IBMs (33) (Figure 1.1G) (details below).

Ragged-red fibers (RRFs), originally identified and named (34) on the basis of Engel-Gomori trichrome staining (28), are important indicators of abnormal mitochondria in human muscle biopsies. RRFs are present in virtually all s-IBM muscle biopsies (16,35,36; Chapters 21 and 22, this volume).

Cytochrome-c-oxidase negative muscle fibers, ultrastructurally abnormal mitochondria containing paracrystalline inclusions (16,35; Chapters 21 and 22, this volume), and multiple mitochondrial-DNA (mtDNA) deletions are also characteristic pathologic features of s-IBM pathology. It has not yet been established with certainty how the s-IBM deletions differ from the mtDNA deletions occurring with "normal" aging; never-

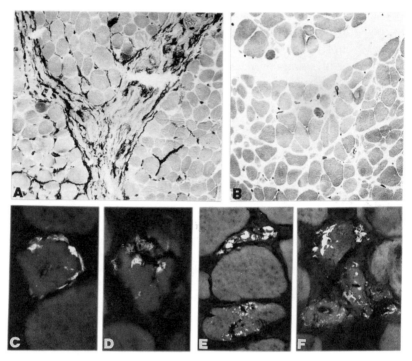

Figure 1.2. Light microscopy of alkaline phosphatase reaction demonstrates strong staining of the perimysial connective tissue in polymyositis (A), whereas in s-IBM muscle the perimysial connective tissue is negative (B). Individual regenerating muscle fibers are positive in both polymyositis and s-IBM (A and B, ×300). C–F: Examples of Congo-red positivity in s-IBM vacuolated muscle fibers, visualized through Texas-red filters (C and D, ×1,320; E and F, ×600).

theless, RRFs are more common in IBM muscle than in same-vintage, "normally aged" muscle without IBM (35; Chapter 22, this volume).

The ultrastructural diagnostic criterion for s-IBM is the presence of cytoplasmic PHFs measuring 15–21 nm, often in clusters ("inclusions") (9) (Figure 1.3). The appearance of PHFs depends greatly on the tissue preparation. In ultra thin sections cut from muscle previously fixed and embedded in a routine manner for electron-microscopic studies, filamentous inclusions appear tubular and may display clear periodicity (Figures 1.3 and 1.4A). However, in ultra thin sections cut from epon-embedded 10-μm cryostat sections of a previously frozen muscle (a technique we routinely use for ultrastructural immunocytochemistry) (7–9), IBM tubulofilaments clearly display a paired helical structure (Figure 1.4B) (9). Our recent studies employing a goniometry stage (R. Alvarez and V.

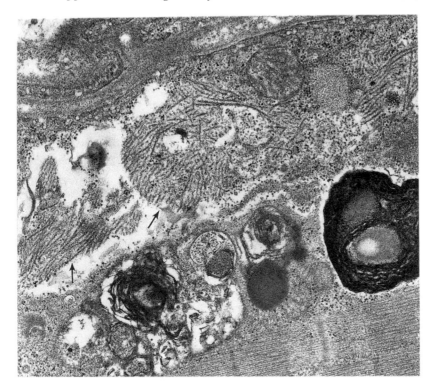

Figure 1.3. Electron microscopy of a portion of an s-IBM vacuolated muscle fiber, routinely fixed and embedded for electron microscopy. In the upper region, there are clusters of 15–21-nm paired helical filaments (PHFs) (arrows), and below there are various lysosomal inclusions including myelin-like whorls (×26,500).

Askanas, unpublished data) demostrated that each tubulofilament is twisted. The widest diameter of IBM PHFs is 15–21 nm, and their twist repeats occur every 40–55 nm. The molecular properties of IBM PHFs and their comparisons with AD PHFs are listed in Table 1.1.

s-IBM vacuolated muscle-fiber cytoplasm also contains collections of 6–10-nm filaments (Figure 1.4C) (7–9), as well as fine flocculomembranous and amorphous material (7,8). Myelin-like whorls and various other lysosomal debris are also present (Figure 1.3).

In s-IBM nuclei there are clusters (inclusions) of 15–21-nm "tubulofilaments" (Figure 1.5), which in favorable sections are also seen to be PHFs (Figure 1.5A,B). Occasionally those filaments may entirely fill a nucleus (Figure 1.5C). Table 1.2 summarizes the most characteristic light- and electron-microscopic features of the s-IBM pathology phenotype.

Table 1.1.

Pathologic aspect	IBM PHFs	AD PHFs
A. Paired helical filaments:		
Widest diameter, nm	15–21	15–22 or 27–34 (depending on tissue prep)
Twist repeat, nm	40–55	65–80
B. Hyper-phosphorylated Tau:		
Antibodies . . .		
Alz-50	+	+
PHF-1	+	+
Tau-1, after dephosphorylation	+	+
AT8	+	+
SMI-31	+	+
SMI-310	+	?
C. Ubiquitin	+	+
D. β-amyloid protein (Aβ)	0	0
E. ApoE	+	+
F. Prion	+	0

All normal proteins situated in a nucleus have been synthesized on ribosomes in the cytoplasm and then move, by virtue of their nucleus-targeting sequences, through the nuclear pores into the nucleoplasm. Inside the nucleus each normal protein has a finite lifetime until it is catabolized (turned over). Normal nuclear proteins include ones having transcription functions and ones having structural functions. Pathologic accumulations of a protein or proteins in nuclei, as occurs in the IBMs, can result from defective control, such as: i) excessive expression; ii) increased transport into the nuclei of a protein that is normally there, or perhaps one not normally there (due to pathologic acquisition of a nucleus-targeting sequence); iii) decreased intranuclear turnover; or iv) "trapping" in pathologic configuration (e.g., the tubulofilament/PHF structures) due to a mechanism (e.g., hyperphosphorylation or glycation, or association with an accessory protein, such as ApoE) that pathologically dis-configures and/or causes pathologic assembly of the accumulated protein(s). Our idea is that the nuclear phenomenon causing the tubulofilaments/PHFs in the IBMs might be parallel to a similar, but yet undefined, pathologic mechanism in the cytoplasm; such a parallelism has been postulated for nuclear rods in adult-onset rod disease of muscle (37,38). (Pathologic accumulations of protein inclusions in nuclei of virus-infested cells are well known, presumably caused by one of the aforementioned mechanisms.)

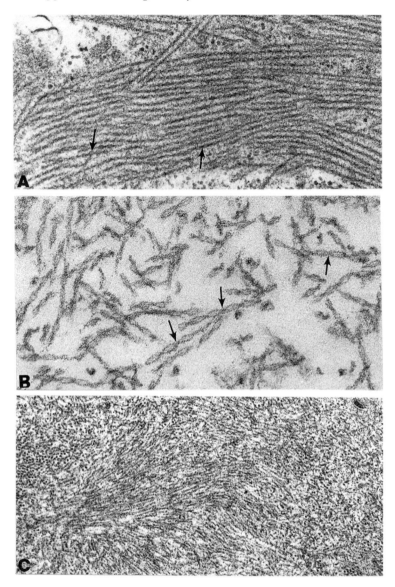

Figure 1.4. Electron microscopy of filamentous inclusions in s-IBM. A: Distinct periodicity and some twists (arrows) are evident in the collection of PHFs in a muscle biopsy routinely fixed and embedded for electron microscopy (×50,000). B: The PHFs display a distinct paired-helical filament pattern (arrows) in a muscle biopsy that was first frozen and subsequently 10-μm cryostat-cut sections of it incubated in phosphate buffered saline (PBS) for 24 hours at 4°C before being fixed and embedded for electron-microscopic studies (×100,000). C: A cluster of many 6–10-nm filaments shows their typical appearance, in both routinely processed and previously frozen specimens (×26,500).

Table 1.2. *Pathologic phenotype of sporadic inclusion-body myositis (s-IBM)*

Vacuolated muscle fibers (VMFs)	+
Inflammation	+
Congo-red positivity within VMFs	+
Ragged-red fibers	+
Cytochrome-c-oxidase-negative muscle-fibers	+
Cytoplasmic paired-helical filaments, 15–21 nm diameter	+
Nuclear paired helical filaments, 15–21 nm diameter	+
Clusters of cytoplasmic 6–10 nm filaments, tightly or loosely packed	+
Various mitochondrial abnormalities, including enlargement, paracyrstalline inclusions, disorganized cristae, and "mushy" matrix	+

Our recent studies of s-IBM muscle biopsies double-labeled with SMI-31 (to visualize PHFs) and with Hoechst reagent (to visualize nuclear DNA) indicate that only a very small percentage of SMI-31-positive inclusions co-localize with the DNA in nuclei (K. Haginoya and V. Askanas, unpublished data). In our opinion, the hypothesis presented by Karpati and Carpenter (ch. 19, this volume) that all s-IBM cytoplasmic PHFs originate in abnormal nuclei seems unlikely. We favor that their genesis is parallel in nuclei and cytoplasm, as noted above.

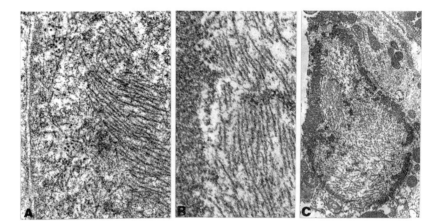

Figure 1.5. Electron microscopy of nuclear PHFs in s-IBM. A and B: The twisted appearance of some PHFs is clearly visible. C: Low-power electron-micrograph demonstrating a nucleus that is virtually completely filled with PHFs (A, ×43,000; B, ×54,000; C, ×9,000).

2. Hereditary inclusion-body myopathies (h-IBMs)

a) Summary of various forms

The h-IBMs encompass several syndromes with very similar muscle pathology but somewhat different clinical manifestations, ages of onset, and genetic patterns. They can be inherited as an autosomal-recessive or autosomal-dominant trait (reviews: 5,16). The exact genetic loci are not yet identified, but in the quadriceps-sparing form among Persian Jews and among other ethnic groups, a linkage to chromosome 9 has recently been reported (see below). The h-IBMs that are inherited differently are likely to be caused by different abnormal genes. It is now known that not all forms having the same mode of inheritance (e.g., autosomal-recessive) are genetically the same. We have proposed in 1995 (16) that the autosomal-recessive IBM of Persian Jews and the quadriceps-sparing Japanese distal myopathy may be the same entity. This has now been confirmed because both groups link to the same locus on chromosome 9p1-q1 (43,43a).

The h-IBMs have many histochemical and ultrastructural abnormalities (described below) similar to those of s-IBM, but characteristically they lack inflammation in the muscle biopsy. (In some patients with autosomal-dominant IBM, a degree of inflammation has been reported (39); we and others have not seen that phenomenon, which might have been produced by recent electromyographic needling or mimicked by foci of phagocytosis.) To emphasize the hereditary aspect and lack of inflammation, we introduced the term "hereditary inclusion-body myopathy" (5). Detailed morphologic differences between s- and h-IBMs are described below and summarized in Tables 1.3 and 1.4.

A. Autosomal-recessive forms of h-IBM

1. Persian (Iranian) Jews. These comprise a distinct subgroup of h-IBM patients, with clinical onset in the second or third decade, or earlier, characterized by progressive lower- and upper-limb muscle weakness (40–42; Chapters 10 and 11, this volume). Distal muscles of the legs are affected early, followed by proximal weakness involving the iliopsoas, hamstring, adductor, and gluteal muscles. The most characteristic feature is relative sparing of the quadriceps muscle (40,42). The lower limbs are affected more severely than the upper limbs. The cranial-nerve muscles usually are not involved, but one of our otherwise typical patients has definite unilateral ptosis (his ptosis and hand weakness respond to edrophonium and pyridostigmine treatment, even though all the other tests to

Table 1.3. *Pathologic phenotype of sporadic inclusion-body myositis (S-IBM), recessive inclusion-body myopathy (R-IBM), and dominant inclusion-body myopathy (D-IBM)*

Pathologic phenotype	S-IBM	R-IBM	D-IBM
Similarities			
Vacuolated muscle fibers (VMFs)	+	+	+
Cytoplasmic paired helical filaments, 15–21 nm diameter	+	+	+
Nuclear paired helical filaments, 15–21 nm diameter	+	+	+
Clusters of cytoplasmic 6–10 nm filaments, tightly or loosely packed	+	+	+
Differences			
Mononuclear-cell inflammation	+	−	−
Congo-red positivity within VMFs	+	− (+[a])	− (+[b])
Ragged-red fibers	+	−	−
Cytochrome-c-oxidase-negative muscle-fibers	+	−	− (+[c])
Various mitochondrial abnormalities, including enlargement, paracrystalline inclusions, disorganized cristae, and "mushy" matrix	+	−	−

[a]In less than 10% of VMFs in 20% of patients
[b]In less than 40% of VMFs
[c]In 2 of 3 patients, 2–5 per biopsy-section

define myasthenia gravis have been negative); our other h-IBM patients have not responded to pyridostigmine treatment.

The parents of these Persian Jewish h-IBM patients are often related (first cousins, frequently). Sometimes there is a "pseudodominant" pattern (e.g., when affected children issue from an affected person married to a cousin who is a carrier) (W. K. Engel and V. Askanas, unpublished data). There are also seemingly sporadic Persian Jewish patients, but their disease could be autosomal-recessive; muscle biopsies of such patients can have the features typical of recessive h-IBM. The abnormal gene has not yet been identified, but linkage to chromosome 9p1-q1 has recently been reported (43; Chapter 11, this volume).

2. Japanese hereditary distal myopathy with rimmed vacuoles. Utilizing a recent review (44), we calculate that autosomal-recessive patients comprise 37% of the Japanese patients having "distal myopathy with rimmed vacuoles" (reviews: 44; Chapter 15, this volume). The onset is in the second or third decade, manifested by weakness mainly of the distal leg muscles,

Table 1.4. *Abnormal accumulation of proteins and their mRNAs*

	Protein			mRNA		
	S-IBM	R-IBM	D-IBM	S-IBM	R-IBM	D-IBM
β-amyloid precursor protein (βAPP, all epitopes)	+	+	+	+	+	+
Prion	+	+	+	+	+	+
Apolipoprotein E	+	+[a]	+[b]	−	−	−
Phosphorylated tau . . . antibody positivity:				−		
• PHF-1	+	+[c]	+[d]			
• SMI-31	+	+	+			
• SMI-310	+	−	−(+[e])			

[a]diffuse staining.
[b]rounded single inclusions.
[c]slight, diffuse staining.
[d]multiple small inclusions, and diffuse.
[e]in less than 20% of VMFs.

followed in a few years by proximal muscle weakness in both lower and upper limbs. Similarly to h-IBM of Persian Jews, the quadriceps muscle was reported to be spared in several Japanese patients (44), and in all the Japanese patients the gastrocnemius and quadriceps muscles were less affected than other muscles (44). In 11% of the Japanese patients without a family history, "consanguinity" was reported, suggesting that their disease might also be autosomal-recessive (44). Muscle biopsies of the Japanese autosomal-recessive patients (review: 44) have the characteristic h-IBM pathology, including: vacuoles; nuclear and cytoplasmic tubulofilamentous inclusions (perhaps these would be seen as PHFs if a different electron microscopic technique would be used); and lack of inflammation. Moreover, "IBM-characteristic" proteins are accumulated in the vacuoles of the Japanese patients (45). In addition, recent studies demonstrated the same 9p1-q1 gene linkage in Japanese patients (43a) as has been reported in Persian Jews (43), confirming what we previously postulated (16), viz. that both ethnic groups have basically the same form of h-IBM.

3. Other forms. Two Mexican brothers of Spanish heritage, whose parents are first cousins, have quadriceps-sparing h-IBM of autosomal-recessive inheritance and muscle-biopsies typical of h-IBM (48; W. K. Engel, V. Askanas, and M. Fardeau, unpublished data). In them the same 9p1q1 genetic linkage recently has been identified (48a). The same 9p1q1 genetic linkage has been identified in other ethnic groups with quadriceps sparing h-IBM (43b), however, our pseudodominant quadriceps sparing Persian Jewish family did not link to this locus (48a).

A Tunisian kindred with a vacuolar neuromuscular disorder, quadriceps sparing, autosomal-recessive inheritance, and symptomatic leukoencephalopathy was reported (46; Chapter 12, this volume). Also described was a kindred having asymptomatic periventricular leukoencephalopathy, but not quadriceps sparing (47). This kindred did not link to chromosome 9p1q1 (43b).

B. Autosomal-dominant forms of h-IBM

1. Welander distal myopathy. This myopathy occurs almost exclusively in Sweden. It was described by Welander in 1951 on the basis of 249 patients from 72 pedigrees (49; Chapter 13, this volume). The clinical onset most commonly is in the third or fourth decade, with symmetrical distal weakness of hand muscles, mainly of the finger extensors (49,50). Eventually the lower limbs also become involved, especially distally (50). Muscle biopsies have the features typical of the h-IBMs (50,51), (described below).

2. Finnish tibial muscular dystrophy. These patients have onset of muscle weakness in the third decade, manifesting severe weakness of the tibialis anterior, causing pronounced foot-drop (52,53; Chapter 14, this volume). Even though red-rimmed vacuoles were described in 28% of the 32 muscle biopsies, tubulofilaments (or PHFs) were not reported. Because often it is quite difficult to find tubulofilaments/PHFs during routine electronmicroscopic examination, especially when the vacuoles are sparse, they should be searched for more extensively by using a recently described electronmicroscopic technique (54), as well as the light-microscopic immunocytochemical technique utilizing the SMI-31 antibody (33).

3. Other examples
a) We have been studying muscle biopsies of three Chicago siblings who have progressive lower- and upper-limb muscle weakness (56). Their father and a paternal cousin also have a similar neuromuscular disorder but have not yet been biopsied. The siblings' muscle biopsies show a pattern characteristic of h-IBM (e.g., vacuoles and lack of inflammation); however, they also show some features (de-

scribed below) of the s-IBM phenotype that are not present in autosomal-recessive forms. (see Tables 1.3 and 1.4)

b) Mainly proximal muscle weakness of both lower and upper limbs was described in two generations of a family from Denver (39). The onset of muscle weakness was in the second or third decade, and the typical h-IBM pathology was present.

c) Other patients with distal myopathy of probable autosomal-dominant inheritance and vacuolated muscle fibers were described in the United States (55). It will be important to revisit their muscle biopsies to seek PHFs.

Our newest classification of h-IBM is presented in Table 1.5.

b) Light-microscopic histochemistry and ultrastructure of the h-IBMs.

In the literature, rimmed vacuoles demonstrable by Engel-Gomori trichrome staining (28), small angular muscle fibers, and lack of inflammation are the typical light-microscopy features described in h-IBM muscle biopsies. Ultrastructural descriptions are less consistent, probably because of differences in techniques and investigators' experience.

Table 1.5. *Classification of hereditary inclusion-body myopathies*

A. Autosomal Recessive, R-IBM
  1. "Quadriceps Spared"
    a. R1a-Chromosome 9p1-q1. Gene = ?
      • Persian (Iranian) Jews
      • Afghani Jews
      • India family
      • Japanese
      • Mexican family
      • Others
    b. R1b-Chromosome ? (Not 9p1-q1). Gene = ?
      • Persian (Iranian) Jewish family – pseudo-dominant (cousin-marriage)
  2. Quadriceps Not-Spared
    a. R2-IBM – Chromosome ?. Gene = ?
      • French-Canadian family, with central nervous system abnormality
      • Others

B. Autosomal Dominant, D-IBM
      • Swedish "distal myopathy"
      • Finnish "tibial muscular dystrophy"
      • Denver family
      • Chicago family
      • Los Angeles, Mexican family
      • Others

In our Center, we have studied muscle biopsies of 38 patients representing several families with autosomal-recessive and autosomal dominant IBM. None of the biopsies showed inflammation. Usually they lack congophilic (or crystal-violet-positive) amyloid. Although some vacuoles are thinly red-rimmed or contain red material demonstrated on Engel-Gomori trichrome staining like in s-IBM, most of the vacuoles, especially in the Persian Jews' biopsies, are large and often appear "empty" Figure 1.6A (following page 104). Pan-esterase-positive small angular muscle fibers, considered indicative of recent denervation, are prominent in all the h-IBM biopsies (Figure 1.6B). In addition to denervation, there is a variable degree of muscle-fiber regeneration, the highest being among the Persian Jews. The regeneration component seems much more pronounced in recessive h-IBM than in s-IBM.

Electronmicroscopically, PHFs are present within the vacuoles and in vacuole-free cytoplasm of all h-IBM muscle biopsies (Figures 1.7A–C and 1.9A). Small clusters of PHFs often are present inside what appears to be an otherwise-healthy muscle fiber (Figure 1.7B,C). Such clusters are not in the neighborhood of nuclei, and the nuclei within those muscle fibers do not have filamentous inclusions. Therefore, it seems unlikely that the cytoplasmic clusters of PHFs in h-IBM are derived by release from broken nuclei (as has been suggested, Karpati et al., Chapter 19, this volume). The size and twist-repeats of h-IBM PHFs are the same as in s-IBM. Tubulofilamentous nuclear inclusions are found in all h-IBM patients (Figures 1.8 and 1.9B). Nuclear tubulofilaments usually have the same size as the cytoplasmic PHFs, but sometimes they appear smaller, depending on the plane of the section. As in s-IBM, some of the nuclear PHFs are clearly twisted, but more commonly their twist is not discernible (probably due to the tight packing of the nuclear tubulofilaments) (Figure 1.8C–E).

Cytoplasmic inclusions of 6–10-nm filaments are also commonly seen in the h-IBMs (Figure 1.10).

Neither ragged-red fibers nor cytochrome-oxidase-negative fibers are present in the h-IBMs (16; Chapter 22, this volume). Also not present in the h-IBMs are mitochondrial paracrystalline inclusions and mitochondrial-DNA deletions (57; Chapter 22, this volume).

To diagnose h-IBM pathologically we recommend the following:

1) Engel-Gomori trichrome staining to visualize vacuolated muscle fibers and determine lack of mononuclear inflammatory cells.

2) Fluorescence-enhanced Congo-red or non-fluorescent crystal-violet staining for amyloid, which is usually absent in most types of h-IBM

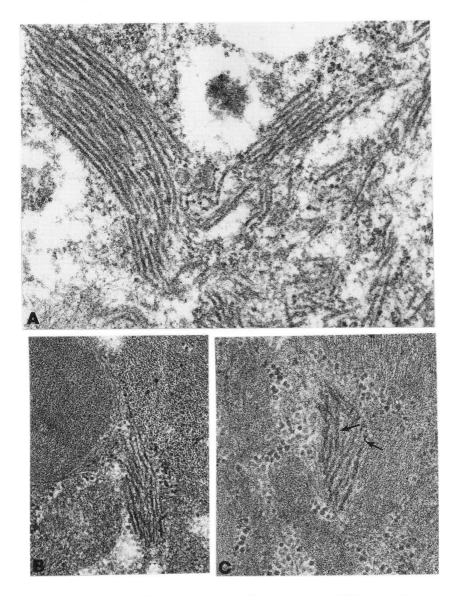

Figure 1.7.   Electron microscopy of muscle-fiber cytoplasmic PHFs in dominant-IBM (i.e., autosomal-dominant h-IBM). A: A large cluster of PHFs, and some smaller groups or individual PHFs, dispersed within the vacuole of a muscle fiber (×67,000). B and C: An otherwise normal-appearing muscle fiber has small clusters of PHFs among normal myofibrils; twists in C are indicated by arrows (B, ×43,000; C, ×67,000).

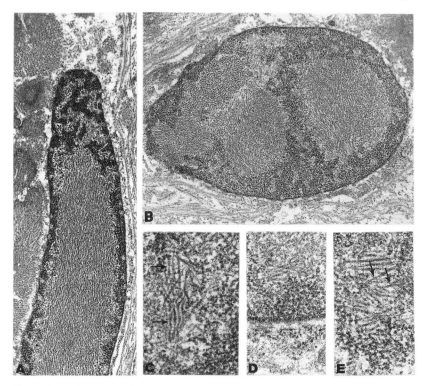

Figure 1.8. Electron microscopy of PHFs in nuclei of dominant-IBM. A and B: Low-power electron micrographs illustrate two nuclei virtually completely filled with collections of PHFs, which would appear as inclusions by light-microscopy (A, ×16,000; B, ×14,000). C–E: Higher-power electron micrographs of nuclear inclusions to illustrate the twisted pattern of nuclear PHFs (arrows) (C–E, ×53,000).

(see below) but is always present in s-IBM muscle biopsies. In autosomal-dominant IBM, occasional muscle fibers contain round congophilic inclusions (56) (Figure 1.6D).

3) Immunocytochemical staining for the presence of PHFs, utilizing the monoclonal antibody SMI-31, which recognizes phosphorylated tau of PHFs in both h-IBM and s-IBM (Figure 1.6C) (33).

4) Immunocytochemical staining utilizing monoclonal antibody SMI-310, which apparently recognizes an epitope of PHF tau different from that recognized by the SMI-31 antibody (58) (see Figure 1.30). The tau epitope recognized by SMI-310 is typically absent from the PHFs of the autosomal-recessive h-IBMs studied (58), and in autosomal-dominant h-IBM it is expressed in only a minority of the abnormal muscle fibers (56). By contrast, essentially all s-IBM PHFs

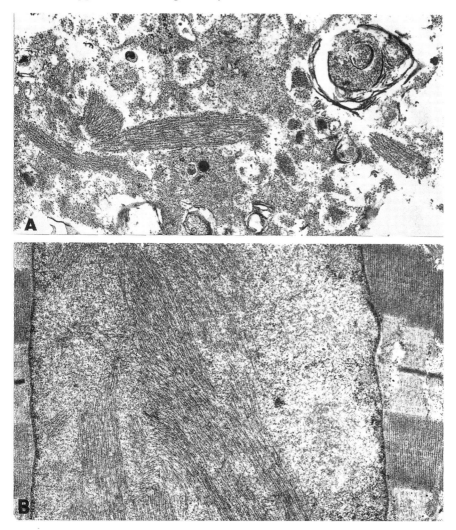

Figure 1.9. Electron microscopy of muscle fibers in recessive-IBM (i.e., autosomal-recessive h-IBM). A: Clusters of cytoplasmic PHFs and various lysosomal inclusions within the vacuole of a muscle fiber (×21,000). B: Clusters of PHFs within the nucleus of another muscle fiber (×14,000).

are strongly labeled with SMI-310 antibody (58). It now appears that these two monoclonal antibodies (both from Sternberger Monoclonal, Inc.) are an excellent diagnostic duo (a "dynamic duo"): SMI-31 to identify both s- and h-IBM, and SMI-310 to distinguish s-IBM from h-IBM.

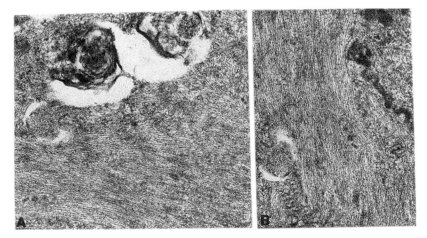

Figure 1.10. Electron microscopy of two clusters of 6–10-nm filaments within a cytoplasmic vacuole (A) and in vacuole-free cytoplasm (B) in recessive-IBM. In A there is a myelin-like whorl (above) adjacent to the filaments (A and B, ×43,000).

II. Unusual Aspects of the Muscle-Fiber Phenotype in s-IBM

A. *Intracellular amyloid deposits*

Classically, "amyloid" denotes the physical configuration of a protein aggregated into β-pleated sheets (β-sheets) that stain with Congo red (i.e. congophilia) and are metachromatically-pink with crystal-violet. A number of different proteins, including the β-amyloid-protein (Aβ) part of β-amyloid precursor protein (βAPP), prion and tau proteins are congophilic, even though their propensity to self-aggregate into β-sheet amyloid has not yet been fully demonstrated; and in the case of tau, such aggregation has been reported not to occur (thus, a conundrum) (59). In 1991 Mendell et al. (6) described wispy, plaque-like Congo-red-positive (green-birefringent) amyloid deposits within s-IBM vacuolated muscle fibers and considered them to be specific for s-IBM. Subsequently we showed that amyloid can be demonstrated in vacuolated IBM muscle fibers by Congo-red, thioflavin-S, and crystal-violet staining (7,8,32,60). The amyloid deposits in IBM muscle fibers often are very small and difficult to see, probably accounting for the occasional publication of "negative" studies (61).

We have developed a new, simple method for enhancing Congo-red-positive amyloid deposits using fluorescence filters and ultraviolet illumination. This allows much easier identification of congophilic amyloid (32). The locations and characteristics of amyloid deposits within vacuolated muscle fibers of s-IBM utilizing this technique are illustrated in Figures 1.1 and 1.2.

Our method of fluorescence-enhanced Congo-red positivity reveals amyloid in all s-IBM patients and, in them, in 60–80% of their vacuolated fibers. Congo-red-positivity in s-IBM fibers appears as squiggly or rod-like deposits. Whereas some of the congophilic amyloid deposits are located deep within the s-IBM muscle fiber, others are subjacent to the plasmalemma, and some appear to have come out of the muscle fiber (review: 5) (Figures 1.1 and 1.2C–F).

Some unresolved questions about the congophilic amyloid in s-IBM relate to its chemical nature and origin, the type of subcellular structure containing it, and its initial location in the muscle fiber. Our current data indicate that PHFs containing hyperphosphorylated tau are congophilic (Figure 1.1); however, it is not known if their congophilia reflects a β-pleated-sheet configuration. As noted earlier, in s-IBM muscle fibers the congophilic amyloid might also be partially due to the abnormally accumulated β-amyloid protein (Aβ) (7,8,60), which is a 39–42-residue polypeptide portion of βAPP (review: 62).

Aβ is considered to be a major component of the 6–10-nm amyloid fibrils in blood vessels and senile plaques in the brain of Alzheimer disease (AD), Down syndrome, and Dutch hereditary cerebrovascular amyloidosis, as well as in persons of very advanced age (62,63). In these conditions, abnormal accumulation of Aβ is considered to be due partly to increased generation of βAPP and partly to abnormal processing of it (62,63). Alzheimer-brain neurofibrillary tangles, composed primarily of hyperphosphorylated tau, also are Congo-red-positive (64). Therefore, in AD it seems that both Aβ and hyperphosphorylated tau contribute to the congophilic amyloidosis. Because injected ubiquitin was reported to induce amyloidogenesis (65), it is possible that the documented increase in ubiquitin within s-IBM muscle fibers (12) can increase amyloid formation there.

Among our many patients with several other non-IBM vacuolar myopathies, including acid-maltase deficiency, hypokalemic periodic paralysis, and undefined types, none had congophilic-amyloid deposits. As in s-IBM, abnormal muscle fibers in some of those disorders can have increased acid-phosphatase staining indicative of increased lysosomal activity; this increased staining is very prominent in acid-maltase deficiency. Because these non-IBM biopsy specimens do not have congophilic amyloid, it is unlikely that the amyloid deposits in s-IBM result simply from a non-specific disturbance of lysosomal function. In our experience to date, the only non-

IBM muscle disorder showing intra-myofiber congophilia is oculo-pharyngeal muscular dystrophy (OPMD). We found congophilia in all four of our American OPMD patients and in two French OPMD biopsies (65a). However, in OPMD, congophilic deposits appear to be smaller than in s-IBM, and usually have a rounded, not a "squiggly," appearance (65a). Whether intra-myofiber congophilia will be convincingly demonstrated in any other muscle disease remains to be seen.

B. Abnormal accumulation of "Alzheimer-characteristic" proteins and prion, and their mRNA's in sporadic inclusion-body myositis

a) Abnormal accumulation of β-amyloid protein (Aβ) and two other epitopes of β-amyloid precursor protein (βAPP)

Aβ was discovered in, and first sequenced from, the amyloid fibrils in cerebral blood vessels of Alzheimer's disease patients (66), and sub-sequently from senile plaques of Alzheimer's-disease brain (67–69). Aβ is a peptide composed of 39–42 aminoacids; it is produced by proteolytic cleavage of the much larger βAPP (reviewed in 62).

βAPP, the product of a chromosome-21 gene, is considered to be a cell-surface glycoprotein. It contains a large extracellular N-terminal domain, a transmembrane Aβ domain, and a short cytoplasmic C-terminal domain (70,71). In normal human muscle, βAPP, apparently full-length because it contains C-terminal, N-terminal, and Aβ epitopes, accumulates promi-nently only at the postsynaptic domain of the neuromuscular junction (NMJ) (Figure 1.11) (72): this suggests that βAPP has an important normal function there. βAPP-mRNA is also increased at human NMJs, indicating that normally-accumulated βAPP is synthesized there (14) (Figure 1.11).

Aβ and βAPP have received considerable attention regarding the pathogenesis of Alzheimer's disease. In addition to the Aβ associated with the dystrophic neurites of senile plaques of AD brains, the C- and N-terminal epitopes of βAPP are also abnormally accumulated there. The accumulation of Aβ in AD brain has been proposed to result from abnormal proteolytic cleavage of βAPP to produce the amyloidogenic fragment Aβ (62,63,68); however, overproduction of βAPP is an addi-tional, or alternative, possibility (62).

Although pathologic accumulations of Aβ and βAPP were previously considered to be confined to the brain and its blood vessels, we have found that Aβ and C- and N-terminal epitopes of βAPP are abnormally accumulated within vacuolated muscle fibers of s-IBM patients (Figure

1.12), wherein these three βAPP-epitopes immuno-colocalize with each other by light-microscopy (7,8). βAPP immunoreactive inclusions are located subplasmalemmally or more internally in the fibers. Occasionally these inclusions extend outside the boundary of a highly vacuolated muscle fiber, (Figure 1.12) (8).

By gold-immuno-electronmicroscopy, Aβ is localized to 6–10 nm amyloid-like fibrils (Figures 1.13, 1.14), irregular clusters of nearly-amorphous dense structures, and to poorly-defined, loose, floccular material (7,8). PHFs do not contain Aβ immunoreactivity (8) (Figure 1.14).

C- and N-terminal epitopes of βAPP are localized to irregular clusters of nearly-amorphous, dense material and to loose floccular material, which are often in close proximity to or adjacent to PHFs (Figure 1.14) (8). However, PHFs themselves never contain immunoreactivity of any of the βAPP epitopes (8) (Figure 1.14). In proximity to the loose floccular material, there are also loosely packed thin fibrils 6–10 nm in diameter, which contain Aβ immunoreactivity but never C- or N-terminal βAPP-epitope immunoreactivity (8).

Abnormal accumulation of βAPP epitopes in s-IBM vacuolated muscle fibers has now been confirmed by others (61,73,74).

It is particularly interesting that muscle fibers in s-IBM patients contain abnormal accumulations of proteins characteristic of Alzheimer-disease brain and that the ultrastructural localization of those proteins is virtually identical in IBM muscle and AD brain (75). For example, in AD brain Aβ is also localized to 6–10-nm fibrils and to amorphous and floccular structures. Moreover, Alzheimer-disease intraneuronal neurofibrillary tangles, composed of PHFs that are morphologically virtually identical to inclusion-body myositis PHFs (9), resemble IBM PHFs in that they do not contain immunoreactive Aβ (71), and do contain hyperphosphorylated tau (see below).

b) Overexpression of the β-APP gene in inclusion-body myositis vacuolated muscle fibers

The βAPP gene normally produces several alternatively-spliced transcripts (76). βAPP-695 mRNA, which lacks the Kunitz-type protease-inhibitor (KPI) epitope, is the predominant βAPP mRNA in normal brain and Alzheimer brain, whereas mRNAs for βAPP transcripts containing the KPI epitope predominate in normal peripheral tissues, including skeletal muscle (and are also present to some extent in normal and AD brain).

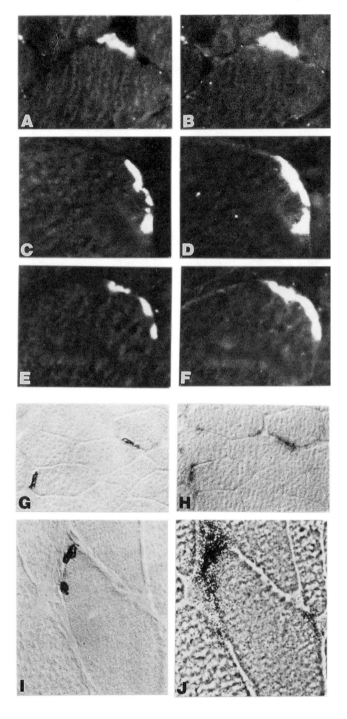

s-IBM vacuolated muscle fibers have increased βAPP-mRNA signal but only for βAPP containing the KPI motif (14). In affected muscle fibers, the increased βAPP-mRNA co-localizes in the same foci as the abnormal accumulations of immunoreactivity for βAPP (including the Aβ epitope) (14) (Figure 1.15). Previously, the only other abnormal human tissues in which βAPP-mRNA was studied were brains of patients with Alzheimer disease and Down syndrome; in them, altered expression of mRNAs of various classes of βAPP were reported (62,77).

We have recently demonstrated that increased βAPP and its mRNA are also present in the human macrophages found in muscle of various muscle diseases (not just the IBMs) (78) (Figures 1.16 and 1.17).

In Alzheimer disease, it has been suggested that the KPI domain of βAPP affects its proteolytic processing, leading to liberation of free Aβ, which then aggregates into the congophilic β-pleated sheets of amyloid fibrils (77). In s-IBM, it is not established which of the several proteins (known and yet to be identified) that accumulate in vacuolated muscle fibers actually form the β-pleated sheets of congophilic amyloid. Possibly the over-produced and accumulated Aβ is one amyloidogenic component. If so, in addition to the demonstrated increase of βAPP synthesis (14), perhaps a) there is abnormal βAPP processing, or b) the excessively-synthesized βAPP simply overloads the normal processing pathway, producing an unmanageable amount of otherwise-trivial Aβ.

c) Abnormal accumulation of prion protein.

Cellular prion protein (PrP^c) is a normal 33–37 kD brain constituent containing 253–254 amino acids. It is considered to be the precursor of the scrapie agent, namely prion protein scrapie, (PrP^{sc}) (reviewed in 79). Hu-

Figure 1.11. Double labeling of normal human individual neuromuscular junctions (NMJs) demonstrates close co-localization of a-bungarotoxin (a-BT) bound to nicotinic acetylcholine receptors with the immunolocalization of three sequences of βAPP (A–J, ×1,375). A, C, and E: a-BT. B: N-terminal region of βAPP (N-βAPP), D: Aβ. F: C-terminal region of βAPP (C-βAPP). The Aβ and C-βAPP immunoreactivities occupy a slightly larger area than those of a-BT and N-βAPP. Punctuate lipofuscin granules are autofluorescent in A, B, and D. H and J: In situ hybridization with the full-length βAPP cRNA probe containing the KPI motif. Normal neuromuscular junctions (NMJs), identified by the acetylcholinesterase reaction (G, I) in sections serial to H and J, have increased βAPP mRNA (H, I) (A–F, ×800; D and E, ×300; I and J, ×1,000). (Reproduced with permission from Askanas et al., *Neurosci. Lett.* 143:96–100, 1992, and from Sarkozi et al., *NeuroReport* 4:815–18, 1993.)

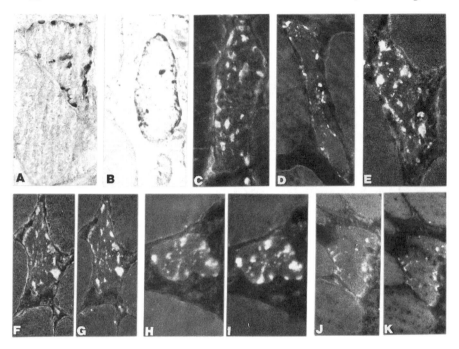

Figure 1.12. Light-microscopic immunocytochemistry of three βAPP sequences in abnormal muscle fibers of s-IBM. A and B: Peroxidase-antiperoxidase (PAP) reaction: (A) N-terminal sequence of βAPP (N-βAPP); (B) C-terminal sequence of βAPP (C-βAPP). C–E: Fluorescence staining: (C) N-βAPP; (D) Aβ; (E) C-βAPP. Abnormal muscle fibers contain clusters of βAPP immunoreactivity scattered within the cytoplasm. In addition, muscle fibers in A and B also have a patchy staining in the peripheral region of the muscle fiber (A and B, ×1,400; C and E, ×1,500; D, ×1,000). Light-microscopic double immunostaining on the same section of abnormal muscle fibers: C-βAPP (F) plus Aβ (G); N-βAPP (H) plus Aβ (I); C-βAPP (J) plus ubiquitin (K). There is close co-localization of N and C epitopes of βAPP with Aβ and with Ub (all, ×1,400). (Reproduced with permission from Askanas et al., *Ann. Neurol.* 34:551–60, 1993.)

man PrP^c is encoded by a single gene, consisting of two exons and one intron, on the short arm of chromosome 20 (79). The normal functions of PrP^c are uncertain. It is considered to be on the outer surface of the cell membrane, with a hypothesized role in cell-cell recognition and/or communication (80). In humans, localization outside the central nervous system of PrP^c and its mRNA has been at the postsynaptic domain of NMJs (80) (Figures 1.18 and 1.21A) and in muscle macrophages (78) (Figure 1.17). PrP^c immunoreactivity has also been reported in "leukocytes" (81).

PrP^{sc} is a 33–37 kD isoform of PrP^c that is resistant to protease-K digestion (note that all β-pleated sheet amyloids, composed of any type of pro-

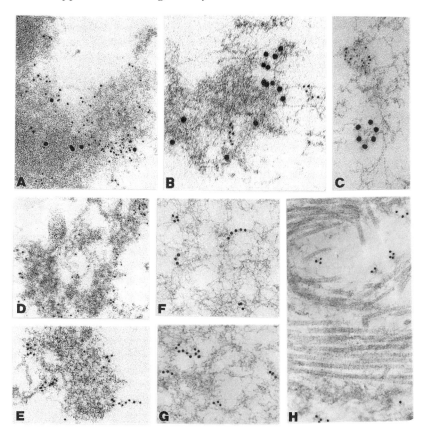

Figure 1.13.   Double (A–C) and single (D–H) gold-immuno-electronmicroscopy of s-IBM muscle. A: *C*-terminal sequence of βAPP (C-βAPP) is marked with 15-nm gold particles, and Aβ is marked with 5-nm gold particles. B: N-terminal sequence of βAPP (N-βAPP) is marked with 15-nm gold particles, and Aβ with 5-nm gold particles. C: N-βAPP is marked with 5-nm gold particles, and Aβ with 15-nm gold particles. While there is close co-localization of N- and C-βAPP with Aβ on the denser amorphous and looser floccular structures in A and B, only Aβ is localized to the loose 6–10-nm fibrillar structures (B, C) (A, ×107,000; B, ×134,000; C, ×128,000). D: C-βAPP is localized to amorphous structures (5-nm gold particles) (×108,000). E–G: Aβ is localized to amorphous structures and to 6–10-nm fibrillar material extending from the amorphous material (E) and organized in loose clusters (F, G) (10-nm gold particles) (E, ×55,000; F and G, ×65,000). H: Anti-C-βAPP-antibody immunodecorated structures are intermingled with collagen fibrils lying slightly outside an abnormal muscle fiber (10-nm gold particles) (×67,000). (Reproduced with permission from Askanas et al., *Ann. Neurol.* 34:551–60, 1993.)

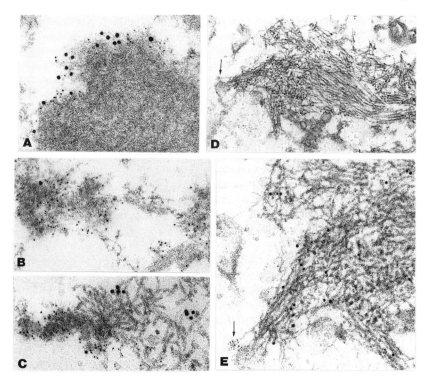

Figure 1.14. Double gold-immuno-electronmicroscopy demonstrating localization of ubiquitin and three epitopes of βAPP in abnormal muscle fibers of s-IBM. Ubiquitin (Ub) is marked with 15-nm gold particles, and βAPP epitopes with 5-nm gold particles. A: Both Ub and Aβ are present on less tightly packed material at the periphery of an amorphous structure. B: Ub and the C-terminal sequence of βAPP (C-βAPP) are present on floccular material (×108,000). C: Ub and the N-terminal sequence of βAPP (N-βAPP) are co-localized at the dense amorphous material (left) adjacent to the 15–21-nm PHFs (center and right), but only Ub is localized to PHFs (×108,000). D and E: Lower- and higher-power magnifications of PHFs immunodecorated by anti-ubiquitin antibody. At the periphery of the collection of PHFs there is a small patch of an amorphous material immunodecorated by anti-Aβ antibody (arrows) (D, ×33,000; E, ×85,000). (Reproduced with permission from Askanas et al., *Ann. Neurol.* 34:551–60, 1993.)

tein, are protease-K resistant). Probably not all protease-K resistant PrPsc is in the form of congophilic amyloid detectable by light-microscopy. PrPsc is thought to be a post-translationally changed PrPc. It is found only in brains of scrapie-infected animals and of patients with sporadic kuru (79), sporadic Creutzfeldt-Jakob disease (CJD), hereditary Gerstmann-

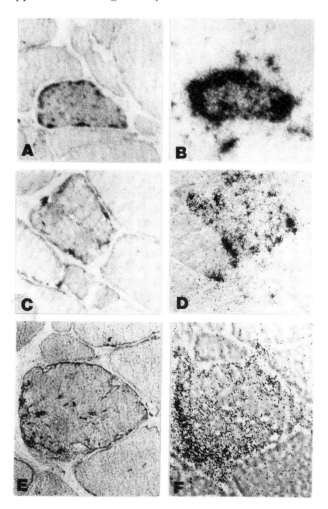

Figure 1.15. Immunocytochemistry of βAPP (A, C, E) and in situ hybridization of βAPP-mRNA (B, D, F) of s-IBM muscle biopsies. In each set, the studies were performed on serial (but not always adjacent) sections. A and C: PAP reaction for Aβ. E: PAP reaction for the C-terminal region of βAPP. D: KPI-specific cRNA probe. B and F: cRNA probe for total βAPP, containing the KPI domain. The sections stained with PAP were photographed in bright-field illumination. The in situ hybridization sections were photographed with interference-contrast polarization optics (B, D) or phase-contrast (F). The IBM muscle fibers that contain abnormal βAPP immunoreactivity express increased βAPP-mRNA. Capillaries in B (below and above the abnormal muscle fiber) and D (adjacent to the lower edge of, and also below, the abnormal muscle fiber) express increased βAPP mRNA (which in capillaries is normal) (A–D, ×900; E and F, ×1,350). (Reproduced with permission from Sarkozi et al., *NeuroReport* 4:815–18, 1993.)

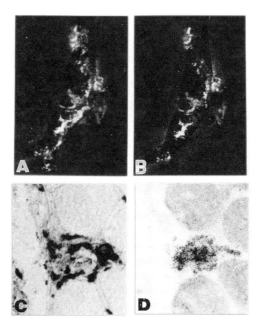

Figure 1.16. Light microscopy of macrophages in morphologically non-specific myopathy: double labeling of macrophages with the specific marker Ber-MAC 3 (A) and with antibody against C-terminal βAPP (B). Macrophages identified by Ber-MAC 3 contain strong βAPP immunoreactivity. D: In situ hybridization of βAPP mRNA. Macrophages identified by Ber-MAC 3 (C) have strong βAPP-mRNA (A and B, ×1,600; C and D, ×800).

Sträussler-Scheinker syndrome (GSS), and hereditary fatal familial insomnia (79,82). PrP^c and PrP^{sc} are encoded by the same gene. The amount of the corresponding PrP-mRNA is the same in scrapie infected brain (79) as in normal brain (whereas PrP-mRNA is increased in s-IBM muscle fibers, see below). Protease-K applied to PrP^{sc} from scrapie-infected brain generates a 27–30 kD digestion-resistant fragment called PrP 27–30, whereas the PrP^c of normal brain is completely digested by protease-K (75). Therefore, PrP 27–30, encoded by a normal cellular gene, is considered to be the disease-characteristic fraction of scrapie brain (79).

In muscle fibers of s-IBM, we have demonstrated PrP immunoreactive inclusions (Figure 1.19) (13). By light-microscopy, PrP closely co-localized with βAPP epitopes and ubiquitin in the s-IBM muscle fibers (Fig. 19D–G). Gold-immuno-electronmicroscopy revealed PrP immunoreactivity on: a) PHFs, b) small and large collections of amorphous material, c) floccular structures, and d) 6–10 nm amyloid-like fibrils (13) (Figure

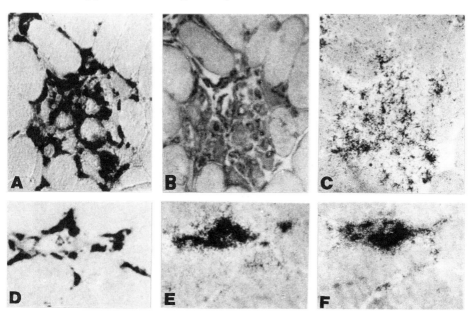

Figure 1.17. Light microscopy of macrophages in morphologically non-specific myopathy: labeling of macrophages with the specific marker Ber-MAC 3 (A, D), prion immunoreactivity (B), prion-mRNA (C, E), and βAPP-mRNA (F). Macrophages contain strong prion immunoreactivity and prion-mRNA. The same cluster of macrophages that contain strong prion-mRNA (E) also contain strong βAPP-mRNA (A–F, ×800).

1.20). This increased accumulation of PrP in s-IBM was recently confirmed by others (74).

d) Overexpression of prion protein gene

We recently demonstrated that PrPc-mRNA is significantly increased in s-IBM muscle fibers, where it co-localizes with the increased PrP-immunoreactivity (15) (Figure 1.21). That increased PrPc-mRNA in IBM vacuolated muscle fibers identifies the first (to our knowledge) human disease manifesting increased PrPc-mRNA. Therefore, PrP abnormally accumulated in IBM muscle fibers probably results, at least partly, from locally increased transcription of PrPc.

Previously, the only abnormal human tissue in which PrP and its mRNA had been studied were brains of patients with prion diseases; however, they did not have increased PrPc mRNA, nor did brains of

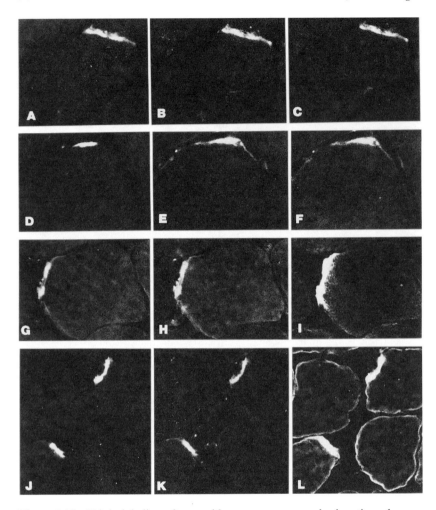

Figure 1.18. Triple-labeling of normal human neuromuscular junctions demonstrates close co-localization of prion (PrP) using polyclonal antiserum against PrP (B, E, H, K), with four postsynaptic-membrane components of human neuromuscular junctions: a-BT (A, D, G, J), desmin (I), ubiquitin (C), and C-βAPP (F). [In addition, dystrophin (L) shows strong localization around the entire perimeter of the muscle fiber.] (all, ×1,000). (Reproduced with permission from Askanas et al., *Neurosci. Lett.* 159:111–14, 1993.)

scrapie-infected animals (79,82). Therefore, our findings in IBM muscle contrast with those of prion brain diseases.

Possibly relevant to our findings is the recent report that transgenic mice carrying high copy numbers of the wild-type (normal) PrP^c gene

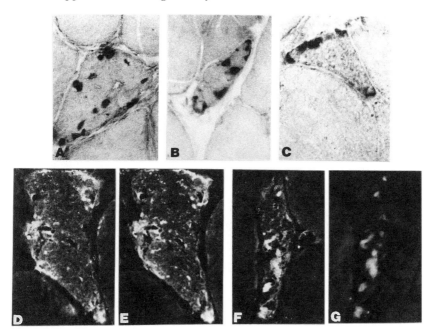

Figure 1.19. Light-microscopy of prion (PrP) immunoreactivity in s-IBM. A–C: PAP immunocytochemistry. Vacuolated muscle fibers have abnormally accumulated PrP deposits demonstrated with three different antibodies against PrP: (A) polyclonal antiserum against PrP (×1,820); (B) polyclonal antiserum against PrP (×1,820); (C) monoclonal antibody against PrP (×1,820). D–G: Double labeling for PrP as in "C" (D, F), for Aβ (E), and for ubiquitin (Ub) (G). There is close co-localization of PrP and Aβ, and of PrP and Ub, in the immunoreactive deposits (E–G, ×2,400). (Reproduced with permission from Askanas et al., *NeuroReport* 5:25–8, 1993.)

developed muscle weakness and histologic evidence of a non-vacuolar myopathy and a neuropathy (83). Even though the mouse myopathy does not resemble IBM morphologically, it is possible that in IBM muscle the increased expression of the PrP^c gene itself may be pathogenic. Because both PrP^c and βAPP mRNAs can, under certain circumstances, be regulated by the same factor, such as nerve-growth factor (84), and both βAPP and prion genes are up-regulated in regenerating muscle fibers (85), it is possible that in IBM there might be a pathologic up-regulation of another, yet-unidentified gene – for example, a gene normally silent in mature muscle fibers that may, through its product acting directly or indirectly as a transcription-factor, up-regulate PrP^c, βAPP, and other genes normally expressed (i) in brain and (ii) focally in mature muscle-fibers at the post-synaptic region of neuromuscular junctions (NMJs)

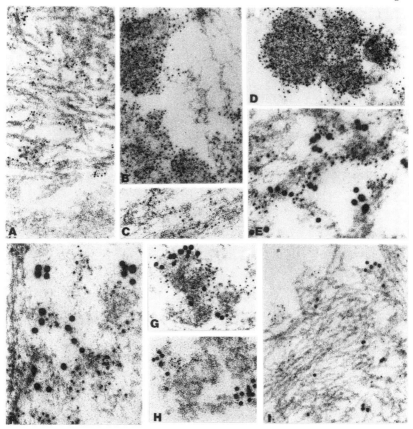

Figure 1.20. Gold-immuno-electronmicroscopy of PrP immunoreactivity in s-IBM vacuolated muscle fibers. A–C: PrP immunolocalization utilizing 5-nm gold particles. A: Only PHFs contain PrP immunoreactivity, while a portion of a myofiber (below) is negative (×145,000). In B, PrP is localized to amorphous material and 6–10-nm filaments, and in C to 6–10-nm filaments (B, ×105,000; C, ×135,000). D–G: Co-localization of PrP (5-nm gold particles) and Aβ (15-nm gold particles); both PrP and Aβ are localized to 6–10-nm filaments and to amorphous material (D, ×105,000; E, ×135,000; F, ×168,000; G, ×130,000). H and I: Co-localization of PrP (15-nm gold particles) and Ub (5-nm gold particles) to amorphous material (H) and PHFs (I) (H, ×107,000; I, ×100,000). (Reproduced with permission from Askanas et al., *NeuroReport* 5:25–8, 1993.)

(but not elsewhere in mature muscle fibers) (see below and Figures 1.11, 1.18, and 1.21). Changes in the abnormal muscle fibers of IBM do not simply reflect regenerative properties because they contain PHFs and other IBM-characteristic features that are not present in otherwise-normal regenerating muscle fibers. Therefore, in the s- and h-IBM, there

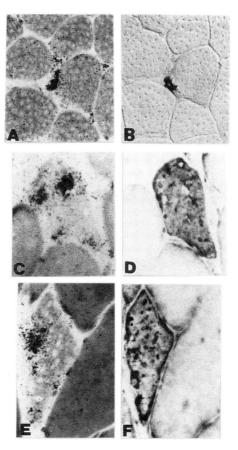

Figure 1.21. In situ hybridization of PrP^c mRNA in human muscle fibers. In normal fibers, PrP^c mRNA is localized only at the NMJ (A), where it is co-localized with acetylcholinesterase (B). In s-IBM, patches of PrP^c mRNA signal (C, E) occur in vacuolated muscle fibers, which also contain immunolocalized PrP in multiple foci (D, F), sometimes corresponding to the PrP^c mRNA patches. Each pair of pictures is from parallel (not necessarily adjacent) sections. All photographs are bright-field, except B (interference-contrast polarization) (A and B, ×700; C–F, ×1,240). (Reproduced with permission from Sarkozi et al., *Am. J. Pathol.* 145:1280–4, 1994.)

seem to be co-existing defects of a) processing (possibly abnormal glycation, for example) and/or b) disposal of prion, and perhaps of some of the other accumulated proteins, along with abnormal polymerization/binding/precipitation of them (which could even be a simple consequence of supply-side exuberance).

e) Abnormal accumulation of a_1-antichymotrypsin (a_1-ACT)

a_1-ACT is a specific inhibitor of serine proteases and belongs to the serpin super-family (reviewed in 86). It forms stable complexes with chymotrypsin, cathepsin G, and mast-cell chymases (86). Even though the physiologic functions of a_1-ACT are not well understood, it is considered a major acute-phase protein associated with inflammatory episodes because its concentration in plasma greatly increases after surgery, burn injuries, and other acute events (86). Proposed functions of a_1-ACT involve control of connective-tissue breakdown and cell-cell interaction, because it has been found to decrease proteoglycan and fibronectin and to inhibit activity of natural-killer T-cells (86).

Previously, abnormal accumulation of a_1-ACT was described in Alzheimer brain, where a_1-ACT was localized in amyloid plaques that also contained Aβ and ubiquitin (87,88). The pathogenic significance of a_1-ACT in AD brain is not certain; because of its ability to tightly associate with Aβ and its presence in Aβ-containing pre-amyloid plaques, it has been proposed to play a pathogenic role in the formation of amyloid fibrils (87–89).

Abnormal accumulation of a_1-ACT has been demonstrated in vacuolated muscle fibers of s-IBM (10). As in AD brain, in IBM muscle a_1-ACT immunoreactivity closely co-localizes with Aβ (10), which a) demonstrates another similarity (in addition to Aβ accumulation) between IBM muscle and AD brain, and b) suggests that the pathogenic mechanisms of both diseases may have commonalities. The origin and role of increased a_1-ACT in s-IBM muscle are not yet known. Our recent studies (unpublished) indicate that a_1-ACT-mRNA is not increased in s-IBM vacuolated muscle fibers. Nevertheless, a_1-ACT may be important in the cascade of pathologic events. Recently, increased accumulation of three serine proteases, cathepsin D, cathepsin G and chymotrypsin, have been described in IBM vacuolated muscle fibers (61,90); their functions there remain to be elucidated.

f) Abnormal accumulation of phosphorylated tau

Tau is a protein belonging to the class of mammalian brain microtubule-associated proteins, and it is found primarily in neural tissue (reviewed in 91–93). Human brain tau is the product of a single gene, whose mRNA is alternatively spliced and whose proteins are variably phosphorylated to generate six isoforms (91,92), all of which are expressed in adult human brain. Some of the 16 exons are constitutively expressed and some are under developmental regulation. Tau-mRNAs have been found only in neurons (91). Hyper-phosphorylated tau is a major constituent of the AD intraneuronal and extracellular PHFs (reviewed in 93,94). All six isoforms of brain tau are abnormally phosphorylated in AD PHFs (95). It has been postulated that abnormal phosphorylation of tau causes significant structural changes of that protein, resulting in alteration of its electrophoretic mobility, molecular size, interaction with microtubules and, possibly, the propensity to self-aggregate into PHFs (96–98). The A68 proteins, also called Alz-50 antigen, are another component of AD PHFs (99–101). Even though the exact molecular composition of A68 proteins is not fully elucidated, they have close similarities, including co-antigenicity, to the tau of PHFs (99,100). In addition to tau protein, AD PHFs also contain ubiquitin (101,102). In AD, it is not understood how PHFs are assembled nor why they accumulate; possible predisposing mechanisms include hyperphosphorylation or abnormal glycation of tau.

Using several highly specific antibodies that react with phosphorylated tau (including SMI-31, Alz-50, PHF-1, AT8, and others), we have demonstrated that vacuolated muscle fibers of s-IBM contain phosphorylated (probably hyperphosphorylated) tau that is localized exclusively to PHFs (9,58) (Figures 1.22–1.24). Table 1.1 shows the similar immunoreactivity in s-IBM of various antibodies that are known to react in AD with PHF phosphorylated tau. Accordingly, it appears that phosphorylated tau participates in the formation of s-IBM PHFs as it does in AD PHFs. Monoclonal antibody SMI-31, which originally was directed against phosphorylated neurofilament heavy-chain but also cross-reacts with epitopes of phosphorylated tau, stains IBM PHFs with such high specificity (Figure 1.24) that we recommend it for the light-microscopic identification of PHFs (33). According to the above findings, the first demonstration of abnormally accumulated tau in diseased tissue other than brain has been provided by our studies showing phosphorylated tau in IBM muscle fibers.

g) Abnormal accumulation of apolipoprotein E (ApoE)

ApoE has recently been linked to the pathogenesis of Alzheimer disease. ApoE is localized immunocytochemically in senile plaques and neurofibrillary tangles (103), it binds to Aβ in vitro (104), and an increased frequency of its E4 allele is associated with earlier clinical onset

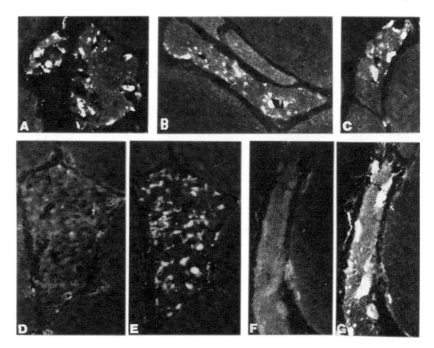

Figure 1.22. Fluorescence-microscopy immunocytochemistry of s-IBM. A–C: Alz-50 immunostaining. The Alz-50 immunoreactive deposits, indicating the presence of phosphorylated tau, are mainly within vacuoles and rarely in what appears to be vacuole-free cytoplasm. D–F: Tau-1 immunoreactivity, without (D, F) and after (E, G) dephosphorylation of adjacent-section pairs (D, E and F, G) of two muscle fibers. The phosphorylated (? hyperphosphorylated) state (D, F) apparently blocks the immunoreactivity of tau with Tau-1 antibody, which is against non-phosphorylated tau (A–C, ×750; D–G, ×1,250). (Reproduced with permission from Askanas et al., *Am. J. Pathol.* 144:177–187, 1994)

of the sporadic and the late-onset-familial forms of Alzheimer disease (105).

ApoE is abnormally accumulated within the vacuoles of s-IBM muscle. Its light-microscopic localization is in the form of intracellular inclusions that closely co-localize with phosphorylated-tau, Aβ, and ubiquitin (106). By electronmicroscopic-immunocytochemistry, ApoE is localized mainly to PHFs (11) (Figure 1.25), and somewhat to the 6–10 nm filaments and amorphous material (137).

Because ApoE-mRNA is not present in IBM vacuolated muscle fibers (137), we postulate that ApoE is transported from the circulation into the vacuolated muscle fibers through its low-density-lipoprotein receptors.

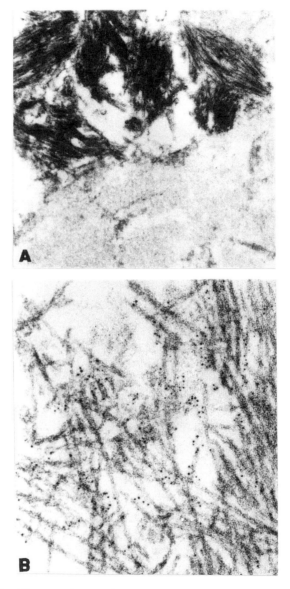

Figure 1.23. Electronmicroscopic-immunocytochemistry of s-IBM cytoplasmic paired-helical filaments (PHFs). A: Low-power electronmicroscopy of Tau-1 immunoreactivity, peroxidase reaction. The dark reaction-product entirely covers the PHFs (above), whereas an adjacent portion of the myofiber (below) is not immunostained (×20,000). B: Higher-power electron micrograph demonstrates the distribution of the 5-nm gold particles on PHFs using Alz-50 antibody (×101,000). (Reproduced with permission from Askanas et al., *Am. J. Pathol.* 144:177–87, 1994.)

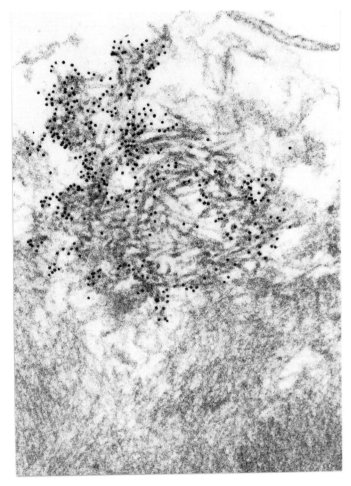

Figure 1.24. s-IBM: electronmicroscopic-immunocytochemistry of SMI-31 anti-body using 10-nm gold particles. SMI-31 exclusively labels PHFs (above); a portion of a myofibril (below) is completely unstained (×85,000).

Because ApoE is known to bind to β-pleated-sheet amyloid of various proteins (107) and to Aβ (104), it is possible that after ApoE is transported into IBM vacuolated muscle-fibers it is captured there by both Aβ and β-pleated-sheet amyloid. Recently, an increased prevalence of the ApoE-4 allele has been reported in 14 s-IBM patients (108; Chapter 9 this volume). But according to a report from Great Britain, the ApoE-4 allele was not preferentially increased in s-IBM patients (109). Our studies

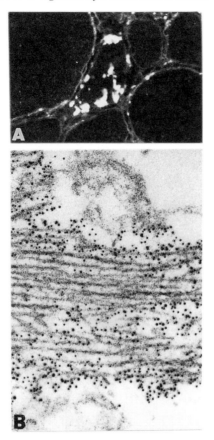

Figure 1.25. Immunolocalization of apolipoprotein E (ApoE) in s-IBM. A: Immunofluorescence staining illustrates strongly immunoreactive ApoE deposits (×1,300). B: Gold-immuno-electronmicroscopy shows accumulation of 5-nm gold particles identifying ApoE on PHFs (×35,000).

indicate that the ApoE-4 allele is not increased in either s- or h-IBM (110). Therefore, a mechanism not specifically requiring an ApoE-4 allele must be responsible for the ApoE accumulation in IBM abnormal muscle fibers.

In both normal and abnormal human muscle biopsies, increased ApoE immunoreactivity is present at the neuromuscular junctions (106,137). Moreover, in various diseases, virtually all regenerating muscle fibers have increased ApoE immunoreactivity, suggesting that this lipoprotein plays a role in the development and repair of normal human muscle fibers (106,137).

h) Abnormal accumulation of Ubiquitin (Ub)

Ubiquitin is a 76-amino-acid, highly-conserved polypeptide present in all eukaryotes. It is thought to regulate degradation of abnormal and short-lived-normal proteins by an ATP-dependent pathway (reviewed in 111,112). The Ub-dependent protein degradation pathway is highly selective; proteins destined for degradation are ligated to Ub and then degraded by a specific protease complex that acts on ubiquitinated proteins (111,112). The transcription regulators p53, cyclins, MATα2 repressor, and oncoproteins are also targets of Ub, indicating a role of Ub in the control of gene expression (111,112). The two quite different proteolytic systems, the Ub system and the lysosomal-autophagic system, were recently found to be functionally related (113).

Ub is of current interest in relation to its proposed role in the pathogenesis of neurodegenerative disorders. Ub is a component of neurofibrillary tangles and senile plaques in Alzheimer-disease brain (101,102), Lewy bodies in Parkinson disease, and abnormal inclusions in lower motor neurons of patients with amyotrophic lateral sclerosis (reviewed in 113).

In 1991 we demonstrated that vacuolated muscle fibers of s-IBM and h-IBM, and of oculopharyngeal muscular dystrophy, contain strongly ubiquitinated inclusions (12) (Figures 1.12, 1.14, and 1.19). The ubiquitinated inclusions in IBM muscle fibers were subsequently confirmed by others (73,114). In normal human muscle fibers, Ubimmunoreactivity is present only at the post-synaptic region of neuromuscular junctions (115).

Our immuno-electromicroscopic finding that Ub was localized to PHFs of IBM muscle (12) (Figures 1.12, 1.18, 1.24) provided the first identification of a molecular component of IBM-PHFs (12). Ub is also localized to 6–10 nm amyloid-like fibrils, floccular material, and amorphous structures; Ub co-localizes with Aβ on all of these except the PHFs (which do not contain Aβ) (7,8).

In IBM muscle, Ub is probably bound to proteins that are abnormally modified post-translationally, and possibly to excessive short-lived normal proteins. It is not known whether ubiquitination in IBM relates to the lysosomal system or is independent of it. It has been shown that Ub can induce amyloidogenesis (65). Of interest is whether this propensity of Ub plays a role in the induction of amyloid deposits within IBM muscle fibers.

Ubiquitination has also been suggested to play a role in immune responses, for example, in activation of the T-cell antigen receptor (116).

Whether this mechanism plays a role in the immune reaction in s-IBM muscle remains to be determined.

i) Abnormal accumulation of nicotinic acetylcholine receptor (nAChR), its mRNA, and 43kD protein

nAChR and its anchoring protein 43 kD are normally present in human and animal muscle fibers only at the postsynaptic domain of the neuromuscular junction (NMJ). We have studied whether they are pathologically expressed in IBM, because other proteins normally present at the postsynaptic domain of the NMJ are abnormally accumulated in IBM vacuolated muscle fibers. We found that nAChR and the 43-kD protein are strongly accumulated in the vacuoles of IBM muscle fibers, where they closely co-localize with each other and with βAPP, PrP, and Ub (117). Those results provided the first demonstration of pathologic accumulation of nAChR and 43-kD protein within human muscle fibers.

j) Abnormal accumulation of superoxide dismutase-1 (SOD1) and overexpression of SOD1 gene

Oxidative stress has been postulated to play a role in AD. Abnormalities of anti-oxidant enzymes were reported in AD brain (118–120), but they were not analyzed in IBM muscle. We therefore studied human muscle biopsies encompassing a wide spectrum of muscle diseases, including the IBMs, for SOD1 immunoreactivity (IR) with monoclonal and polyclonal isoform-specific antibodies, and for SOD1-mRNA by in situ hybridization with a full-length cRNA probe. Of s-IBM vacuolated muscle fibers 60–70% had SOD1-IR present as strong focal accumulations within the vacuoles, and sometimes more diffusely in the vacuole-free cytoplasm. The SOD1-mRNA signal was also very strong in vacuolated muscle fibers (121). Regenerating muscle fibers, in all biopsies that contained them, showed, in a diffuse pattern, positive SOD1-IR and SOD1-mRNA signal (121; V. Askanas et al., unpublished data). Strong SOD1-IR was also present at all neuromuscular junctions in normal and pathologic muscle biopsies (117). Our studies demonstrated for the first time that: a) SOD1 is overexpressed in IBM-vacuolated muscle fibers, which suggests that oxidative-stress might play a role in IBM pathogenesis (as has also been proposed in AD). Moreover, SOD1 probably plays a role in normal neuromuscular-junction biology and in ordinary muscle-fiber regeneration. Our newest, yet-unpublished observations, indicate abnormal accumulation of heme oxygenase-1 in s-IBM vacuolated muscle fibers, providing additional evidence that oxidative stress may play a role in IBM pathogenesis. (The role of nitric oxide induced oxidative stress in s- and h-IBM is described below in "Update on the Newest Results.")

Table 1.6 describes all the proteins and their mRNA's found to be abnormally accumulated in s-IBM. Table 1.7 lists proteins that we have studied and found not to be accumulated in IBM vacuolated muscle fibers.

III. Phenotypic Differences and Similarities Between Sporadic and Hereditary Forms of IBM

A. *Intracellular amyloid deposits*

In autosomal-recessive h-IBM, fluorescence-enhanced Congo-red positivity of vacuolated fibers occurs in less than 10% of our patients and in them, in only 10–25% of their vacuolated fibers (16), whereas Congo-red positivity occurs in 100% of our s-IBM patients and in the majority of their vacuolated fibers. In the four autosomal-dominant h-IBM patients we studied, fluorescence-enhanced Congo-red-positive amyloid deposits were present in three siblings from the Chicago family described above,

Table 1.6. *Sporadic inclusion-body myositis vacuolated muscle fibers contain:*

Abnormal Accumulations of . . .
- Ubiquitin
- β-amyloid protein (Aβ)
- N- and C-terminal epitopes of β-amyloid precursor protein
- a_1-antichymotrypsin
- Apolipoprotein E
- Prion
- Hyperphosphorylated tau
- Nicotinic acetylcholine receptor
- 43-kD protein, rapsyn
- SOD1

Increased mRNA of . . .
- β-amyloid precursor protein
- Prion protein, cellular type
- Nicotinic acetylcholine receptor
- SOD1

No Increase of mRNA of . . .
- Apolipoprotein E
- a-antichymotrypsin
- Tau

Table 1.7. *Proteins not accumulated in IBM vacuolated muscle fibers*

Dystrophin	Cytokeratins
Vinculin	Nonphosphorylated tau
Titin	Big tau
Vimentin	Tubulin α and β
Desmin	Nonphosphorylated neurofilament
Lamin B	Phosphorylated low-kD neurofilament

and it was not detectable in one unrelated patient. The amyloid deposits of the Chicago family were much less frequent than in s-IBM but more than in autosomal-recessive IBM (56) (Table 1.3).

In the few h-IBM patients and their few muscle fibers that contain amyloid deposits, those deposits are more rounded (Figure 1.6) than in s-IBM; the h-IBM congophilic amyloid does not occur in the form of the small linear "squiggles" that are typical of s-IBM amyloid (the s-IBM squiggles probably represent PHFs containing β-pleated-sheet hyper-phosphorylated-tau) (Fig. 1.1). s-IBM muscle also has some of the rounded amyloid deposits; we propose that in both s- and h-IBM the rounded deposits may represent Aβ associated with collections of 6–10 nm filaments (see above) (V. Askanas et al., unpublished data).

B. Light-microscopic abnormal accumulations of "Alzheimer-characteristic" proteins and prion, and their mRNA's.

As in s-IBM, within the vacuolated muscle fibers of h-IBM there are abnormal accumulations of: a) *prion protein* (PrP) and PrP-mRNA (13,119) (Figure 1.26; and b) several proteins typically accumulated in Alzheimer brain, namely (i) *Aβ* (7), (ii) *N-and C-terminal* epitopes of *βAPP* (8) (Figure 1.27), (iii) α_1-*antichymotrypsin* (α_1-ACT) (10) (Fig. 28), (iv) *apolipoprotein E* (ApoE) (11), and (v) *ubiquitin* (12) (Figure 1.27). This total ensemble of proteins that we have found accumulated in s-IBM and h-IBM muscle fibers appears to be unique for these diseases, in our experience to date. Whether this will remain true as more muscle diseases are analyzed in similar detail remains to be determined. A partial exception is oculopharyngeal muscular dystrophy (OPMD), an autosomal-dominant disease having some features in common with the IBMs, namely accumulation in the rare vacuolated muscle fibers of ubiquitin (12,73), βAPP (60), and phosphorylated tau (33, and V. Askanas et al.,

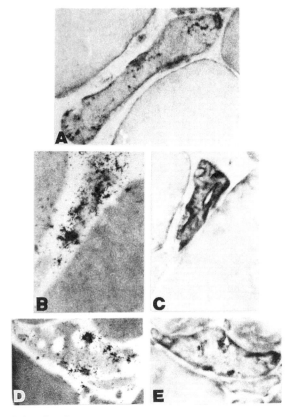

Figure 1.26. Prion (PrP) immunoreactivity. In vacuolated muscle fibers of recessive h-IBM there is increased PrP immunoreactivity (A, C, E) and increased PrP-mRNA (B, D). Reactions on B-C and D-E were performed on parallel, but not immediately adjacent, cross-sections (A, ×1,650; B–E, ×1,240). (Reproduced with permission from Askanas et al., *NeuroReport* 5:25–8, 1993, and Sarkozi et al., *Am. J. Pathol.* 145:1280–4, 1994.)

unpublished data). The other "IBM proteins" have not been studied in detail in OPMD muscle.

βAPP-mRNA, encoding βAPP containing the Kunitz-type protease-inhibitor (KPI) sequence (14), is also increased within vacuolated h-IBM muscle fibers, suggesting that the abnormal accumulation of the corresponding protein is generated, at least partly, by locally-increased transcription.

However, h-IBM is *different* from s-IBM regarding phosphorylated tau. Phosphorylated-tau identified by tau-1 monoclonal antibody is, in an individual 10 μm thick transverse section, abnormally accumulated

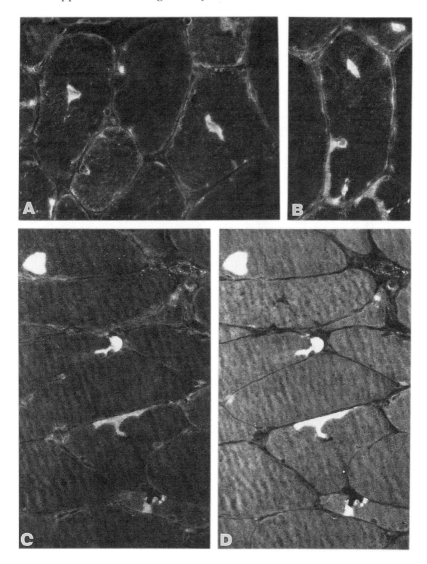

Figure 1.27. Fluorescence staining of βamyloid precursor protein (βAPP) epi-topes in a muscle biopsy of recessive h-IBM. A and B: Muscle fibers have large interior cytoplasmic inclusions immunoreactive with antibody against a C-termi-nal sequence of βAPP; a muscle fiber in "B" also has a strong subsarcolemmal immunoreactivity, part of which extends toward the interior of the fiber (×1,050). C and D: Double immunostaining for Aβ (C) and ubiquitin (Ub) (D) in the same tissue-section. Aβ is localized with Texas red and Ub with green FITC (×813). There is identical co-localization between Aβ and Ub. (Reproduced with permission from Askanas et al., *Ann. Neurol.* 34:551–60, 1993, and Askanas et al., *Am. J. Pathol.* 141:31–6, 1992.)

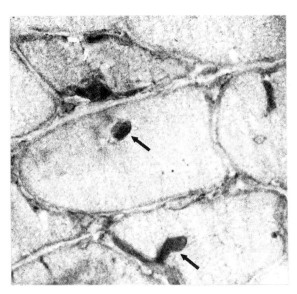

Figure 1.28. PAP reaction identifying abnormal accumulation of α_1-antichymotrypsin in recessive h-IBM ($\times 1,800$).

in 60–80% of the vacuolated muscle fibers of s-IBM, but it is abnormally accumulated in only 24% of the h-IBM vacuolated muscle fibers that are immunoreactive for the other excessive proteins (9). The monoclonal antibody *SMI-31* (which originally was directed against phosphorylated neurofilament heavy-chain but also cross-reacts with epitopes of phosphorylated-tau) is abundantly immunoreactive in both s-IBM and h-IBM (33,56) (Figure 1.6). At the subcellular level, in h-IBM as in s-IBM, the SMI-31 exclusively immunolabels PHFs (33) (Figure 1.29). By contrast, immunoreactivity with monoclonal antibody *SMI-310* (which originally was directed against phosphorylated heavy-chain neurofilament but also cross-reacts with another still-unknown epitope of phosphorylated-tau) is not detected at all in the h-IBM vacuolated muscle fibers, whereas it is strongly positive in 60–80% of the s-IBM vacuolated muscle fibers (58). *SMI-310,* by ultrastructural immunocytochemistry, exclusively labels PHFs, but only in s-IBM; it is not at all reactive with h-IBM PHFs (Figure 1.30). Accordingly, in h-IBM vacuolated muscle fibers, the paucity of both congophilic amyloid and several epitopes of phosphorylated-tau, plus the apparently-absolute qualitative difference in phosphorylated-tau epitopes in their lack of reaction with

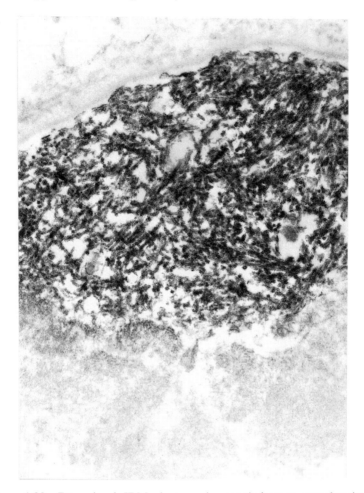

Figure 1.29. Recessive h-IBM electronmicroscopic-immunocytochemistry of SMI-31 antibody using the indirect horseradish-peroxidase method. SMI-31 exclusively labels paired helical filaments (above); a portion of the myofiber is completely unstained (below) (×25,000).

SMI-310, provide a subtle but clear distinction from the muscle-fiber phenotype of s-IBM.

Regarding the tau protein, we propose that its pathologic state evolves, namely that when the tau epitope in s-IBM-PHFs (9) becomes antigenically and configurationally reactive with the SMI-310 antibody it becomes congophilic. Accordingly, we propose that in autosomal-recessive h-IBM the PHF-tau, which typically reacts with SMI-31 but not with SMI-310 and

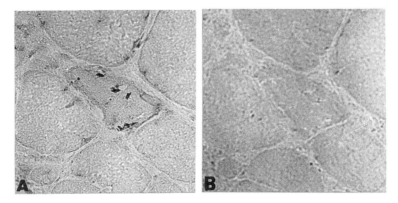

Figure 1.30. Immunoreactivity of SMI-31 (A) and SMI-310 (B) in recessive h-IBM. Stainings were performed in closely adjacent parallel sections. The same vacuolated muscle fiber in the middle of each microphotograph (arrow) has positive SMI-31 inclusions, but is not immunoreactive with SMI-310 (A and B, ×1,000).

is not congophilic: a) is in a putatively earlier state of molecular modification; and b) does not evolve beyond that stage because of a subtle, unknown difference in the pathogenesis as compared with s-IBM.

The status of the Aβ accumulated in IBM might also evolve, and in autosomal-recessive h-IBM it might be remaining in an earlier stage of modification. In our s-IBM patients, double-fluorescence studies revealed that some vacuolated muscle fibers were Aβ-immunoreactive but Congo-red negative (7–9), a finding similar to Aβ in Congo-red-negative "diffuse-plaques" of Alzheimer-disease brain (122) – we conclude that, in them, the Aβ is not in Congophilic β-pleated sheets. In autosomal-recessive h-IBM, virtually all vacuolated muscle fibers are Aβ-positive but Congo-red negative; and so we also postulate that in these fibers Aβ is not in β-pleated-sheets and thus may be in an earlier stage of the pathogenic process (as has also been suggested for Alzheimer diffuse-plaques).

Proteins that we have studied, which are not accumulated in either s- or h-IBM are listed in Table 1.6.

IV. Neuropathy in S-IBM and H-IBM

In transverse sections of every s-IBM and h-IBM biopsy there are small angular muscle fibers, darkly stained with the pan-esterase and NADH-tetrazolium-reductase (NADH-TR) reactions; such fibers are considered to have been recently denervated. On electromyography (EMG), nearly all IBM patients have a definitely neurogenic pattern reflecting both a) recent denervation (fibrillations and positive sharp waves), and b) previous denervation followed by established-reinnervation (polyphasics of normal and longer duration, and often increased amplitude) (123; W.K. Engel et al., unpublished data) (note that denervation of a muscle fiber can result from a neurogenous or occasionally a myogenous process [124]). The s- and h-IBM patients also usually have *b*rief-duration *s*mall-amplitude overly *a*bundant motor-unit action-*p*otentials (BSAPs), often *p*olyphasic (BSAPPs). BSAPs and BSAPPs indicate fractionation of motor units and can be caused by a disorder of distal axonal twigs, neuromuscular junctions, or muscle fibers. They are *not diagnostic* of a myopathic process (125,126).

In h-IBM, the histochemical evidence of denervation, in the form of small dark (with NADH-TR and pan-esterase stainings) angular muscle fibers, sometimes greatly predominates over the vacuolated fibers or other definitely myopathic features, such that we are tempted to call it "hereditary inclusion-body myopathy-neuropathy." For example, two Persian Jewish brothers, whose cousin had many vacuolated muscle fibers, did not have any vacuoles in their initial biopsies, which looked like only pronounced ordinary denervation. Because of their family history they were rebiopsied, and only one vacuolated muscle fiber was found in one of the patients and none in the other (W.K. Engel and V. Askanas, unpublished data). In s-IBM, we propose that the neuropathic component may not be responsive to immunosuppression treatment.

V. Tissue Culture of h-IBM Muscle

When muscle fibers of autosomal-recessive Persian-Jewish type of h-IBM were cultured aneurally, they expressed a partial IBM phenotype, in the form of vacuoles, as well as accumulations of βAPP and prion protein (V. Askanas and J. McFerrin, unpublished data). When the cultured h-IBM muscle fibers were innervated by motor neurons of cocultured fetal rat spinal-cord to become rather well-differentiated, they showed even more of the IBM phenotype, namely PHFs (127; V. Askanas et al., unpublished data). Because these characteristic IBM features have been reproduced in cultured h-IBM muscle, probably the abnormal h-IBM gene is responsible for their expression in the h-IBM patient. Therefore, this culture model can provide genetically and morphologically abnormal living tissue that is readily accessible for a wide range of molecular studies, including therapeutic trials. One therapeutic possibility would be to use adenovirus vectors carrying βAPP or prion cDNA in antisense orientation, both of which we have recently constructed in our laboratory. However, in the patient the antisense might impair not only their pathologic functions but also the normal functions of βAPP or prion, for example at neuromuscular junctions and in the brain.

VI. Induced Overexpression of the βAPP Gene Conveyed by Adenovirus Vector into Cultured Normal Human Muscle

To determine whether abnormally accumulated βAPP in IBM muscle is at least partially responsible for development of the IBM phenotype, we transferred the βAPP-751 gene, using adenovirus vector, into cultured normal human muscle (128,129). Cultured human muscle overexpressing the βAPP gene had strongly increased amounts of both βAPP-mRNA and βAPP protein by Northern blot, immunoblot, in situ hybridization, and immunocytochemistry (Figures 1.31 and 1.32).

Like s-IBM biopsied muscle fibers, the βAPP-overexpressing cultured muscle fibers were vacuolated (Figure 1.33) and had patches of Congored-positive amyloid (128). Electronmicroscopy revealed 15–21 nm nuclear tubulofilaments, 6-10 nm cytoplasmic filaments, and lysosomal inclusions (128,128a). These studies (which were the first to utilize the adenovirus vector for transferring the βAPP gene) provided the novel demonstration that overexpression of the βAPP gene in muscle can produce several aspects of the IBM cellular phenotype.

It is also of particular interest that βAPP-overexpressing cultured muscle fiber had abnormal mitochondria with paracrystalline inclusions by electronmicroscopy and were cytochrome-c-oxidase (cox)negative histochemically (129) (Figures 1.34–1.36). These findings demonstrated that overexpression of the βAPP gene and the resultant overproduction of βAPP in human muscle fibers can cause decreased COX enzymatic activity and structural abnormalities of mitochondria, with the degree of abnormality correlating with the duration of βAPP overexpression. Decreased COX activity preceded the mitochondrial structural abnormalities. These changes were not caused simply by the adenovirus itself, because there were no mitochondrial abnormalities in our controls, which consisted of cultured human muscle infected with a) recombinant wild adenovirus, b) adenovirus carrying βAPP cDNA in antisense orientation, and c) adenovirus carrying β-galactosidase reporter-gene (129).

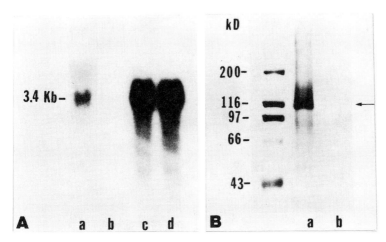

Figure 1.31. A: Autoradiograph of northern blot of RNA extracted from cultured control human muscle (lanes a and b) and sister cultures infected for 5 days (lane c) and 10 days (lane d) with adenovirus carrying the βAPP gene. Ten micrograms of total RNA were loaded in each lane. Lanes b–d were exposed for 10 minutes. Lane a is the same as lane b, but exposed for 5 hours. There is strikingly increased βAPP-mRNA signal in the βAPP-gene-infected muscle cultures. B: Immunoblots of proteins isolated from βAPP-overexpressing muscle (lane a) and cultured control sister muscle (lane b) probed with antibody against the C-terminal epitope of βAPP. There is a strong band corresponding to 116-kDa βAPP in the βAPP-overexpressing cultures (lane a), but only a very faint band (indicated by arrow) in the control cultures (lane b). Cultures were infected 10 days previously with the adenovirus carrying the βAPP gene. The left lane displays molecular-weight standards. (Reproduced with permission from Askanas et al., *Proc. Natl. Acad. Sci. USA* 93:1314–19, 1996.)

Mitochondrial COX deficiency and structural abnormalities were not secondary to the other recognized aspects of βAPP-induced muscle degeneration, because the mitochondrial changes were present earlier, in muscle fibers lacking other signs of degeneration, as well as later in vacuolated muscle fibers.

As in s-IBM, abnormalities of the COX system have been described in AD. For example, COX enzymatic activity and the mRNA for a mitochondrial-encoded COX II subunit were reported to be decreased in AD brain (130–132).

The cause of mitochondrial abnormalities in IBM muscle and AD brain is not known. Our study demonstrated a relationship between βAPP overexpression and the abnormalities of COX and mitochondrial structure. Whether the βAPP effect on mitochondria was direct or indi-

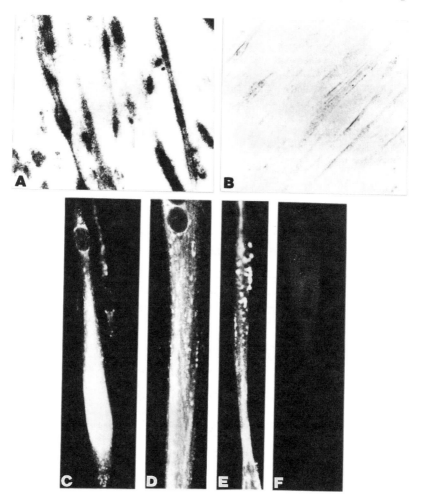

Figure 1.32.   A and B: In situ hybridization with βAPP-751 antisense cRNA of 3-week-old cultured human muscle 7 days after infection with an adenovirus vector carrying the βAPP gene (A), and of uninfected control sister culture (B). Autoradiographic exposure time was 3 hours (A), or 8 hours (B). There is strikingly increased βAPP-751-mRNA signal in the βAPP-gene-infected culture (A), emphasized by the very dark image (A) despite the much shorter auto-radiographic-exposure time compared to the control (B) (×510). C–F: Im-munofluorescence with antibodies against Aβ (C), and C-terminal (D) and N-terminal (E) epitopes of βAPP, in βAPP-overexpressing cultured human mus-cle fibers; and against C-terminal portion of βAPP in an uninfected sister control muscle fiber (F). The βAPP-overexpressing cultures show strikingly increased immunoreactivity of all βAPP epitopes (C–E), whereas the uninfected control (F) is negative. (In all other control cultures, stainings with antibodies against Aβ and N-terminal βAPP were also negative.) (Reproduced with permission from Askanas et al., *Proc. Natl. Acad. Sci. USA* 93:1314–19, 1996.)

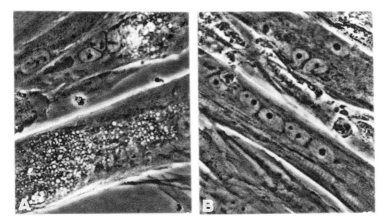

Figure 1.33. Phase-contrast micrographs of 4-week-old cultured human muscle 2 weeks after βAPP gene transfer (A) and a non-infected sister control cultured human muscle (B). There are various degrees of vacuolization in the βAPP-over-expressing cultured muscle fibers, whereas same-age control muscle fibers are healthy and cross-striated (A and B, ×2,400). (Reproduced with permission from Askanas et al., *Proc. Natl. Acad. Sci. USA* 93:1314–19, 1996.)

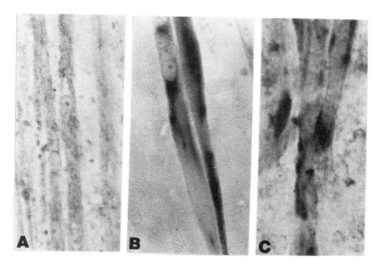

Figure 1.34. Light microscopy of cytochrome oxidase (COX) staining of cul-tured human muscle. A: The COX reaction is negative in the βAPP-overexpress-ing cultured human muscle fibers 15 days after βAPP-gene transfer, whereas sister-cultured muscle fibers infected with the recombinant wild adenovirus vec-tor (B), and uninfected control sister-cultured muscle fibers (C), have very strong COX staining (A–C, ×560). (Reproduced with permission from Askanas et al., *Proc. Natl. Acad. Sci. USA* 93:1314–19, 1996.)

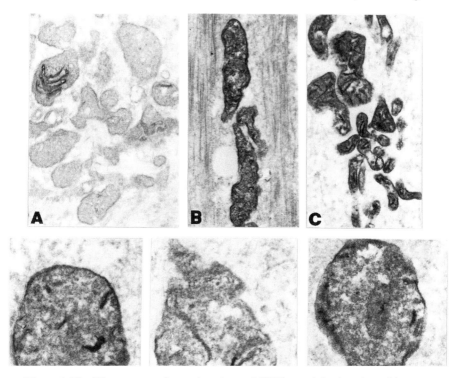

Figure 1.35. Ultrastructural cytochemistry of COX reactivity in cultured human muscle 4 days after βAPP-gene transfer (A), in a sister-cultured muscle infected with the recombinant wild adenovirus vector (B), and in a sister noninfected-control cultured muscle (C). There is strong COX reactivity in the mitochondria of muscle fibers in both controls (B, C), whereas the βAPP-overexpressing muscle mitochondria are devoid of COX reactivity (except for one mitochondrion at upper left), although they do not yet manifest major structural abnormalities. D–F: Examples of abnormal mitochondria in which COX activity is located only in patches on a few remaining cristae (D, E) or on the inner mitochondrial membrane (F) (A, ×8,400; B and C, ×7,700; D and E, ×18,900; F, ×14,700). (Reproduced with permission from Askanas et al., *Proc. Natl. Acad. Sci. USA* 93:1314–19, 1996.)

rect is not known. Perhaps increased βAPP can affect DNA stability, repair, or transcription.

Our model of human-muscle tissue culture offers several advantages for studies of overexpression of βAPP and other genes. For example, it enables culturing, to a rather mature state, the human cells primarily affected by the disease, namely, the muscle fibers (reviewed in 133). And because human muscle fibers can be cultured for several weeks, it is possible to study chronologically the changes consequent to gene over-

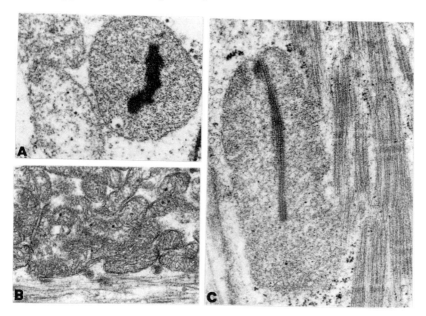

Figure 1.36. Electron microscopy of abnormal mitochondria in βAPP-over-expressing cultured muscle fibers. Three weeks after βAPP-gene transfer, mito-chondria have lost their normal cristae pattern and contain paracrystalline inclusions (A, C), while a control uninfected sister culture (B) has normal mito-chondria (A, ×26,000; B, ×27,000; C, ×43,000). (Reproduced with permission from Askanas et al., *Proc. Natl. Acad. Sci. USA* 93:1314–19, 1996.)

expression, in both a) aneurally cultured human muscle fibers, and b) ones innervated and driven to more complete maturity (including transy-naptically-generated contractions) by co-cultured fetal-rat spinal-cord motor-neurons (133).

By demonstrating that βAPP-gene transfer causes decreased COX activity and structural abnormality of mitochondria, our study suggests that overexpressed βAPP may play a key role in the induction of those abnormalities, both in IBM and in AD, and provides an excellent experi-mental model for further molecular studies of various abnormalities due to βAPP overexpression. For example, our newest studies indicate that the SOD1 gene is upregulated in cultured muscle fibers overexpressing the βAPP-gene (117), indicating that increased βAPP accumulation may contribute, directly or indirectly, to the evidence of oxidative stress we have observed in biopsied IBM muscle fibers (see below).

VII. Speculations on the Yet-Unknown Pathogenesis of s-IBM and h-IBM

A. How a Cascade of Self-Perpetuating Muscle Fiber Destruction Might Start

We have previously proposed that *increased* expression of genes is at least one component underlying the demonstrated increase of the IBM-characteristic proteins (16). It is possible that one gene-product (protein) might start a detrimental cascade by acting, directly or indirectly, as a transcription factor activating genes for some of the other "IBM-proteins." For example, βAPP or prion (PrPc), or one of their products, could have this effect, as might another yet-unidentified protein. Our theoretical model of h-IBM and s-IBM is presented in Figure 1.37. The model incorporates several hypotheses. One hypothesis concerns a fundamental role of mono-specific (box 2a) enhanced transcription of βAPP mRNA (box 3a), or PrPc-mRNA (box 3b). This could be caused in h-IBM (box 1a) by i) an inherited alteration of the gene for a putative transcription factor (TF) or a factor controlling it, or ii) an inherited alteration of a promoter/enhancer of the βAPP or PrPc gene. In s-IBM (box 1b), a viral DNA integrated into the cell genome (and/or an immunologic abnormality) could lead to production of a protein TF (or a factor controlling it) – or perhaps serves as a template for directly transcribing βAPP or PrPc. The increased βAPP, or PrPc, (boxes 3a and 3b) might then i) produce a partial IBM phenotype (box 5, left short bracket) or complete phenotype (box 5, left long bracket), or ii) directly or indirectly increase transcription of some of the other "IBM-proteins" (boxes 4a and 4b) resulting in a full (box 5, left long bracket) or partial (box 5, left short bracket) phenotype. Other "IBM proteins" that do not show detectable evidence of transcription either in IBM muscle or in normal muscle, e.g. ApoE, tau, and a_1-ACT (V. Askanas and W.K. Engel, unpublished data), would be accumulated by other mechanisms, perhaps i) increased uptake, ii) increased adhesion to Aβ, PrPc or another protein, or iii) decreased catabolism (box 5, lower part).

Alternatively, the fundamental phenomenon in h- or s-IBM might be an increase of a Group-Specific Transcription Factor/Mechanism (box 2b) that more directly activates transcription of two or more of the IBM proteins (box 4c), resulting in the IBM-phenotype; this mechanism might be less likely in view of the effect of induced βAPP overexpression (see above). (The putative Group-Specific TF (box 2b) could have similarities to a) what occurs at normal neuromuscular junctions (NMJs) involving a hypothetical "junctionalization TF" (2b), or b) to what occurs to some degree in regenerative muscle fibers (2b); or, it is also possible that an increase of βAPP expression is an early step of a cascade leading to accumulation of various other characteristic proteins at the NMJs.)

Conceivably, the most fundamental detrimental cellular effect in IBM might be a pathologically *decreased* expression of yet-undelineated genes that have a direct or indirect suppressor effect on the expression of other genes, such that those other genes become pathologically overexpressed.

The actual starting mechanism for s-IBM might be a still-to-be-discovered virus infestation that alters gene transcription. The clinical onset of s-IBM in later-adult life suggests that possibly a component of "normal aging" of muscle-fibers is a necessary background co-factor required for s-IBM to develop and progress.

For h-IBM, the cause presumably is a mutated gene producing a protein having either a loss-of-function or an aberrant gain-of-function. Because the clinical manifestation begins in young-adulthood even though the gene-mutation was present from birth, it is possible that full-maturity or very-early-aging changes in muscle fibers provide a necessary cellular environment for instigation of the progressive cellular damage.

B. Putative Junctionalization of Non-Junctional Regions of Muscle Fibers

Several of the accumulated "IBM-proteins" and the increased "IBM-mRNAs" are ones normally found accumulated in the muscle-fiber only at the post-synaptic region of the neuromuscular junction (NMJ). "Junctionalization" is a term we introduced (16) to include the normal phenomena of protein and mRNA accumulation at the NMJ. Junctionalization is induced by the contacting motor-neuron axonal-tip and presumably is governed (at least partially) through enhanced expression of the junctional-protein genes within the muscle-fiber nuclei that are located immediately post-synaptically ("junctional nuclei"). Normally in the innervated mature muscle fiber, those "junctional-protein" genes are concurrently downregulated in the non-junctional nuclei located elsewhere throughout the muscle fiber. Because we have demonstrated in IBM that most of the accumulated "IBM-proteins" (e.g. βAPP (72), prion (81), a_1ACT (134), fibroblast growth factor (135), transforming growth factor beta (136), ubiquitin (115), AChR and the 43 kD protein (117) are those same "junctional proteins," we proposed (16) that in s-IBM and h-IBM there is a pathologic "junctionalization" of extrajunctional regions of the IBM muscle-fiber, causing altered gene expression

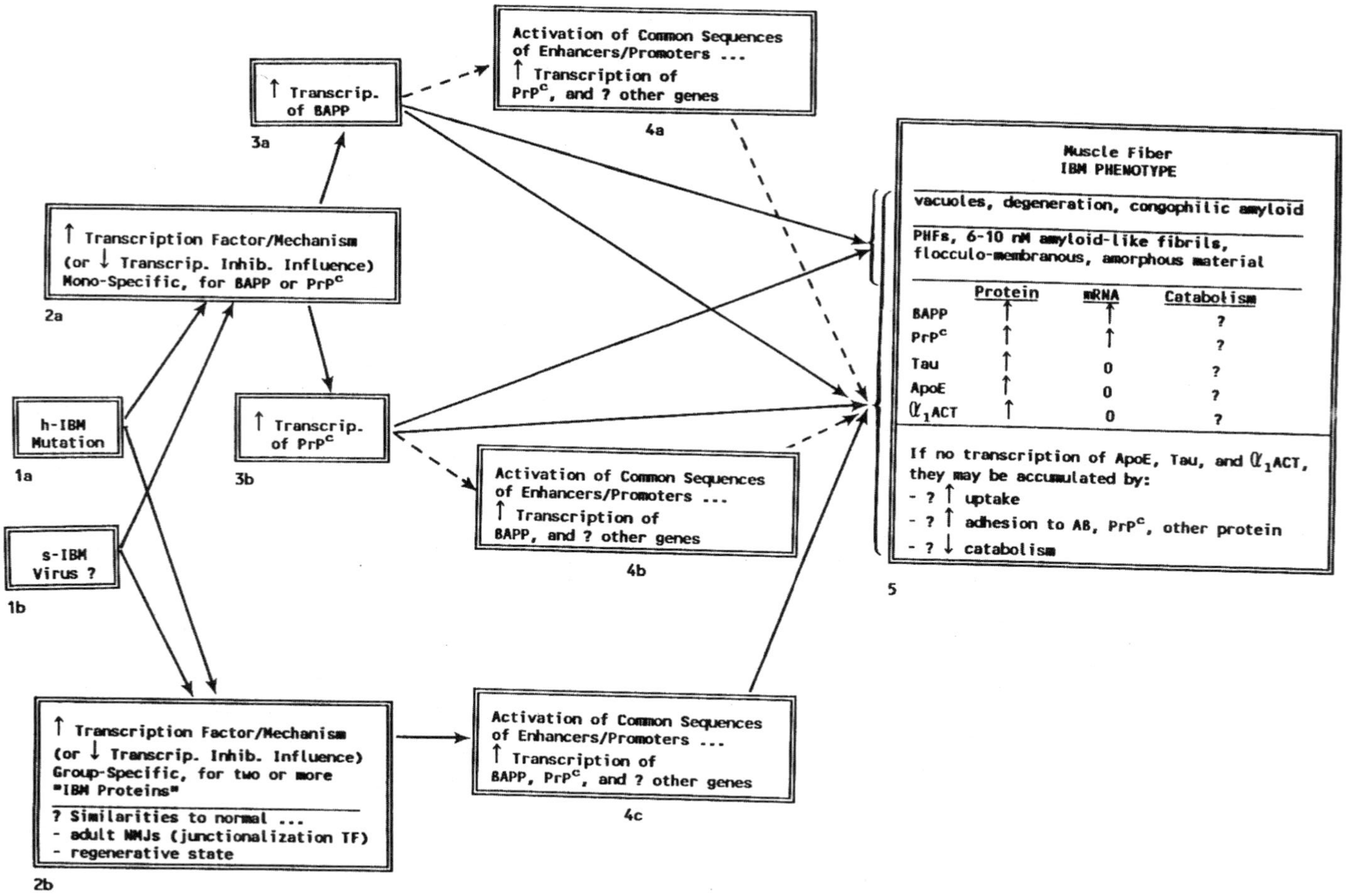

Figure 1.27 Theoretical model of h-IBM and s-IBM

Muscle Fiber IBM PHENOTYPE

vacuoles, degeneration, congophilic amyloid

PHFs, 6-10 nM amyloid-like fibrils, flocculo-membranous, amorphous material

Protein		mRNA	Catabolism
BAPP	↑	↑	?
PrP^c	↑	0	?
Tau	↑	0	?
ApoE	↑	0	?
α_1ACT	↑	0	?

If no transcription of ApoE, Tau, and α_1ACT, they may be accumulated by:
- ? ↑ uptake
- ? ↑ adhesion to AB, PrP^c, other protein
- ? ↓ catabolism

5

Activation of Common Sequences of Enhancers/Promoters ...
↑ Transcription of PrP^c, and ? other genes

4a

Activation of Common Sequences of Enhancers/Promoters ...
↑ Transcription of BAPP, and ? other genes

4b

Activation of Common Sequences of Enhancers/Promoters ...
↑ Transcription of BAPP, PrP^c, and ? other genes

4c

↑ Transcription of BAPP

3a

↑ Transcription of PrP^c

3b

↑ Transcription Factor/Mechanism (or ↓ Transcrip. Inhib. Influence) Mono-Specific, for BAPP or PrP^c

2a

↑ Transcription Factor/Mechanism (or ↓ Transcrip. Inhib. Influence) Group-Specific, for two or more "IBM Proteins"
? Similarities to normal ...
- adult NMJs (junctionalization TF)
- regenerative state

2b

h-IBM Mutation

1a

s-IBM Virus ?

1b

of the "IBM-junctionalized" (previously non-junctional) nuclei. This junctionalization could be induced, directly or indirectly, or by a putative virus in s-IBM or by the mutated-gene protein in h-IBM (Figure 1.34).

VIII. Possible Relevance to Alzheimer-Disease Pathogenesis

Because the same proteins accumulate within the s- and h-IBM muscle fibers and in the brain in sporadic and hereditary forms of Alzheimer disease (AD), these muscle diseases might have pathogenic analogies to AD, and knowledge of one might help to elucidate the other. Within each organ-disease group, the sporadic and hereditary forms are morpho-chemical phenocopies of each other. Between the two muscle-disease and two brain-disease groups, perhaps: a) the sporadic forms involve parallel pathogenic mechanisms (possibly provoked by a viral and/or autoimmune process); and b) the two hereditary forms might involve similar mechanisms eventuating in accumulation of identical proteins. A facilitatory substratum of ordinary cellular "aging" might be involved, especially in the sporadic forms of each.

One protein, prion, is not accumulated in the AD brain but is accumulated in the brain of sporadic and hereditary prion diseases (13). In the prion brain diseases, prion mRNA is not increased, but instead a unique mechanism of prion accumulation has been proposed (78). Because the muscle fibers of the IBMs do have a pathologic accumulation of prion-mRNA, they are different from the prion brain diseases; we suggest that, in the IBM muscle-fiber, increased prion protein is related to an enhanced mRNA-directed synthesis and the prion accumulation is like that occurring normally at NMJs (77). Phenotypic similarities between s-IBM muscle and AD brain are illustrated in Table 1.8.

Biopsy provides relatively easy access to s-IBM and h-IBM muscle. And in contrast to adult human neurons of Alzheimer and prion-disease brain, s-IBM and h-IBM human muscle can be cultured and maintained in a rather mature state for an extended period of time. These aspects make this a valuable system for further study of the pathogenesis of these degenerative muscle diseases, which might have some cellular pathogenic mechanisms fundamentally analogous to ones of the degenerative brain diseases.

IX. Update on the Newest Results

The update relates to our new results obtained while this book was in press.

Table 1.8.

Cellular phenotype	Inclusion body myositis, muscle fibers	Alzheimer-disease, brain
CONGHOPHILIA, associated with Amyloid-βeta (Aβ)	Small-Plaques, intra-cellular	Large Plaques, extra-cellular
Aβ in FILAMENTS	6–10 nm	6–8 nm
Other βAPP epitopes, accumulated	YES	YES
751-βAPP-mRNA, increased	YES	YES?
PHF bundles are		
Congophilic	YES	YES, Neurofibrillary, Tangles
PHFs in bundles, contain:		
• TAU-Phosphorylated	YES	YES
• Ubiquitin	YES	YES
• Apolipoprotein E (APO E)	YES	YES
a_1-Antichymotrypsin (ACT), accumulated	YES	YES
a_1-ACT-mRNA, increased	NO	YES, in astrocytes
APO E-mRNA, increased	NO	NO
SOD1, accumulated	YES	YES
SOD1 mRNA, increased	YES	?
Mitochondrial abnormalities, including COX deficiency	YES	YES
NON-ALZHEIMER accumulations:		
• Prion (probably normal cellular type)	YES	NO
• Prion-mRNA (normal cellular type)	YES	NO

A. Nitric oxide Induced Oxidative Stress

1. Background

a. Nitric oxide (NO). NO is a short-lived reactive gas. It is formed by *nitric oxide synthetase* (NOS) directly from the guanidino nitrogen of L-arginine (reviewed in 138). NO is considered to be an intercellular and intracellular messenger, having diverse normal functions: playing a role in vasodilation; mediating anti-microbial toxicity of macrophages; serving as an inter-neuronal messenger; and possibly inducing transcriptional and post-transcriptional regulation of genes (reviewed in 138,139). Excessive production of NO is postulated to play an important role in various diseases, including neurodegenerative, inflammatory and immunological processes (138,140,141). Previously, its role in diseased human muscle has not been studied.

b. Nitric oxide synthetases (NOS). There are three forms of human NOS, *neuronal (nNOS), inducible (iNOS),* and *endothelial (endothelial NOS).* These have been cloned and are encoded by different genes on chromosomes 12,17 and 7, respectively (reviewed in 138,139,142). nNOS and endothelial-NOS are constitutive, and are stimulated mainly by intracellular Ca^{2+} via calmodulin (138,139,142). Even though their activation does not require new enzyme synthesis, new synthesis of nNOS has been demonstrated under certain circumstances (reviewed in 138). iNOS, present especially in activated macrophages, can be induced in various other cells (138,142). iNOS is transcriptionally regulated (139,142). Its increased synthesis can be stimulated by cytokines, inflammation and other pathologic processes (139,142).

c. Superoxide dismutase 1 (SOD1). The *superoxide ion* O^{2-} is a product of normal cell metabolism, especially mitochondrial oxidations. Superoxide is toxic by itself, and it readily combines with NO to form the even more toxic *peroxynitrite* (140,141). The enzyme SOD1 generally provides a protective mechanism by converting superoxide to peroxide (H_2O_2). However, the peroxide must be inactivated by conversion to H_2O by a peroxidase (such as glutathione peroxidase) or catalase; otherwise, excess H_2O_2 can also lead to toxic free radicals of oxygen.

4. Nitrotyrosine. Increased nitric oxide (NO) combines rapidly with superoxide to form the powerful oxidizing agent *peroxynitrite,* which nitrates tyrosine groups of protein to form the stable compound *3-nitrotyrosine (nitrotyrosine)* (140,141). Nitration of proteins can disturb their functions and cause various pathologic processes.

2. Results

nNOS, iNOS, and *nitrotyrosine* are abnormally accumulated in vacuolated muscle fibers of both s-IBM and h-IBM (143,144). These abnormalities were not present in any of the disease-control muscle biopsies of patients with polymyositis, dermatomyositis, morphologically nonspecific myopathies, or amyotrophic lateral sclerosis, as they were in s-

and h-IBM. These studies were the first to demonstrate increased amounts of nNOS, iNOS, and nitrotyrosine in abnormal human muscle.

We have also demonstrated that SOD1 and SOD1-mRNA are abnormally accumulated in vacuolated muscle fibers of s- and h-IBM (121).

Comment

Even though we do not know whether all the immunoreactive NOS in all the subcellular sites is enzymatically active, the presence of nitrotyrosine in IBM vacuolated muscle fibers allows the hypothesis that abnormal accumulation of NOSs in IBM leads to overproduction of NO and subsequently to the NO-induced "oxidative stress." Possibly this mechanism contributes to the vacuoles and other degenerative aspects of IBM muscle, including loss of cytochrome-c-oxidase and structural abnormalities of mitochondria which are known to be initiated by NO (145).

The possible role of SOD1 in tyrosine nitration in IBM is not yet established. The increase of SOD1 in IBM vacuolated muscle fibers (121) may have occurred independently of NO mechanisms, or it initially may have been an attempted protective response to decrease ambient superoxide and the consequent formation of peroxynitrite, i.e., to protect the muscle fiber against "oxidative stress." However, in conditions of overwhelming amounts of NO and peroxynitrite, SOD1 can actually catalyse protein nitration to facilitate nitrotyrosine production (141).

B. *Immunolocalization of Interleukins 1α, 1β and 6*

1. Results

We have recently found by immunolocalization that interleukins (ILs) 1α, IL1β and IL6 are abnormally accumulated in vacuolated muscle fibers of s-IBM, typically in the form of small "squiggles" and patches (146). By immuno-electronmicroscopy, all three ILs were virtually exclusively present on paired helical filaments (PHFs). In addition, interstitial macrophages and ones phagocytosing muscle fibers were positive with antibodies against these three ILs and with the macrophage marker, Ber-MAC3. Regenerating muscle fibers (in all s-IBM and other biopsies that contained them) had positive immunoreactivity of these three ILs in a diffuse pattern but not in squiggles. At the postsynaptic zone of all normal neuromuscular junctions (NMJs) immunoreactivities of IL-1α, IL-1β and IL-6 were also accumulated.

2. Comment

Our studies indicate that IL-1α, IL-1β and IL-6 may play a role in a) s-IBM pathogenesis, and b) in normal muscle biology, namely, regeneration and NMJ function.

C. Overexpression of β-amyloid Precursor Protein (APP) Gene in Cultured Normal Human Muscle Transferred by Adenovirus Vector Prevents Formation of Neuromuscular Junctions (NMJs) and Functional Innervation: Relevance to Inclusion-Body Myositis (s-IBM)

1. Background and Technique

In normal adult human muscle fibers, βAPP and its mRNA are present only at the postsynaptic domain of NMJs (14,72). In s-IBM, muscle fibers contain vacuoles having abnormal focal accumulations of βAPP and βAPP-mRNA scattered diffusely in non-junctional regions (8,14). Because denervation of muscle fibers in s-IBM is evidenced both morphologically and electrophysiologically, we investigated whether abnormally accumulated βAPP may, at least partially, be responsible for a "myogenous" impairment of innervation of s-IBM muscle fibers.

To produce muscle fibers with excessive βAPP, a 3-kb human 751-βAPP cDNA was transferred into cultured normal young human myotubes (immediately after myoblast fusion), using a replication-deficient recombinant adenovirus (RDRA) vector (as described above and in 129). Three days after βAPP gene transfer, βAPP-overexpressing and sister-control muscle were co-cultured with fetal rat spinal cord (having dorsal root ganglia attached) as described (147).

Results

Control innervated muscle fibers became fully cross-striated, were continuously and rhythmically contracting, and had acetylcholinesterase (AChE) and acetylcholine receptors (AChRs) accumulated only at the NMJs, as in our previous studies (147, reviewed in 133). In contrast, the same-age βAPP-overexpressing muscle fibers resembled our human muscle fibers cultured aneurally (i.e. without co-cultured spinal-cord neurons). They were not cross-striated and not contracting. AChE on them was in large and diffuse patches, and only 2–3% of the fibers had AChR clusters (148). Although the cultured control muscle fibers were contacted by axons outgrowing from the spinal-cord explants and stopping at individual muscle fibers, the βAPP-overexpressing fibers appeared to be passed over by axons that seemed not to recognize that they should stop on the muscle fibers and induce the NMJs (148). That impaired innervation was not due to an influence on spinal cord neurons of βAPP fragments released to the medium because treatment of control cultures with the conditioned medium did not influence innervation.

Comment

This is the first demonstration that overexpression of βAPP in muscle fibers inhibits their innervation. This mechanism could prevent IBM muscle fibers from remaining properly innervated or regenerating IBM muscle fibers from becoming correctly innervated – if so, this would be a "myogenous-deinnervation" (a concept introduced by one of us (W.K.E.) (149,150)). If it would be established that the experimentally excessive βAPP inhibits proper innervation, presumably the moderate increase present in normal generating or regenerating muscle fibers is not inhibitory.

Acknowledgments

Studies described in this review were supported in part by the National Institutes of Health, Muscular Dystrophy Association, the Alzheimer Association, and the Sheldon Katz, Helen Lewis, and Ron Stever Research Funds. We thank our research-team colleagues R. B. Alvarez, E. Sarkozi, J. McFerrin, M. Mirabella, M. Bilak, S. Baqué, P. Serdaroglu, K. Haginoya, and C. C. Yang, who participated in various aspects of the studies described. Assistance in photographic processing by M. Baburyan, histochemical preparations by T. Nguyen, and preparation of the manuscript by L. Martinez is appreciated. We also thank our Clinical Fellows who over the past several years have participated in the care of our patients. We are grateful to our physician colleagues who graciously referred to us their patients, and to the very cooperative patients themselves, without whom these studies would not have been possible and for whose ultimate benefit these studies aspire.

References

1. Yunis EJ, Samaha FJ. Inclusion body myositis. *Lab Invest* 25:240–248, 1971.

2. Carpenter S, Karpati G, Heller I, Eisen A. Inclusion body myositis: a distinct variety of idiopathic inflammatory myopathy. *Neurology* 28:8–17, 1978.

3. Tomé FMS, Fardeau M, Lebon P, Chevallay M. Inclusion body myositis. *Acta Neuropathol* 7:287–291, 1981.

4. Lotz BP, Engel AG, Nishino H, Stevens JC, Litchy WJ. Inclusion body myositis: observations in 40 patients. *Brain* 112:727–747, 1989.

5. Askanas V, Engel WK. New advances in inclusion-body myositis. *Curr Opin Rheumatol* 5:732–741, 1993.

6. Mendell JR, Sahenk Z, Gales T, Paul L. Amyloid filaments in inclusion body myositis. *Arch Neurol* 48:1229–1234, 1991.

7. Askanas V, Engel WK, Alvarez RB. Light- and electronmicroscopic localization of β-amyloid protein in muscle biopsies of patients with inclusion-body myositis. *Am J Pathol* 141:31–36, 1992.

8. Askanas V, Alvarez RB, Engel WK. Abnormal accumulations of β-amyloid precursor epitopes in muscle fibers of inclusion body myositis. *Ann Neurol* 34:551–560, 1993.

9. Askanas V, Engel WK, Bilak M, Alvarez RB, Selkoe DJ. Twisted tubulofilaments of inclusion-body myositis muscle resemble paired helical filaments of Alzheimer brain and contain hyperphosphorylated tau. *Am J Pathol* 144:177–187, 1994.

10. Bilak M, Askanas V, Engel WK. Strong immunoreactivity of α_1-antichymotrypsin colocalizes with β-amyloid protein and ubiquitin in vacuolated muscle fibers of inclusion-body myositis. *Acta Neuropathol* 85:378–382, 1993.

11. Askanas V, Mirabella M, Engel WK, Alvarez RB, Weisgraber KH. Apolipoprotein E immunoreactive deposits in inclusion-body muscle diseases. *Lancet* 343:364–365, 1994.

12. Askanas V, Serdaroglu P, Engel WK, Alvarez RB. Immunolocalization of ubiquitin in muscle biopsies of patients with inclusion body myositis and oculopharyngeal muscular dystrophy. *Neurosci Lett* 130:73–76, 1991.

13. Askanas V, Bilak M, Engel WK, Alvarez RB, Tomé FMS, Leclerc A. Prion protein is abnormally accumulated in inclusion-body myositis. *NeuroReport* 5:25–28, 1993.

14. Sarkozi E, Askanas V, Johnson SA, Engel WK, Alvarez RB. β-amyloid precursor protein mRNA is increased in inclusion-body myositis muscle. *NeuroReport* 4:815–818, 1993.

15. Sarkozi E, Askanas V, Engel WK. Abnormal accumulation of prion protein mRNA in muscle fibers of patients with sporadic inclusion-body myositis and hereditary inclusion-body myopathy. *Am J Pathol* 145:1280–1284, 1994.

16. Askanas V, Engel WK. New advances in the understanding of sporadic inclusion-body myositis and hereditary inclusion-body myopathies. *Curr Opin Rheumatol* 7:486–496, 1995.

17. Mikol J, Engel AG. Inclusion body myositis. In: Engel AG, Franzini-Armstrong C (eds), *Myology: Basic and Clinical,* vol. 2. McGraw-Hill, New York, 1994, pp. 1384–1398.

18. Riminton DS, Chambers ST, Parkin PJ, Pollock M, Donaldson IM. Inclusion-body myositis presenting solely as dysphagia. *Neurology* 43:1241–1243, 1993.

19. Schlesinger I, Soffer D, Lossos A, Meiner Z, Argov Z. Inclusion body myositis: atypical clinical presentations. *Eur Neurol* 36:89–93, 1996.

19a. Engel WK, Haginoya K, Alvarez RB, Sabetian K, Bajoghli M, Askanas V. Sporadic inclusion-body myositus (s-IBM) in an HTLV-I-positive Iranian Muslim. *Neurology* 48:124, 1997.
20. Abarbanel JM, Lichtenfeld Y, Zirkin H, Louzon Z, Osimani A, Farkash P, Herishanu Y. Inclusion body myositis in post-poliomyelitis muscular atrophy. *Acta Neurol Scand* 78:81–84, 1988.
21. Hund E, Heckl R, Goebel HH, Meinck H-M. Inclusion body myositis presenting with isolated erector spinae paresis. *Neurology* 45:993–994, 1995.
22. Ytterberg SR, Roelofs RI, Mahowald ML. Inclusion body myositis and renal cell carcinoma: report of two cases and review of the literature. *Arthritis Rheumatol* 36:416–421, 1993.
23. Askanas V, Engel WK, Mirabella M. Idiopathic inflammatory myopathies: inclusion-body myositis, polymyositis, and dermatomyositis. *Curr Opin Neurol* 7:448–456, 1994.
24. Oddis CV. Therapy for myositis. *Curr Opin Rheumatol* 5:742–748, 1993.
25. Sayers ME, Chou SM, Calabrese LH. Inclusion-body myositis: Analysis of 32 cases. *J Rheumatol* 19:1385–1389, 1992.
26. Soueidan SA, Dalakas MC. Treatment of inclusion-body myositis with high-dose intravenous immunoglobulin. *Neurology* 43:876–879, 1993.
27. Amato AA, Barohn R, Kissel JT, Sahenk Z. Inclusion-body myopathy: treatment with intravenous immunoglobulin. *Neurology* 44:130, 1994.
28. Engel WK, Cunningham GG. Rapid examination of muscle tissue: an improved trichrome method for fresh-frozen biopsy sections. *Neurology* 13:919–923, 1963.
29. Engel AG, Arahata K. Monoclonal antibody analysis of mononuclear cells in myopathies: II. Phenotypes of autoinvasive cells in polymyositis and inclusion body myositis. *Ann Neurol* 16:209–215, 1984.
30. Dalakas MC, Illa I. Common variable immunodeficiency and inclusion body myositis: a distinct myopathy mediated by natural killer cells. *Ann Neurol* 37:806–810, 1995.
31. Hopkinson ND, Hunt C, Powell RJ, Lowe J. Inclusion body myositis: an underdiagnosed condition? *Ann Rheum Dis* 52:147–151, 1993.
32. Askanas V, Engel WK, Alvarez RB. Enhanced detection of Congo-red-positive amyloid deposits in muscle fibers of inclusion-body myositis and brain of Alzheimer disease using fluorescence technique. *Neurology* 43:1265–1267, 1993.
33. Askanas V, Alvarez RB, Mirabella M, Engel WK. Use of anti-neurofilament antibody to identify paired-helical filaments in inclusion-body myositis. *Ann Neurol* 39:389–391, 1996.
34. Engel WK. "Ragged-red fibers" in ophthalmoplegia syndromes and their differential diagnosis. *Intl Congr Ser Excerpta Med* 237:28, 1971.
35. Oldfors A, Moslemi A-R, Fyhr I-M, Holme E, Larsson N-G, Lindberg C. Mitochondrial DNA deletions in muscle fibers in inclusion body myositis. *J Neuropathol Exp Neurol* 54:581–587, 1995.
36. Rafai Z, Welle S, Kamp C, Thornton CA. Ragged-red fibers in normal aging and inflammatory myopathy. *Ann Neurol* 37:24–29, 1995.
37. Engel WK, Oberc MA. Abundant nuclear rods in adult-onset rod disease. *J Neuropathol Exp Neurol* 34:119–132, 1975.
38. Engel WK. Rod (nemaline) disease. In: Goldensohn ES, Appel SH (eds), *Scientific Approaches to Clinical Neurology*. Lea & Febiger, Philadelphia, 1977, pp. 1667–1691.

39. Neville HE, Baumbach LL, Ringel SP, Russo Jr LS, Sujansky E, Garcia CA. Familial inclusion body myositis: Evidence for autosomal dominant inheritance. *Neurology* 42:897–902, 1992.
40. Argov Z, Yarom R. "Rimmed vacuole myopathy" sparing the quadriceps: A unique disorder in Iranian Jews. *J Neurol Sci* 64:33–43, 1984.
41. Massa R, Weller B, Karpati G, Shonbridge E, Carpenter S. Familial inclusion body myositis among Kurdish-Iranian Jews. *Arch Neurol* 48:519–522, 1991.
42. Sadeh M, Gadoth N, Hadar H, Ben-David E. Vacuolar myopathy sparing the quadriceps. *Brain* 116:217–232, 1993.
43. Mitrani-Rosenbaum S, Argov Z, Blumenfeld A, Seidman CE, Seidman JG. Hereditary inclusion body myopathy maps to chromosome 9p1-q1. *Hum Mol Genetics* 5:159–163, 1996.
43a. Ikeuchi T, Asaka T, Saito M, Tanaka H, Higuchi S, Tanaka K, Saida K, Uyama E, Mizusawa H, Fukuhara N, Nonaka I, Takamori M, Tsuji S. Gene locus for autosomal recessive distal myopathy with rimmed vacuoles maps to chromosome 9. *Ann Neurol* 41:432–437, 1997.
43b. Argov Z, Tiran E, Eisenberg I, Sadeh M, Seidman CE, Seidman JG, Karpati G, Mitrani-Rosenbaum S. Various types of hereditary inclusion body myopathies map to chromosome 9p1-q1. *Ann Neurol* 41:548–551, 1997.
44. Sunohara N, Nonaka I, Kamei N, Satoyoshi E. Distal myopathy with rimmed vacuole formation: A follow-up study. *Brain* 112:65–83, 1989.
45. Murakami N, Ihara Y, Nonaka I. Muscle fiber degeneration in distal myopathy with rimmed vacuole formation. *Acta Neuropathol* 89:29–34, 1995.
46. Hentati F, Ben Hamida C, Tomé FMS, Queslati S, Fardeau M, Ben Hamida M. "Familial inclusion body myositis" sparing the quadriceps with asymptomatic leukoencephalopathy in a Tunisian kindred. *Neurology* 41:422, 1991.
47. Cole AJ, Kuzniecky R, Karpati G, Carpenter S, Andermann E, Andermann F. Familial myopathy with changes resembling inclusion body myositis and periventricular leukoencephalopathy: a new syndrome. *Brain* 111:1025–1037, 1988.
48. Fardeau M, Askanas V, Tomé FMS, Engel WK, Alvarez RB, McFerrin J, Chevallay M. Hereditary neuromuscular disorder with inclusion-body myositis-like filamentous inclusions: clinical, pathological, and tissue culture studies. *Neurology* 40:120, 1990.
48a. Middleton LT, Christodoulou K, Askanas V, Engel WK, McFerrin J, Kyriakides T, Zamba E, Papadopoulou E. Molecular genetics of autosomal-recessive hereditary inclusion-body myopathy (AR-IBM). *Ann Neurol*, 42:414, 1997.
49. Welander L. Myopathia distalis tarda hereditaria. *Acta Med Scand* 141:1–124, 1951.
50. Lindberg C, Borg K, Edström L, Oldfors A. Inclusion body myositis and Welander distal myopathy: a clinical neurophysiological and morphological comparison. *J Neurol Sci* 103:76–81, 1991.
51. Borg K, Tomé FMS, Edström L. Intranuclear and cytoplasmic filamentous inclusions in distal myopathy (Welander). *Acta Neuropathol* 82:102–106, 1991.
52. Udd B, Partanen J, Halonen P, Falck B, Hakamies L, Heikkilä H, Ingo S, Kalimo H, Kääriäinen H, Laulumaa V, Paljärvi L, Rapola J, Reunanen M, Sonninen V, Somer H. Tibial muscular dystrophy: late adult-

onset distal myopathy in 66 Finnish patients. *Arch Neurol* 50:604–608, 1993.

53. Partanen J, Laulumaa V, Paljärvi L, Partanen K, Naukkarinen A. Late onset foot-drop muscular dystrophy with rimmed vacuoles. *J Neurol Sci* 125:158–167, 1994.

54. Askanas V, Alvarez RB. Fast and reliable method for electronmicroscopic identification of cytoplasmic tubulo-filaments in muscle biopsies of patients with inclusion-body myositis. *Acta Neuropathol* 84:335–336, 1992.

55. Markesbery WR, Griggs RC, Herr B. Distal myopathy: electron microscopic and histochemical studies. *Neurology* 27:727–735, 1977.

56. Alvarez RB, Mirabella M, Sarkozi E, Heller S, Engel WK, Askanas V. Partial expression of cellular phenotype of sporadic inclusion-body myositis in autosomal dominant inclusion-body myopathy. *Neurology* 46:487, 1996.

57. Paquis V, Paul R, Askanas V, Engel WK, Desnuelle C. mtDNA deletions in muscle of sporadic inclusion-body myositis (S-IBM) and hereditary inclusion-body myopathy (H-IBM). *Neurology* 45:445, 1995.

58. Mirabella M, Alvarez RB, Bilak M, Engel WK, Askanas V. Difference in expression of phosphorylated tau epitopes between sporadic inclusion-body myositis and hereditary inclusion-body myopathies. *J Neuropathol Exp Neurol* 55:761–773, 1996.

59. Schweers D, Schönbrunn-Hanebeck E, Marx A, Mandelkow E. Structural studies of tau protein and Alzheimer paired helical filaments show no evidence of β-structure. *J Biol Chem* 269:24290–24297, 1994.

60. Askanas V, Engel WK, Alvarez RB, Glenner GG. β-amyloid protein immunoreactivity in muscle biopsies of patients with inclusion-body myositis. *Lancet* 339:560–561, 1992.

61. Villanova M, Kawai M, Lubke U, Oh SJ, Perry G, Six J, Ceuterick C, Martin J-J, Cras P. Rimmed vacuoles of inclusion body myositis and oculopharyngeal muscular dystrophy contain amyloid precursor protein and lysosomal markers. *Brain Res* 603:343–347, 1993.

62. Selkoe DJ. Normal and abnormal biology of the β-amyloid precursor protein. *Annu Rev Neurosci* 17:489–517, 1994.

63. Marz J. Boring in on β-amyloid's role in Alzheimer's. *Science* 255: 688–689, 1992.

64. Ksiezak-Reding H, Dickson DW, Davies P, Yen S-H. Recognition of tau epitopes by anti-neurofilament antibodies that bind to Alzheimer neurofibrillary tangles. *Proc Natl Acad Sci USA* 84:3410–3414, 1987.

65. Alizadeh-Khiavi K, Normand J, Chronopoulos S, Ali-Khan Z. Alzheimer's disease brain-derived ubiquitin has amyloid-enhancing factor activity: behavior of ubiquitin during accelerated amyloidogenesis. *Acta Neuropathol* 81:280–286, 1991.

65a. Askanas V, Alvarez RB, Sarkozi E, Bilak M, Mirabella M, Tomé FMS, Fardeau M, Engel WK. Partial expression in oculopharyngeal muscular dystrophy (OPMD) muscle fibers of the intracellular phenotype of sporadic inclusion-body myositis (s-IBM). *Neurology* 48:331, 1997.

66. Glenner GG, Wong CW. Alzheimer's disease. Initial report of the purification and characteristics of a novel cerebrovascular amyloid protein. *Biochem Biophys Res Commun* 120:885–890, 1984.

67. Masters CL, Simms G, Weinman NA, Multhaup G, McDonald BL, Beyreuther K. Amyloid plaque core protein in Alzheimer's disease and Down's syndrome. *Proc Natl Acad Sci USA* 82:4245–4249, 1985.

68. Selkoe DJ, Abraham CR, Podlisny MB, Duffy LK. Isolation of low molecular weight proteins from amyloid plaque fibers in Alzheimer's disease. *J Neurochem* 146:1820–1834, 1986.

69. Joachim CL, Selkoe DJ. The seminal role of β-amyloid in the pathogenesis of Alzheimer disease. *Alz Dis & Assoc Disord* 6:7–34, 1992.

70. Kang J, Lermaine HG, Unterbeck A, Salbaum JM, Masters CL, Grzeschik KH, Multhaup G, Beyreuther K, Muller-Hill B. The precursor of Alzheimer's disease amyloid A4 protein resembles a cell-surface receptor. *Nature* 325:733–736, 1987.

71. Robakis NK, Ramakrishna N, Wolfe G, Wisniewski HM. Molecular cloning and characterization of a cDNA encoding the cerebrovascular and neuritic plaque amyloid peptides. *Proc Natl Acad Sci USA* 84:4190–4194, 1987.

72. Askanas V, Engel WK, Alvarez RB. Strong immunoreactivity of β-amyloid precursor protein, including the β-amyloid protein sequence, at human neuromuscular junctions. *Neurosci Lett* 143:96–100, 1992.

73. Leclerc A, Tomé FMS, Fardeau M. Ubiquitin and β-amyloid-protein in inclusion-body myositis (IBM), familial IBM-like disorder and oculopharyngeal muscular dystrophy: an immunocytochemical study. *Neuromusc Disord* 3:283–291, 1993.

74. Yang SL, Wong K, Westaway D, Prusiner SJ, DeArmand SJ. Inclusion-body myositis: a prion protein overexpression myopathy? *Brain Pathol* 4:568, 1994.

75. Tabaton M, Cammarata S, Maucardi G, Manetto V, Autilio-Gambetti L, Perry G, Gambetti P. Ultrastructural localization of β-amyloid, τ and ubiquitin epitopes in extracellular neurofibrillary tangles. *Proc Natl Acad Sci USA* 88:2089–2102, 1991.

76. Ponte R, Gonzalez-DeWhitt P, Schilling J, Miller J, Hsu D, Greenberg B, Davis K, Wallace W, Lieberberg I, Fuller F, Cordell B. A new A4 amyloid mRNA contains a domain homologous to serine proteinase inhibitors. *Nature* 331:525–527, 1988.

77. Tanzi RE, Hyman BT. Studies of amyloid beta-protein precursor expression in Alzheimer's disease. *Ann NY Acad Sci* 640:149–154, 1991.

78. Askanas V, Sarkozi E, Bilak M, Alvarez RB, Engel WK. Human muscle macrophages express β-amyloid precursor and prion proteins and their mRNAs. *NeuroReport* 6:1045–1049, 1995.

79. Prusiner SB. Molecular biology of prion and diseases. *Science* 252:1515–1522, 1991.

80. Askanas V, Bilak M, Engel WK, Leclerc A, Tomé FMS. Prion protein is strongly immunolocalized at the postsynaptic domain of human normal neuromuscular junctions. *Neurosci Lett* 159:111–114, 1993.

81. Cashman NR, Loertscher R, Nalbantoglu J, Shaw I, Kascsak RJ, Bolton DC, Bendheim PE. Cellular isoform of the scrapie agent protein participates in lymphocyte activation. *Cell* 61:185–192, 1990.

82. Prusiner SB, Hsiao KK. Human prion diseases. *Ann Neurol* 35:385–395, 1994.

83. Westaway D, DeArmond SJ, Cayetano-Canlas J, Groth D, Foster D, Yang S-L, Torchia M, Carlson GA, Prusiner SB. Degeneration of skeletal muscle, peripheral nerves, and the central nervous system in transgenic mice overexpressing wild-type prion proteins. *Cell* 76:117–129, 1994.

84. Mobley WC, Neve RL, Prusiner SB, McKinley MP. Nerve growth factor increases mRNA levels for the prion protein and the β-amyloid precur-

sor protein in developing hamster brain. *Proc Natl Acad Sci USA* 85:9811–9815, 1988.

85. Askanas V, Sarkozi E, Bilak M, Engel WK. Expression of β-amyloid precursor protein, prion, acethylcholine receptor and their mRNAs in human muscle fibers regenerating in vivo. *Brain Pathol* 4:322, 1994.

86. Carrell RW, Travis J. Serpins: the superfamily of plasma serine protease inhibitors. In: Barret A, Salvesen G (eds), *Protease Inhibitors.* Elsevier, Amsterdam, 1987, pp. 403–420.

87. Abraham CR, Selkoe DJ, Potter H. Immunochemical identification of the serine protease inhibitor a_1-antichymotrypsin in the brain amyloid deposits of Alzheimer's disease. *Cell* 52:487–501, 1988.

88. Abraham CR, Shirahama T, Potter H. a_1-antichymotrypsin is associated solely with amyloid deposits containing the β-protein. Amyloid and cell localization of a_1-antichymotrypsin. *Neurobiol Aging* 11:123–239, 1990.

89. Rozemuller JM, Stam FC, Eikelenboom P. Acute phase proteins are present in amorphous plaques in the cerebral but not in the cerebella cortex of patients with Alzheimer's disease. *Neurosci Lett* 119:75–78, 1990.

90. Bilak M, Askanas V, Engel WK. Abnormalities of the serine proteases chymotrypsin (CT) and cathepsin G and their inhibitor (serpin) a_1-antichymotrypsin (a_1-ACT) in muscle biopsies of inclusion-body myositis. *J Neuropathol Exp Neurol* 52:277, 1993.

91. Goedert M, Crowther RA, Garner CC. Molecular characterization of microtubule-associated proteins tau and MAP2. *TINS* 14:193–199, 1991.

92. Kosik KS. The molecular and cellular biology of tau. *Brain Pathol* 3:39–43, 1993.

93. Trojanowski JQ, Schmidt ML, Shin R-W, Bramblett GT, Rao D, Lee VM-Y. Altered tau and neurofilament proteins in neurodegenerative diseases: diagnostic implications for Alzheimer's disease and Lewy body dementias. *Brain Pathol* 3:45–54, 1993.

94. Mandelkow EM, Mandelkow E. Tau as a marker for Alzheimer's disease. *Trends Biochem Sci* 18:480–483, 1993.

95. Goedert M, Spillantini MG, Cairns NJ, Crowther RA. Tau proteins of Alzheimer paired helical filaments: abnormal phosphorylation of all six brain isoforms. *Neuron* 8:159–168, 1992.

96. Kosik KS, Orredchio LD, Binder L, Trojanowski JQ, Lee VM-Y, Lee G. Epitopes that span the tau molecule are shared with paired helical filaments. *Neuron* 1:817–825, 1988.

97. Ksiezak-Reding H, Yen SH. Structural stability of paired helical filaments requires microtubule-binding domains of tau: a model of self-association. *Neuron* 6:717–728, 1991.

98. Lee VM-Y, Trojanowski JQ. The disordered neuronal cytoskeleton in Alzheimer's disease. *Curr Opin Neurobiol* 2:653–656, 1992.

99. Wolozin BL, Pruchnicki A, Dickson DW, Davies P. A neuronal antigen in the brains of Alzheimer patients. *Science* 232:648–650, 1986.

100. Lee VM-Y, Balin BJ, Otvos Jr L, Trojanowski JQ. A68: A major subunit of paired helical filaments and derivatized forms of normal tau. *Science* 251:675–678, 1991.

101. Mori H, Kondo J, Ihara Y. Ubiquitin is a component of paired helical filaments in Alzheimer's disease. *Science* 235:1641–1644, 1987.

102. Perry G, Friedman R, Shaw G, Chan V. Ubiquitin is detected in neurofibrillary tangles and senile plaque neurites of Alzheimer disease brains. *Proc Natl Acad Sci USA* 84:3033–3036, 1987.

103. Namba Y, Tomonaga M, Kawasaki H, Otomo E, Ikeda K. Apolipoprotein E immunoreactivity in cerebral amyloid deposits and neurofibrillary tangles in Alzheimer's disease and kuru plaque amyloid in Creutzfeldt-Jakob disease. *Brain Res* 541:163–166, 1991.

104. Strittmatter WJ, Weisgraber KH, Huang DY, Dong L-M, Salvesen GS, Pericak-Vance M, Schmechel D, Saunders AM, Goldgaber D, Rose AD. Binding of human apolipoprotein E to synthetic amyloid β peptide: isoform-specific effects and implications for late-onset Alzheimer disease. *Proc Natl Acad Sci USA* 90:8098–8102, 1993.

105. Saunders AM, Strittmatter WJ, Schmechel D, St. George-Hyslop PH, Pericak-Vance MA, Joo SH, Rosi BL, Gusella JF, Crapper-MacLachlan DR, Alberts MJ, Hulette C, Crain B, Goldgaber D, Roses AD. Association of apolipoprotein E allele ε4 with late-onset familial and sporadic Alzheimer's disease. *Neurology* 43:1467–1472, 1993.

106. Mirabella M, Askanas V, Engel WK, Weisgraber KH. Immunocytochemical localization of apolipoprotein E (ApoE) in inclusion body myositis (IBM). *Neurology* 44:347, 1994.

107. Wisniewski T, Frangione B. Apolipoprotein E: a pathological chaperone protein in patients with cerebral and systemic amyloid. *Neurosci Lett* 135:235–238, 1992.

108. Garlepp MJ, Tabarias H, van Bockxmeer FM, Zilko PJ, Laing B, Mastaglia FL. Apolipoprotein E ε4 in inclusion body myositis. *Ann Neurol* 38:957–959, 1995.

109. Harrington CR, Anderson JR, Chan KK. Apolipoprotein E type E4 allele frequency is not increased in patients with sporadic inclusion-body myositis. *Neurosci Lett* 183:35–38, 1995.

110. Askanas V, Engel WK, Mirabella M, Weisgraber KH, Saunders AM, Roses AD, McFerrin J. Apolipoprotein E alleles in sporadic inclusion-body myositis and hereditary inclusion-body myopathy. *Ann Neurol* 40:264, 1996.

111. Hershko A, Ciechanover A. The ubiquitin system for protein degradation. *Annu Rev Biochem* 61:761–807, 1992.

112. Jentsch S. Ubiquitin-dependent protein degradation: A cellular perspective. *Trends Cell Biol* 2:98–103, 1992.

113. Lowe J, Mayer RJ, Landon M. Ubiquitin in neurodegenerative diseases. *Brain Pathol* 3:55–65, 1993.

114. Albrecht S, Bilbao JM. Ubiquitin expression in inclusion-body myositis. *Arch Pathol Lab Med* 117:789–793, 1993.

115. Serdaroglu P, Askanas V, Engel WK. Immunocytochemical localization of ubiquitin at human neuromuscular junctions. *Neuropathol App Neurobiol* 18:232–236, 1992.

116. Cenciarelli C, Hou D, Hsu K-C, Rellahan BL, Wiest DL, Smith HT, Fried VA, Weissman AM. Activation-induced ubiquitination of the T cell antigen receptor. *Science* 257:795–797, 1992.

117. Askanas V, Alvarez RB, Bilak M, Froehner S, Engel WK. Muscle nicotinic acetylcholine receptor (nAChR) and its associated protein 43 kD (43K) are highly accumulated in vacuolated muscle fibers (VMFs) of inclusion body myositis (IBM). *Neurology* 44:131, 1994.

118. de Haan JB, Cristiano F, Iannello RC, Kola I. Cu/Zn-superoxide dismutase and glutathione peroxidase during aging. *Biochem Mol Biol Intl* 35:1281–1297, 1995.

119. Beal MF. Aging, energy, and oxidative stress in neurodegenerative diseases. *Ann Neurol* 38:357–366, 1995.

120. Dickinson MJ, Singh I. Down's syndrome, dementia, and superoxide dismutase. *Brit J Psych* 162:811–817, 1993.

121. Askanas V, Sarkozi E, Alvarez RB, McFerrin J, Siddique T, Engel WK. Superoxide-dismutase-1 (SOD1) gene and protein in vacuolated muscle fibers of sporadic inclusion-body myositis (s-IBM), hereditary inclusion-body myopathy (h-IBM), and in cultured human muscle after β-amyloid precursor protein (βAPP) gene transfer. *Neurology* 46:487, 1996.

122. Yamaguchi H, Hirai S, Morimatsu M, Shoji M, Harigaya Y. Diffuse type of senile plaques in the brains of Alzheimer-type dementia. *Acta Neuropathol* 77:113–119, 1988.

123. Eisen A, Berry K, Gibson S. Inclusion body myositis (IBM): Myopathy or neuropathy? *Neurology* 33:1109–1114, 1983.

124. Engel WK. Integrative histochemical approach to the defect of Duchenne muscular dystrophy. In: Rowland LP (ed), *Pathogenesis of the Human Muscular Dystrophies.* American Elsevier, New York, 1977, pp. 277–309.

125. Engel WK. Myopathic EMG – nonesuch animal. *N Engl J Med* 289:486, 1973.

126. Engel WK. Brief, small, abundant motor-unit action potentials. *Neurology* 25:173–176, 1975.

127. Alvarez RB, Fardeau M, Askanas V, Engel WK, McFerrin J, Tomé FMS. Characteristic filamentous inclusions reproduced in cultured innervated muscle fibers from patients with familial "inclusion body myositis." *J Neurol Sci* 98:178, 1990.

128. Askanas V, McFerrin J, Baqué S, Engel WK, Sarkozi E, Alvarez RB. Overexpression of β-amyloid precursor protein (βAPP) gene in cultured normal human muscle using adenovirus vector induces aspects of inclusion-body myositis (IBM) phenotype. *Neurology (suppl 4)* 45:208–209, 1995.

128a. Askanas V, McFerrin J, Alvarez RB, Baqué S, Engel WK. βAPP gene transfer into cultured human muscle induces inclusion-body myositis aspects. *NeuroReport* 8:2155–2158, 1997.

129. Askanas V, McFerrin J, Baqué S, Alvarez RB, Sarkozi E, Engel WK. Transfer of β-amyloid precursor protein gene using adenovirus vector causes mitochondrial abnormalities in cultured normal human muscle. *Proc Natl Acad Sci USA* 93:1314–1319, 1996.

130. Chandrasekaran K, Giordano T, Brady DR, Stoll J, Martin LJ, Rapoport SI. Impairment in mitochondrial cytochrome oxidase gene expression in Alzheimer disease. *Mol Brain Res* 24:336–340, 1994.

131. Simonian NA, Hyman BT. Functional alterations in Alzheimer's disease: selective loss of mitochondrial-encoded cytochrome oxidase mRNA in the hippocampal formation. *J Neuropathol Exp Neurol* 53:508–512, 1994.

132. Mutisya EM, Bowling AC, Beal MF. Cortical cytochrome oxidase activity is reduced in Alzheimer's disease. *J Neurochem* 63:2179–2184, 1994.

133. Askanas V, Engel WK. Cultured normal and genetically abnormal human muscle. In: Rowland LP, DiMauro S (eds), *Handbook of Clinical Neurology.* Elsevier, Armsterdam, 1992, pp. 85–116.

134. Bilak M, Askanas V, Engel WK. Alpha-1 antichymotrypsin is strongly immunolocalized at normal human and rat neuromuscular junctions. *Synapse* 16:280–283, 1994.

135. Bilak M, Askanas V, Engel WK, Alvarez RB. Twisted tubulofila-ments (TTFs) in inclusion body myositis (IBM) muscle contain fibroblast growth factor (FGF) and its receptor (FGF-R). *Neurology* 44:130, 1994.

136. Mirabella M, Askanas V, Engel WK. Transforming growth factor-Beta 1 is abnormally accumulated in vacuolated muscle fibers of sporadic inclu-sion-body myositis and hereditary inclusion-body myopathy. *Ann Neurol* 36:320–321, 1994.

137. Mirabella M, Alvarez RB, Engel WK, Weisgraber KH, Askanas V. Apolipoprotein E and apolipoprotein E messenger RNA in muscle of inclusion-body myositis and myopathies. *Ann Neurol* 40:864–872, 1996.

138. Dawson TM, Snyder SH. Gases as biological messengers: Nitric oxide and carbon monoxide in the brain. *J Neurosci* 14:5147–5159, 1994.

139. Nathan C, Xie Q-W. Regulation of biosynthesis of nitric oxide. *J Biol Chem* 269:13725–13728, 1994.

140. Beckman JS, Chen J, Crow JP, Ye YZ. Reactions of nitric oxide, super-oxide and peroxynitrite with superoxide dismutase in neurodegenera-tion. In: Seil FJ (ed) *Progress in Brain Research, Neural Regeneration,* Vol. 103, pp 371–380. Elsevier Science BV, Amsterdam, 1994.

141. Crow JP, Beckman JS. The role of peroxynitrite in nitric oxide-mediated toxicity. In: Kaprowski H, Maeda H (eds) *Current Topics in Microbiol-ogy and Immunology, The Role of Nitric Oxide in Physiology and Patho-physiology,* Vol. 196, pp 57–73. Springer-Verlag, Berlin, 1995.

142. Förstermann U, Closs EI, Pollock JS, Nakane M, Schwarz P, Gath I, Kleinert H. Nitric oxide synthase isozymes: Characterization, purification, molecular cloning, and functions. *Hypertension* 23:1121–1131, 1994.

143. Yang C-C, Alvarez RB, Engel WK, Askanas V. Increase of nitric oxide synthases and nitrotyrosine in inclusion-body myositis. *NeuroReport* 8:153–158, 1996.

144. Yang C-C, Alvarez RB, Engel WK, Askanas V. Nitric-oxide induced oxi-dative stress in muscle fibers of hereditary inclusion-body myopathy (h-IBM) and sporadic inclusion-body myositis (s-IBM). *Neurology* 48:331–332, 1997.

145. Brown GC. Nitric oxide regulates mitochondrial respiration and cell func-tions by inhibiting cytochrome oxidase. *FEBS Lett* 369:136–139, 1995.

146. Haginoya K, Alvarez RB, Engel WK, Askanas V. Light- and electron-mi-croscopic immunolocalization of interleukins 1α, 1β and 6 in vacuolated muscle fibers of sporadic inclusion-body myositis (s-IBM). *Neurology* 48:126, 1997.

147. Askanas V, Kwan H, Alvarez RB, Engel WK, Kobayashi T, Martinuzzi A, Hawkins EF. De novo neuromuscular junction formation on human muscle fibers cultured in monolayer and innervated by fetal rat spinal cord: Ultrastructural and ultrastructural-cytochemical studies. *J Neurocy-tol* 16:523–537, 1987.

148. McFerrin J, Price SM, Baqué S, Engel WK, Askanas V. Overexpression of ςamyloid precursor protein (APP) gene in cultured normal human muscle using adenovirus vector prevents formation of neuromuscular junctions (NMJs) and functional innervation: Relevance to inclusion-body myositis (s-IBM). *Neurology* 48:332, 1997.

149. Ringel SP, Engel WK, Bender AN. Extrajunctional acetylcholine receptors on myogenously de-innervated muscle fibers. *J Histochem Cytochem* 24:1033–1034, 1976.
150. Ringel SP, Bender AN, Engel WK. Extrajunctional acetylcholine receptors. Alterations in human and experimental neuromuscular diseases. *J Histochem Cytochem* 24:1033–1041, 1976.

Part II

Historical Perspective

2

Evolving Concepts of Inclusion-Body Myositis

GEORGES SERRATRICE

Is Inclusion-Body Myositis a Misnamed Disease?

Inclusion-body myositis (IBM) is a term applied by Yunis and Samaha (1) in 1971 to a slowly progressive myopathy that clinically mimicked a chronic polymyositis. However, pathologically, they observed vacuoles containing cytoplasmic degradation products. Ultrastructural study showed tubulofilamentous nuclear inclusions and filamentous inclusions 15–18 nm in diameter. Yunis and Samaha, emphasizing the relationship between inclusions and paramyxovirus capsids, suggested the use of a myositis designation.

Now there are increasing doubts that this disease is actually a primary muscle inflammatory disease, in spite of the few overlaps in the clinical and pathologic findings in the three major inflammatory myopathies: dermatomyositis, polymyositis, and IBM. Those doubts are based on several findings: (i) In a significant number of cases inflammatory infiltrates are lacking. (ii) Other cellular pathologic findings have been reported that cannot be explained by a primary dysimmune process. (iii) An anti-dysimmune treatment has shown no consistent efficacy. (iv) Similar myopathologic conditions without inflammation can be observed in familial diseases recently cited as inclusion-body myopathies. Thus the question arises: Is IBM a degenerative muscle disease? Moreover, is IBM an entity?

A Pathologic Definition

The definition of IBM is based mainly on the pathologic findings. IBM is not a disease, but a syndrome. Specific clinical symptoms and signs – if they exist – are related to a common pathologic abnormality: cytoplasmic and nuclear inclusions of filaments.

IBM filaments are 16–18 nm in external diameter and 6 nm in internal diameter – twisted, rectilinear, composed of globular units, parallel or disseminated, cytoplasmic and sometimes nuclear. Light microscopy reveals rimmed vacuoles, single or multiple, invading 2–70% of fibers;

they can be peripheral or central, in normal fibers or in atrophic fibers. They contain basophilic granulations that stain with Sudan black, osmium tetroxide, or acid phosphatase. Amyloid deposits are other characteristic findings. Another important morphologic change that is not fully understood is the inconstant presence of lymphohistiocytic inflammation. Numerous other abnormalities are frequent, although not specific.

Corresponding to this definition of the disease are some clinical findings, not specific, but relatively frequent in sporadic cases: frequency in old age (50 years and older), more often among males; progressive onset of weakness and amyotrophy, often asymmetrical, and predominant in the distal upper or lower limbs, but proximal too, with mixed myogenic and neurogenic electromyographic (EMG) findings; frequent areflexia, sometimes myalgias and dysphagia; relentless course in spite of dysimmune treatment. Serum creatine kinase study and ancillary examinations are not conclusive.

In fact, the disease is usually primary and sporadic; it is sometimes hereditary, without uniform inheritance, and in some cases secondary, probably as an epiphenomenon developing in well-defined neuromuscular diseases. Recent identification of kindreds with hereditary IBM (termed h-IBM, that is, hereditary inclusion-body myopathy, in contrast to the sporadic forms, termed s-IBM) (2) suggests that IBM may sometimes be a genetic disease. There are some significant pathologic differences between the two forms of the disease (3). Inflammatory changes are almost invariably found in s-IBM, but only rarely encountered in h-IBM, as in the secondary cases observed with several neuromuscular diseases.

The history of IBM has been punctuated with several evolving concepts since (and before) the first description of the disease in 1971 (1).

Early Studies

The first case of IBM to be reported in the literature appears to have been a myopathy with cellular inclusions reported by Adams, Kakulas, and Samaha (4) in 1965.

In 1967, Chou (5) observed virus-like particles in the muscle tissue of a patient with chronic polymyositis and in 1968 emphasized a viral hypothesis for polymyositis in reporting the case of a 66-year-old man with dysphagia, progressive proximal muscle weakness, fiber necrosis and regeneration, and inflammation. Ultrastructural study revealed both intranuclear and intracytoplasmic tubular filamentous structures, giant mitochondrias, and membranous bodies. Those filaments were similar to paramyxoviruses in structure, and it was suggested that polymyositis could result from a chronic viral infection.

In 1970, Carpenter, Karpati, and Wolfe (6) reported on a patient who had a chronic myopathy. Muscle biopsy showed vacuoles, phospholipid accumulations, and eosinophilic cytoplasmic inclusions, and electron microscopy revealed intracytoplasmic and intranuclear filaments. They postulated that the disease might be due to a myxovirus.

In 1971, Sato et al. (7) reported another case of polymyositis with nuclear and cytoplasmic inclusions. The viral study failed to show any evidence of viral infection.

IBM: a Distinct Disease

The term IBM was coined by Yunis and Samaha (1) in 1971 to describe a distinct clinicopathologic entity. They observed eosinophilic fibrillar inclusions in the sarcoplasm and nuclei of muscles in a 26-year-old woman who had a 5-year history of progressive muscle weakness typical of chronic polymyositis. Electron-microscopic examination showed that the eosinophilic inclusions consisted of aggregates of straight, hollow filaments with diameters ranging from 15 to 17 nm. The morphology of those filaments was similar to that of the myxovirus nucleocapsid; however, they could also have represented altered thick myosin filaments. The clinical and pathologic similarities between their case and the cases previously reported prompted Yunis and Samaha to distinguish such cases of chronic polymyositis with filamentous inclusions as a third form of myositis (in addition to acute dermatomyositis and chronic polymyositis), which they called IBM.

Following their description, several cases were reported by Hudson et al. (8) in 1971, Jerusalem et al. (9) in 1972, Hughes and Esiri (10) in 1975, Oteruelo (11) in 1976, and Ketelsen et al. (12) in 1977.

In a conclusive study in 1978, Carpenter et al. (13) presented their findings from a group of 6 patients who had been thoroughly studied both clinically and pathologically. They proposed to classify IBM as a variety of inflammatory muscle disease, distinguishable from the other varieties not only by its pathologic features but also by some clinical characteristics, among them the ineffectiveness of immunosuppressive treatments.

IBM: Third Form of Inflammatory Myopathy

Many subsequent reports have substantiated and reemphasized the findings of Carpenter et al. (13). Matsubara and Mair (14) described ultrastructural changes in IBM, and several cases have been reported by Kula et al. (15), Lisson et al. (16), Hubner and Pongratz (17), and Tomé et al. (18). In 1982, Danon et al. (19) reported 7 cases that were polymyositis-like, but corticosteroid-resistant, which tended to suggest distinct primary disease. The same year, Mikol et al. (20) isolated an adenovirus type 2 in a muscle biopsy specimen, but no similar cases were subsequently reported.

Study of paraffin sections is of little use in establishing the diagnosis. In paraffin sections the typical rimmed vacuoles are seldom recognized. Three main alterations are seen, but not constantly: structural abnormalities, small angular fibers, and inflammation.

There are marked variations in muscle-fiber diameters, in some cases with hypertrophied fibers (never observed in polymyositis), longitudinal splitting, central nuclei, abundant nuclei, and ring fibers. Necrosis of various degrees is observed, sometimes in isolated fibers, and sometimes in 5% of fibers, but less frequently than in polymyositis. Macrophage invasion of fibers is frequently observed. Regeneration with basophilic fibers and prominent nuclei is rare. Fibrosis and fatty infiltrations are frequent.

Small groups of angular fibers are very frequently reported (9,21,22). Ringel et al. (22) noted their presence in 1–5% of fibers in 3 cases, 5–10% in 8 cases, and more than 10% in 8 cases. Type grouping is rare (9,10,12,13,20,21,23,24). In some cases only nuclear bags are observed. Reversely target fibers have rarely been reported (21,25). These aspects might suggest a neurogenic atrophy; however, intramuscular nerves, muscle spindles, and motor endplates are not markedly abnormal.

The extent of inflammation is highly variable. Theoretically it characterizes s-IBM; however, there are some exceptions. The infiltration is sometimes profuse. It is only endomysial. There is a partial invasion of non-necrotic fibers (13,26,27). The inflammatory cells are mainly lymphocytes and macrophages. In some cases infiltrates are moderate. Inflammation is almost invariably found in s-IBM, but is only rarely encountered in h-IBM and is never seen in neuromuscular diseases with rimmed vacuoles.

Cryostat sections point to the diagnosis, showing rimmed vacuoles. Vacuoles can occur subsarcolemmaly or in the center of the fiber. They are round or irregular in shape, 3–30 µm in diameter and 10–100 µm in longitudinal section. They are rimmed by basophilic granular material. This ab-

normal material is also present in their lumina and in the adjacent sarcoplasm. The basophilic granules stain positively with Sudan black, acid hematoxylin, and osmium tetroxide. Reactivity with acid phosphatase is
sometimes noted, but only in some fibers, thus differentiating rimmed
vacuoles from autophagic vacuoles (in which all the vacuoles have a strong
reaction with acid phosphatase). Single or multiple rimmed vacuoles are
present in 2–90% of fibers, either evenly distributed between type I and
type II fibers or prominent in type I fibers (28). Eosinophilic inclusions are
found in the cytoplasm, usually contiguous to the vacuoles. Atrophy can
involve either type I or type II fibers. Ragged red fibers are frequent, as are
cytochrome-oxidase-negative fibers. But similar findings are common in
polymyositis. Finally, three findings predict the detection of the filamentous inclusions of IBM by electron microscopy: (i) rimmed vacuoles, (ii)
groups of angulated atrophic fibers, (iii) endomysial inflammation.

Filament Identification

Ultrastructural study will show filamentous inclusions in the cytoplasm or
in the nuclei or in both. The filaments have a mean outer diameter of 18
nm and mean inner diameter of 6 nm. The lengths of filaments range
from 1 to 5 μm or more (11). Some smaller and larger diameters have
been observed: 10–20 nm, outer diameter; 3–8 nm, inner diameter (13,
14). Inclusions are rectilinear, sometimes with striations of 5 nm along the
long axis (6,7,18). At high resolution, the longitudinally oriented filaments appear to be composed of a mosaic of globular units 3–4.5 nm wide
(20). The cytoplasmic filaments are parallel. They can be concentrically
aggregated in clusters or randomly distributed. They are sometimes intermingled with disorganized myofibrils. The intranuclear filaments can
be arranged in parallel or at random. They are surrounded by chromatin.
Some of them perforate the envelope of the nucleus. They are extruded
into the cytoplasm. The cytoplasmic filaments are easy to find and identify. The intranuclear filaments have been detected in only about 40% of
cases. Cytoplasmic tubulofilaments in s-IBM were reported by Askanas
et al. (29) to be associated with pairs of twisted filaments measuring 15–21
nm in inner diameter, with the twisting occurring every 45–55 nm. The
paired helical filaments in IBM muscle closely resemble the paired helical
filaments of Alzheimer-disease brain (30).

The filaments are often surrounded by autophagic vacuoles containing
degradation products. Myelinlike whorls and various other kinds of
lysosomal and cellular debris are present. Glycogen granules and degen-

erating mitochondria are observed. However, the vacuoles are different from "true autophagic vacuoles." They are not fully surrounded by membranes, and only some of them show acid phosphatase positivity. Dilatation of triads is sometimes observed. These autophagic vacuoles correspond to the vacuoles observed by light microscopy (13).

Various nonspecific structural abnormalities of muscle have been reported. A lot of muscle fibers show no pathologic changes. Focal loss of myofilaments occurs in some damaged fibers. Z-band streaming, numerous cytoplasmic bodies (25), desmine, a T-tubule system, and honeycombs (20) have occasionally been observed. Mitochondria are often increased in number and in size (23,31,32). Some contain crystalline inclusions (13, 25). These abnormalities are consistent with the ragged red fibers and cytochrome-c-oxidase-negative fibers detected in cryostat sections. Carpenter et al. (13) and Matsubara and Mair (14) reported concentric laminated bodies and annulated lamellae. Satellite cells are abundant.

The number of nuclei is increased in atrophic fibers. The nuclei are indented with vacuoles encircled by membrane, clusters of thin filaments, and invagination of organelles and cytoplasmic bodies into the nucleus. The number of capillaries is significantly increased. Carpenter et al. (13) evaluated the number of capillaries relative to the number of muscle fibers in transverse semithin epon sections. The increase in capillaries is in contrast to the capillary loss in dermatomyositis. The capillary endothelial cells are often prominent and show active pinocytosis. A negative sign is the absence of tubuloreticular inclusions in endothelial cells, except in a case reported by Chad et al. (33) with Sjögren syndrome and a case reported by Sato and Tsubaki (34) associated with a connective-tissue disease.

Finally, no changes within the muscle fiber appear to be specific. Only the filamentous inclusions are typical of the disease in electron-microscopic study.

Nerve abnormalities have seldom been described. Sural nerve biopsy was performed in some patients (9,13,19). The findings were normal (9,19,25) or showed axonal degeneration (13,25) or polyglucosan bodies (13). Motor endplates were normal, except in two reports (25,35).

Frequency and Etiology

The true frequency of IBM is difficult to estimate, for several reasons. In spite of a stringent definition, many cases reported as IBM are not true IBM, but more probably are neuromuscular diseases with rimmed vacuoles. Conversely, there are frequent reports of distal myopathy with rimmed vacuoles in Japan, in contrast with other countries, where reports of IBM are much more common. According to Satoyoshi et al. (36), some cases of distal myopathy are misdiagnosed as IBM. However, it seems that both are the same disorder. Pathologically, rimmed vacuoles displayed on frozen sections are variable in distribution and are not detected in paraffin-embedded muscle specimens. Thus the frequency could be underestimated in some patients. Usually, ultrastructural study is not carried out for all muscle specimens. Therefore the filaments may not be detected.

Finally, the incidence of IBM among adult idiopathic inflammatory myopathies has varied in the different series reported, between one-fifth and one-third of cases. For example, the frequency is 15–17% in some series (13,19) and 28% in another (27).

A characteristic feature is the late onset of the disease. IBM appears primarily in middle-age persons, with 50% between the ages of 50 and 70 years. That is in contrast to the findings in large series of polymyositis, in which an earlier age of onset has been observed. The ages have, however, ranged from 16 to 84 years, with 20% between 10 and 30 years. Eisen et al. (21) suggested a bimodal distribution, with a small group significantly younger, in the range of 15–40 years. Some childhood cases have been reported (21,37,39).

An important consideration is the delay between the onset and the diagnosis. The mean duration of weakness before diagnosis is 6–7 years. The duration of symptoms before biopsy has varied from 4 months to 36 years in various reports (13,27,35,37,39).

The onset is usually insidious, with a slow progression. This insidious onset of IBM differs from that of polymyositis, in which symptoms and signs usually evolve over weeks or months.

In the different series there has been a 3 : 1 male predominance. The reason for that male preponderance is unknown. No hormonal factor has been found.

Therefore, IBM is considered by Askanas and Engel (40) to be the most common muscle disease in patients aged 55 years or older, especially in males.

Clinical Characteristics of s-IBM

Clinically, s-IBM is characterized by progressive muscle weakness and amyotrophy. But the distribution of the muscular weakness varies, especially at the time of the diagnosis – sometimes distal, sometimes proximal, sometimes asymmetrical, with or without dysphagia.

In fact, the weakness can be generalized or localized to the limbs. The first symptoms can involve the upper or, more frequently, the lower limbs, simultaneously or successively. In at least half of the cases, prominent symmetrical or asymmetrical muscle wasting and weakness occur in the distal limbs, usually with some proximal limb weakness. In some cases the weakness remains confined to the upper limbs (24) or to the lower limbs (13,41). The main severely affected muscles are the quadriceps, the wrist and finger extensors or flexors, the tibialis anterior, the iliopsoas, the biceps, and the triceps. In some patients, focal quadriceps involvement has been noted, as well as sternomastoid amyotrophy. Atrophy of the affected muscles is frequent and in the majority of cases proportional to the weakness. Facial atrophy is rare. Isolated erector spinae paresis was reported by Hund et al. (42), corresponding to a bent-spine syndrome (43).

Areflexia is frequent even without severe muscle weakness. At the beginning, tendon reflexes are often normal. They are reduced in 40% of cases. Ankle and knee reflexes are often abolished in the absence of amyotrophy.

Myalgias are predominant in 20% of cases, and the clinical features resemble those of polymyositis, especially when dysphagia is present. In other cases transient myalgias are occasionally noted at the beginning or during the evolution of the disease, but are not predominant.

The natural history of the disease is not well documented, except for the slowly progressive onset, as previously mentioned. The course of the symptoms after biopsy has been described in several series. Lotz et al. (27) observed 28 patients during a mean period of 72 months. They reported a slow, relentless progression of the disease. The 6 patients in their series who were observed for 15 years or longer became severely disabled. Usually IBM develops relentlessly. Some patients remain valid for many years after the onset of the disease. It is often after the biopsy diagnosis that their condition becomes more severe and they become disabled. Some patients are confined to wheelchairs. In some patients s-IBM is a severe neuromuscular disease.

IBM: a Nonhomogeneous Disease

Julien et al. (44) did not recognize IBM as an entity, taking into account the clinical, biological, and electrophysiologic heterogeneity and the frequency of associated diseases like mesenchymoma or scleroderma.

Moreover, they cited similar inclusions in Paget disease, as previously reported by Rebel et al. (45) and Mills and Singer (46).

In considering the question whether IBM was a myopathy or neuropathy, Eisen et al. (21) described 6 patients in whom the electrophysiologic and morphologic features were more in keeping with a neurogenic disorder than a myopathic disorder. Distal predominance, loss of tendon reflexes, normal serum creatine kinase (CK), neurogenic EMG findings, increased density of single fibers at EMG, fiber-group atrophy, and angular fibers could favor a neurogenic disease, as previously suggested by Jerusalem et al. (9). Of special interest from the study of Eisen et al. (21) is the report of a familial case in a 23-year-old patient with distal muscle weakness, atrophy, and areflexia. His older brother was similarly but more severely affected. Similar familial cases were observed in 1983 by Matsubara and Tanabe (31), formerly considered to represent hereditary distal myopathy with filamentous inclusions.

More recently, numerous cases have been described with inhomogeneous clinical, electrophysiologic, and pathologic findings (22,41,47–49). Three clinical subgroups have been suggested (37): multifocal amyotrophies, pseudopolymyositis, and pseudodegenerative forms.

The forms in first subgroup, asymmetrical and multifocal amyotrophies, are the most frequent. A slowly progressive weakness appears, involving the biceps, brachioradialis, and wrist extensors and/or flexors on one side and the peroneal muscles, but also the lower girdle muscles. In other patients, proximal weakness is associated with asymmetrical distal weakness and atrophy. In rare cases there is an isolated quadriceps myopathy. Sternomastoid-muscle atrophy is present in some cases (37). Interestingly, IBM and myotonic dystrophy are the only neuromuscular diseases having sternomastoid atrophy. Several similar cases were reported by Jerusalem et al. (9), Lisson et al. (16), and Tomé et al. (18), as well as cases 1, 4, 5, and 6 of Eisen et al. (21).

Other cases of pseudopolymyositis appear as treatment-resistant polymyositis (41). The patients observed by Sato et al. (7), Matsubara and Mair (14), Chad et al. (33), and Danon et al. (19) presented features similar to those of a chronic cortico-resistant polymyositis. Such cases of treatment-resistant pseudopolymyositis are characterized by high serum CK concentrations, dysphagia, myalgias, and sometimes symmetrical weakness without marked wasting. In some cases a dysimmune disease is associated: scleroderma (35), Sjögren syndrome (33), connective-tissue diseases (24), thrombocytopenia (50), or chronic inflammatory demyelinating neuropathy (37).

The pseudodegenerative forms of the third subgroup can mimic either progressive spinal atrophies or muscular dystrophies. The duration of the disease before diagnosis tends to be particularly long. These pseudo-degenerative forms are illustrated by the cases of Ketelsen et al. (12) and cases 2 and 7 of Eisen et al. (21).

Tentative Criteria

Taking into account these different forms, some tentative diagnostic criteria have been proposed. The clinical data and laboratory findings are characteristic in many IBM patients. However, the diagnosis is more difficult in numerous atypical cases. For this reason, precise criteria are necessary to assess cases of s-IBM.

In 1994, Serratrice et al. (51) proposed the following list of criteria:

1. Features required for the diagnosis:
    Morphologically: rimmed vacuoles, inflammation, amyloid deposits, inclusions
    Progressive and chronic asymmetrical muscle weakness and amyotrophy
    Absence of other neurologic signs or clearly defined neuromuscular disease
2. Features highly suggestive of the diagnosis:
    Morphologically: same as for item 1, plus neurogenic atrophy, congophilic deposits, and partial invasion of fibers
    Clinical features: old-age onset, male predominance, disseminated or multifocal amyotrophy, focal amyotrophy (e.g., quadriceps, sternomastoid, wrist flexor or extensor weakness,), myalgias, dysphagia, areflexia, progressive course over 6 months, unresponsive to treatment
    Ancillary examinations: neurogenic and myogenic EMG findings, high serum CK concentration   (no more than 10-fold) with normal erythrocyte sedimentation rate (ESR), ragged muscle on CT scan of muscle
3. Features casting doubt on the diagnosis:
    Morphologically: absence of inflammation, presence of ragged red fibers (in great number)
    Clinical features: isolated proximal muscle weakness, prominent myalgias and dysphagia, cutaneous abnormalities, diffuse weakness without amyotrophy, sensory disturbances, improvement with corticosteroids

Ancillary examinations: high ESR, normal EMG findings, dystrophic type of muscle CT scan
4. Features that rule out the diagnosis:
Morphologically: less than 2% rimmed vacuoles, absence of inclusions in ultrastructural study
Clinical features: features consistent with a clearly defined neuromuscular disease (e.g., facioscapulohumeral dystrophy, progressive spinal atrophy)
Ancillary examinations: antiganglioside antibodies, normal muscle CT scan

Finally the following scheme was proposed: IBM is the diagnosis if all the significant morphologic criteria are present and they are the only changes observed, in the absence of any other neuromuscular disease. IBM is considered probable if, in addition to filamentous inclusions, there is an atypical amyotrophy (asymmetrical, focal), even with areflexia. IBM is possible in the presence of myalgias and dysphagia and in the absence of biological (and sometimes morphological) inflammation. IBM is to be ruled out if any definite neuromuscular disease is present. However, a question remains in hereditary cases. There are no criteria to differentiate hereditary IBM from certain hereditary muscular dystrophies in the absence of a genetic study.

More recently, Mendell has proposed a new list of criteria (2). With reference to Mendell's list of criteria (see Chapter 3), s-IBM can be the definitive diagnosis in a patient with characteristic muscle biopsy findings. Conversely, in the absence of typical inclusions, s-IBM can be possible when the following features pointed out among the criteria are observed in the patient: 6-month duration of the disease, age of 30 years or more, typical muscle weakness, characteristic inflammatory EMG findings.

Neuromuscular Diseases with Rimmed Vacuoles

Rimmed vacuoles can be observed in various neuromuscular diseases, either sporadic or hereditary. The best examples of sporadic cases are the post-poliomyelitic syndrome (52,53), progressive spinal atrophy, and amyotrophic lateral sclerosis. Rimmed vacuoles are also present in glycogenosis, McArdle syndrome, and progressive spinal atrophy.

In several muscular dystrophies, especially in facioscapulohumeral dystrophy, rimmed vacuoles are present. Oculopharyngeal muscular dystrophy represents a special case in which 8.5-nm-diameter myonuclear filaments are specific. But 15–18-nm myonuclear and cytoplasmic filaments can be found. This association could contribute to a better evaluation of s-IBM filaments, because oculopharyngeal muscular dystrophy is a hereditary disease with a locus in chromosome 14.

IBM and Dysimmunity

The association with several dysimmune diseases is frequently observed: Raynaud and Buerger syndromes (5), coeliac disease (10), malignant mesenchymoma (13), scleroderma (35), sarcoidosis (19), Paget disease (19), thrombocytopenia (50), collagen vascular disease (24,54). In a report of 40 patients, Lotz et al. (27) described a significant association with an autoimmune disease in 15% of cases, with diabetes mellitus in 20% of cases.

In their cases involving cellular inflammation, Arahata and Engel (55–58) evaluated the nature of the inflammatory exudate. The exudate was predominantly endomysial, with T cells and macrophages. There was a partial invasion of non-necrotic muscle fibers. The endomysial inflammatory cells had surrounded and invaded non-necrotic muscle fibers. The majority of T cells were CD8 cytotoxic cells. However, the same partial invasion of fibers is seen in chronic polymyositis and thus probably is nonspecific.

Immuno-electron microscopy has confirmed that the fibers are invaded by immune finger-like extensions of T8+ cells and macrophages that are surrounded by non-necrotic fibers. At a slightly more advanced age, T8+ cells appear in a small cavity in the superficial region of the muscle fiber. Later on, the cavity can include 5–20 cells. These cells replace or displace the fiber. At a more advanced stage of destruction, few myofibrils are still observed. Surprisingly, the macrophages contain but few heterophagic vacuoles. Their activity appears more cytotoxic than phagocytic. Ultimately, segments of the muscle fiber are completely replaced by the invading cells.

Whether it is a primary or a dominant process that induces muscle loss remains unknown, and the atrophy could be related to a dysimmune state. This fact may explain why s-IBM cannot be treated with immunosuppressive drugs.

In s-IBM there is an oligoclonal pattern of arrangement of T-cell-receptor (TCR) genes, but the heterogeneity of the CDR3-domain sequence suggests that the primary T-cell response is not mounted against a muscle-specific antigen, but could be triggered by a superantigen (59).

Amyloid Deposits and Brain-specific Proteins in IBM

New advances in our understanding of the pathogenic mechanisms have been published by Mendell et al. (60) and in several works by Askanas et al. (61–64). Askanas has progressively identified amyloid deposits and other abnormally accumulated substances: ubiquitin, β-amyloid protein, β-amyloid precursor protein, a_1-antichymotrypsin, hyperphosphorylated τ protein, and prion protein (65). Thus there are striking similarities between the pathologic findings in IBM and Alzheimer disease in regard to accumulations of the same proteins in the muscle in IBM and in the brain in Alzheimer disease. The presence of an amyloidopathy raises the question of a primary or a secondary effect. A possible role of zinc in the fibrillogenesis should also be considered.

The Nucleus Hypothesis

The pathologic process involves not only the cytoplasm but also the nucleus. In some cases, Carpenter and Karpati (66), using electron microscopy, observed disintegration of the nuclei in IBM muscle fibers. The myonuclear content is discharged into the cytoplasm, and that could induce the rimmed vacuoles. This process may result in temporary inappropriate expression of non-muscle molecules by the extranuclear genome that escaped the normal intranuclear regulatory control of gene expression. The progressive depletion of nuclei, exceeding the compensatory capacity of satellite cells, could lead to fiber atrophy and loss. An unknown process could incite a cytotoxic reaction against muscle fibers. It is also possible that an alteration of the nuclear gene could alter the mitochondrial DNA. The nuclear matrix could be a target of the pathogenetic factor, resulting in aberrant gene expression.

In s-IBM patients (but not in controls) a single-strand-DNA-binding protein accumulates in many myonuclei (67), but it differs from replication protein A (34-kDa subunit), another single-strand-DNA-binding protein that is also increased in many myonuclei in s-IBM and polymyositis. The number of myonuclei that exhibit the unidentified abnormal, single-strand-DNA-binding protein is far greater than the number of those showing ultrastructural abnormalities. This could suggest that the biochemical abnormality of myonuclei precedes structural alterations.

The Concept of h-IBM

In addition to the previously cited familial IBM cases, the concept of hereditary inclusion-body myopathy (h-IBM) has received increasing attention (40). It occurs in a group of patients with varied clinical features and varied inheritance, either autosomal-recessive or autosomal-dominant. There are two main differences between h-IBM and s-IBM: h-IBM's lack of inflammation in muscle biopsy specimens, and sometimes some unusual distribution of atrophy, sparing the quadriceps muscle. Several Japanese cases of distal myopathy with rimmed vacuoles probably belong in this group.

Vacuolated fibers are free of congophilic amyloid deposits in h-IBM, but contain large accumulations of β-amyloid protein and prion. Thus they could represent an early change.

As is the case for s-IBM, the diagnosis of h-IBM is based mainly on morphologic changes. There are abnormalities similar to those of s-IBM, exclusive of the inflammatory infiltrates. The clinical picture for h-IBM is different and variable, with h-IBM usually occurring in childhood or young adulthood, frequently sparing the quadriceps muscles and in some cases associated with brain abnormalities. h-IBM can occur as either an autosomal-recessive or autosomal-dominant inheritance. The genetic locus is not known, except in a few cases. Its nosologic place is poorly understood.

Several syndromes with different clinical presentations have been reported. The most characteristic are the autosomal-recessive forms that spare the quadriceps. Thirty members of 9 families sharing the same features were observed by Argov and Yarom (68), Massa et al. (69), and Sadeh and Gadoth (70). All of them were of Iranian Jewish origin. The disease occurred in early childhood, childhood, or young adulthood. It involved axial and limb muscles, but spared the quadriceps, even at a very advanced stage. Less constantly, biceps brachii and triceps brachii were spared. Areflexia was frequent. EMG findings were neurogenic, except in Sadeh and Gadoth's case (70). Serum CK concentrations were normal or moderately increased. Muscle CT scan showed hypodensity of limbs and paraspinal muscles. The evolution of the disease was slowly progressive, but relentless. Ten years after onset, the patient became disabled, mainly because of inability to walk. A subgroup was reported in a Tunisian kindred with a relatively, quadriceps-sparing amyotrophy, inflammation, and asymptomatic leukoencephalopathy (71). The 9 cases of Argov and Yarom (68) presented an early scapuloperoneal predominance of weakness. The preservation of the quadriceps was not only clinical; there were no rimmed vacuoles seen at quadriceps muscle biopsy.

There have also been several reports of hereditary forms without sparing of the quadriceps. The first (21) concerned a 23-year-old man with symptoms since early childhood: globally distributed muscle weakness and wasting that were marked distally, with foot-drop and areflexia. An older brother was more severely affected. A family with an autosomal-dominant inheritance limited to males was observed by Neville et al. (72). The clinical features were proximal lower-limb and facial weakness. In 3 families with autosomal-dominant inheritance (73) there was a symmetrical generalized amyotrophy. Proximal and distal weakness of late onset, with dominant inheritance and inflammatory myopathy with rimmed vacuoles, was observed by Klingman et al. (74). Except for the mode of inheritance, those previous cases shared the same features: The disease had a juvenile or adult onset. Weakness and atrophy were proximal and distal, with involvement of axial muscles. Facial muscles were slightly involved in one family.

Another form is h-IBM with leukoencephalopathy. Cole et al. (75) investigated a family of 6 male siblings, 5 of them having progressive IBM and asymptomatic leukoencephalopathy. Cranial CT scans showed hypodensity of cerebral white matter. MRI of the brain showed increased signal density from cerebral white matter, including periventricular white matter and the corona radiata, but sparing the subcortical U system. The clinical features differed from the usual presentation of IBM: onset in early childhood, and proximal weakness. The mode of inheritance was not determined. The cases reported by Hentati et al. (71) involved similar leukoencephalopathy, but with relative quadriceps sparing.

Misappreciated h-IBM

Some familial distal myopathies are difficult to differentiate from h-IBM, particularly Welander late-onset distal myopathy, late-onset dominant distal myopathy, and Japanese cases of distal myopathies with rimmed vacuoles.

In 1951, Welander (76) described 249 cases of distal myopathy in 72 families (149 men, 100 women). The mean age of onset was 47 years. The age of onset of symptoms ranged from 20 to 77 years. Thus Welander myopathy has been regarded as a myopathy of late-adult onset. The inheritance pattern was autosomal-dominant, with incomplete penetrance. Signs began in the distal upper limbs in 89% of the cases, in the distal lower limbs in 8%, and simultaneously in 3%. The initial symptom was clumsiness of the fingers. At times the process could be asymmetrical. Weakness was marked in the fingers and small muscles of the hand. Proximal weakness was uncommon. Tendon reflexes were normal. The course was benign. EMG findings were myogenic. The histologic changes were myogenic. Vacuoles were "sometimes observed" by Welander. In fact, rimmed vacuoles are frequently found in the muscle fibers, and filamentous inclusions have been observed by Thornell et al. (77) and Borg et al. (78). Lindberg et al. (79) compared the pathologic findings in 5 cases of Welander disease and 5 cases of IBM. They found cytoplasmic inclusions in all cases, but no nuclear inclusions in Welander disease. EMG findings were neurogenic and myogenic in all cases. Small angular muscle fibers were present. Inflammatory infiltrates were absent in Welander disease, and inflammation was the main pathologic feature that differentiated s-IBM from Welander myopathy. Finally, Welander myopathy could represent a benign, very slowly progressive, distal form of h-IBM, without inflammation.

Several cases of "distal myopathies with rimmed vacuoles" have been described in Japan (31,36,80–87). They are sometimes cited as being of the "Nonaka type." Nonaka et al. (85,88) reviewed 37 cases in Japan, which they described as "distal myopathy with rimmed vacuole formation." Among those patients, 25 were females, and 12 males. The mean age of onset was 26 years. In 12 patients there was an autosomal-recessive inheritance. In most patients, the onset of weakness and atrophy occurred in the peroneal muscles, associated with foot-drop and steppage gait. A few patients had gastrocnemius weakness. Late proximal weakness developed, but the quadriceps muscles generally were not involved. The finger and hand muscles were moderately weak. Neck flexors were weak in some cases. Serum CK concentrations were normal or slightly raised. EMG findings were myogenic and neurogenic. Muscle biopsy showed multiple or single rimmed vacuoles in numerous muscle fibers, both in the center and at the periphery of fibers. Rimmed vacuoles were more common in type I muscle fibers. In addition, there was marked variation in muscle-fiber size, but no inflammatory cells. Necrotic fibers were rare. Filamentous nuclear or cytoplasmic inclusions were found in 8 cases. The course was progressive. Proximal muscles became severely weak, as did the neck flexor muscles. Some patients became unable to raise their heads when in the supine position. A follow-up study (87) showed the prognosis to be extremely poor. Severe, generalized skeletal-muscle involvement appeared in the advanced stages. In the initial stage, the leg muscles were more prominently affected. In the advanced stage, weakness of the proximal muscles was predominant. In spite of the opinion of Sunohara et al. (87), who considered those cases to represent a different disease, Japanese cases are difficult to differentiate from h-IBM or s-IBM.

Markesbery et al. (89) observed another type of distal myopathy in a French-English family. There was autosomal-dominant inheritance. In 7 adults, the onset of weakness occurred in the ankle dorsiflexor muscles between the ages of 43 and 51 years. Later the weakness involved the fingers and wrist extensors. Finally the proximal muscles were affected. The onset in the lower limbs was in contrast to the situation with Welander myopathy, in which weakness begins in the hands. EMG findings were neurogenic and myogenic. Muscle biopsy revealed a dystrophic process, with variability of fiber size, necrosis, central nuclei, an increase in connective tissue, and fatty infiltration. The most striking change was the presence of numerous vacuoles.

Tibial muscular dystrophy, common in Finland (90), is similar to the Markesbery distal myopathy, with distal onset in the anterior compartment of muscles.

Other types of distal myopathies have been observed. In the older literature, the two Gowers cases (91) probably represented a myotonic dystrophy and a scapuloperoneal syndrome. The cases reported by Milhorat and Wolff (92) could represent a desmine myopathy. The cases reported by Sumner et al. (93) were close to the Markesbery type. The "Miyoshi type," probably different, is an autosomal-recessive distal muscular dystrophy. The onset occurs in the posterior compartment of the legs, with atrophy of the gastrocnemius muscles. Serum CK concentrations are raised from 20 to 150 times normal. Muscle biopsy shows necrotic and regenerating fibers, variability of fiber size, and small angular fibers, but never rimmed vacuoles. These last types of familial distal myopathies are different from h-IBM. In fact, it seems justified to maintain the Welander type and the Japanese cases of distal myopathy in the framework of h-IBM.

Mitochondria and IBM

Ragged red fibers are sometimes present in IBM muscle, and some proportion of muscle fibers will show an absence or low levels of cytochrome-c-oxidase (COX) activity, in spite of high succinate dehydrogenase activity. Ragged red fibers and COX-negative fibers are present more frequently than can be accounted for considering the patients' ages. Usually more than 1% of fibers are affected. Ultrastructural studies frequently show increases in the number and size of mitochondria. Some mitochondria contain crystalline inclusions.

These findings have prompted the search for mitochondrial DNA (mtDNA) deletions in IBM. Oldfors et al. (94) detected large mitochondrial deletions in skeletal-muscle specimens from 3 patients with IBM, ages 39, 60, and 71 years. In all 3 cases, 2–5% of muscle fibers showed an absence or low levels of COX activity. When in situ hybridization was performed, deleted mtDNA was accumulated in COX-deficient muscle fibers, with deletions affecting the region corresponding to an ND4 probe. Southern-blot analysis revealed a 16.5-kb fragment corresponding to normal mtDNA in the 3 cases. Thus muscle fibers with deficient COX activity are more common in patients with IBM than in controls of similar age. Finally, in IBM, DNA deletions affect only the COX-negative fibers. Deletions of various sizes are seen. In a similar study, Santorelli et al. (95) confirmed that multiple mtDNA deletions occurred with high frequency in patients with IBM. They studied 30 IBM patients and detected mtDNA deletions by Southern-blot analysis in 53% of patients, and by polymerase chain reaction in 70% of patients.

The pathogenesis of accumulation of deleted mtDNA with secondary COX deficiency in muscle fibers in IBM is unknown. But a pathogenetic role is arguable for several reasons. The major reason is that in mitochondrial encephalomyopathies, filamentous inclusions have never been observed. Another one is that ragged red fibers are found in common polymyositis. Likewise, COX-negative muscle fibers are observed in normal aged individuals, and mtDNA deletions in muscle may occur with increasing age. Oldfors et al. (94) suggested that COX-negative fibers in IBM are fibers that have undergone regeneration. After necrosis, the satellite cells and their mitochondria proliferate. Deleted mtDNA could be present in some satellite cells, and their deleted mtDNA could be accumulated in regenerating muscle. It is also possible that mtDNA deletion may be induced during the replication of mtDNA in regenerating muscle fiber or that impaired communication between nuclear and mitochondrial genomes causes multiple DNA deletions.

It is probable that mtDNA deletions are not of pathogenetic significance in IBM. It is rather a secondary phenomenon. Moreover, there is no clear correlation between the number of COX-negative fibers and the degree of muscle weakness or the disease duration.

Is IBM a Disease Entity?

This provocative question seems irrelevant. However, because IBM is defined on the basis of morphologic changes, the clinical assessment remains doubtful, and the clinical expression can be typical or atypical. Amyotrophy and muscle weakness are variable: asymmetrical or multifocal, proximal or distal, chronic or progressive, sometimes pseudopolymyositic, sometimes pseudodystrophic. Hereditary forms are either recessive or dominant, with variable semiology. Moreover, IBM is frequent in various specific neuromuscular diseases: facioscapulohumeral dystrophy, oculopharyngeal myopathy, glycogenosis, progressive spinal atrophy, and other diseases. So the question is raised: Are the filamentous inclusions responsible for the clinical features? Do they represent primary or secondary processes in different diseases?

In fact, s-IBM could be a distinct entity in which specific pathologic features are consistently associated with a constellation of clinical findings, whereas h-IBM is probably different.

IBM: an Untreatable Disease?

There is no effective treatment for IBM. Considering the inflammatory changes, many immunosuppressive drugs have been tried without success (96). IBM appears as a cortico-resistant inflammatory myopathy (19). In rare cases, some slight improvement has been reported with prednisone treatment or with immunosuppressive drugs. Pathologically, the inflammatory changes disappear, but there is no clinical or pathologic improvement. The aggravation of the disease suggests that the invasion by cytotoxic T cells could be a secondary rather than a primary process. Intravenous immunoglobulin seems to improve muscle strength in rare cases, but subjective assessment could be responsible. Finally, none of the drugs tested has produced anything more than minor improvement, and that in a minority of patients. At the present time, until further advances are made, IBM remains an untreatable disease.

This chapter has reviewed the main questions raised by IBM. All these points will be developed more extensively in the following chapters of this book.

References

1. Yunis EJ, Samaha FJ. Inclusion body myositis. *Lab Invest* 1971, 25:240.
2. Griggs RC, Askanas V, DiMauro S, et al. Inclusion body myositis and myopathies. *Ann Neurol* 1995, 38:705–713

3. Askanas V, Engel WK, Mirabella M. Idiopathic inflammatory myopathies: inclusion body myositis, polymyositis and dermatomyositis. *Curr Opin Neurol* 1994, 7:448–456.
4. Adams RD, Kakulas BA, Samaha FA. A myopathy with cellular inclusions. *Trans Am Neurol Assoc* 1965, 90:213.
5. Chou SM. Myxovirus-like structures in a case of human chronic polymyositis. *Science* 1967, 158:1453.
6. Carpenter S, Karpati G, Wolfe L. Virus-like filaments and phospholipid accumulation in skeletal muscle study of a histochemically distinct chronic myopathy. *Neurology* 1970, 20:889–903.
7. Sato T, Walker DL, Peters HA, et al. Chronic polymyositis and myxovirus-like inclusions: electronmicroscopic and viral studies. *Arch Neurol* 1971, 24:409–418.
8. Hudson AJ, Oteruelo FT, Haust MD. Unusual generalized myopathy of late onset: clinical and morphological study. In Serratrice G, Roux H (eds), *Actualités de Pathologie Neuromusculaire*. Paris, l'Expansion Scientifique Française, 1971.
9. Jerusalem F, Baumgartner G, Wyler R. Virus-ähnliche Einschlüsse bei chronischen neuromuskulären Prozessen Elektronenmikroskopische Biopsiebedunde von 2 fällen. *Arch Psychiatr Nerven Kr* 1972, 215:148.
10. Hughes JT, Esiri MM. Ultrastructural studies in human polymyositis. *J Neurol Sci* 1975, 25:347–360.
11. Oteruelo FT. Intranuclear inclusions in a myopathy of late onset. *Virchows Arch B Cell Pathol* 1976, 20:319–324.
12. Ketelsen UP, Beckman H, Zimmerman MS, et al. Inclusion body myositis: a "slow virus" infection of skeletal musculature. *Klin Wochenschr* 1977, 55:1063–1066.
13. Carpenter S, Karpati G, Heller I, Eisen A. Inclusion body myositis: a distinct variety of idiopathic inflammatory myopathy. *Neurology* 1978, 28:8.
14. Matsubara S, Mair WGP. Ultrastructural changes in polymyositis. *Brain* 1979, 102:701.
15. Kula RW, Sher JH, Shafiq SA, et al. A chronic neuromuscular disease with basophilic inclusion material in muscle. *Neurology* 1979, 29:595 (abstract).
16. Lisson G, Pongratz D, Hubner G, et al. Ultrastructural and clinical studies in inclusion body myositis. *Fortschr Neurol Psychiatr* 1980, 48:121–127.
17. Hubner G, Pongratz D. Inclusion body myositis. *Biol Cell* 1980, 39:283.
18. Tomé FMS, Fardeau M, Lebon P, et al. Inclusion body myositis. *Acta Neuropath* 1981, suppl 7:287–291.
19. Danon MJ, Reyes MG, Perurena OH, et al. Inclusion body myositis (IBM): myopathy or neuropathy? *Neurology* 1983, 33:1109.
20. Mikol J, Felten-Papaiconomou A, Ferchal F, et al. Inclusion body myositis: clinicopathological studies and isolation of an adenovirus type II from muscle biopsy specimen. *Ann Neurol* 1982, 11:576.
21. Eisen A, Berry K, Gibson G. Inclusion body myositis (IBM): myopathy or neuropathy? *Neurology* 1983, 333:1109.
22. Ringel SP, Kenny CE, Neville HE, et al. Spectrum of inclusion body myositis. *Arch Neurol* 1987, 44:1154.
23. Fidzianska A. Virus-like structures in muscle in chronic polymyositis. *Acta Neuropathol* 1973, 23:23.

24. Lane RJM, Fulthorpe JJ, Hudgson P. Inclusion body myositis: a case with associated collagen vascular disease responding to treatment. *J Neurol Neurosurg Psychiatry* 1985, 48:270.
25. Figarella-Branger D. La myosite à inclusions. Une trop grande hétérogénéité. Etude clinicopathologique. A propos de 21 observations. Medical thesis, Marseille, 1988
26. Arahata K, Engel AG. Monoclonal antibody analysis of mononuclear cells in myopathies. I. Quantification of subsets according to diagnosis and sites of accumulation and demonstration and counts of muscle fibers invaded by T cells. *Ann Neurol* 1984, 16:193.
27. Lotz BP, Engel AG, Nishino H, et al. Inclusion body myositis: observations of 40 patients. *Brain* 1989, 112:727.
28. Figarella-Branger D, Pellissier JF, Pouget J, et al. Myosites à inclusions et maladies neuromusculaires avec vacuoles bordées. *Rev Neurol* 1992, 148:281–290.
29. Askanas V, Engel WK, Alvarez RB, Glenner GG. β-amyloid protein immunoreactivity in muscle of patients with inclusion body myositis. *Lancet* 1992:339–560.
30. Askanas V, Engel WK, Bilak M, et al. Twisted tubulofilaments of inclusion body myositis muscle resemble paired helical filaments of Alzheimer brain contain hyperphosphorylated tau. *Am J Pathol* 1994, 144:177–187.
31. Matsubara S, Tanabe H. Hereditary distal myopathy with filamentous inclusions. *Acta Neurol Scand* 1982, 65:363.
32. Chou SM. Prospects of viral etiology in polymyositis. In: Kakulas BA (ed), *Proceedings of the Second International Congress on Muscle Diseases.* Amsterdam, Excerpta Medica, 1972, pp. 17–28.
33. Chad D, Good P, Adalman L, et al. Inclusion body myositis associated with Sjögren's syndrome. *Arch Neurol* 1983, 39:186.
34. Sato T, Tsubaki T. Characteristics of virus-like structures in polymyositis. In: Kakulas BA (ed), *Proceedings of the Second International Congress on Muscle Diseases.* Amsterdam, Excerpta Medica, 1972, pp. 29–35.
35. Salama J, Tomé FMS, Lebon P, et al. Myosite à inclusions. Etude clinique, morphologique et virologique concernant une nouvelle observation associée à une sclérodermie généralisée et à un syndrome de klinefelter. *Rev Neurol* 1980, 136:863.
36. Satoyoshi E, Murakami N, Takemitu N, Nonaka I. Significance of rimmed vacuoles in various neuromuscular disorders. In: Serratrice G, Pellissier JF, Pouget J, et al. (eds), *Système nerveux, muscles et maladies systémiques: acquisitions récentes.* Paris, Expansion Scientifique Française, 1993, pp. 83–92.
37. Serratrice G, Pellissier JF, Pouget J, et al. Formes cliniques des myosites à inclusions: 12 cas. *Rev Neurol (Paris)* 1989, 145:781.
38. Lake BD, Payan P, Pike M, et al. Inclusion body myositis and peripheral axonal neuropathy in a 14-year old boy. *J Neurol Sci (suppl)* 1990, 98:179.
39. Verma A, Bradley WG, Adesina AM, et al. Inclusion body myositis with cricopharyngeus muscle involvement and severe dysphagia. *Muscle and Nerve* 1991, 14:470.
40. Askanas V, Engel VK. New advances in inclusion body myositis. *Curr Opin Rheumatol* 1993, 5:737–741.
41. Calabrese LH, Mitsumoto H, Chou SM. Inclusion body myositis presenting as treatment-resistant polymyositis. *Arthritis Rheum* 1987, 30:397.

42. Hund E, Heckl R, Goebel HH, Meinck HM. Inclusion body myositis presenting with isolated erector spinae paresis. *Neurology* 1995, 45:993–994.
43. Serratrice G, Pouget J, Pellissier JF. Bent spine syndrome. *J Neurol Neurosurg Psychiatry* 1996, 60:51–54.
44. Julien J, Vital CL, Vallat JM, et al. Inclusion body myositis: clinical biological and ultrastructural study. *J Neurol Sci* 1982, 55:15.
45. Rebel A, Malkani K, Basle M, et al. Osteoclast ultrastructure in Paget's disease. *Calcif Tissue Res* 1976, 20:187–199.
46. Mills BG, Singer R. Nuclear inclusions in Paget's disease of bone. *Science* 1976, 194:201–202.
47. Serratrice G. Inclusion body myositis: an inflammatory disease? *Acta Cardiomyol* 1991, 2:11–116.
48. Sawchak JA, Kula RW, Sher JH, et al. Clonicopathologic investigations in patients with inclusion body myositis (IBM). *Neurology (suppl)* 1983, 33:237.
49. Tateishi J, Nagara H, Ohta M, et al. Intranuclear inclusions in muscle, nervous tissue and adrenal gland. *Acta Neuropathol (Berlin)* 1984, 63:24.
50. Riggs JF, Schochet SS, Gutman L, et al. Inclusion body myositis and chronic immune thrombocytopenia. *Arch Neurol* 1984, 41:93.
51. Serratrice G, Pouget J, Pellissier JP. Inclusion body myositis. Semiology and criteria. *J Rééduc Fonct* 1995, 9:23.
52. Abarbanel JM, Lichtenfeld Y, Zirkin H, et al. Inclusion body myositis in post-poliomyelitis muscular atrophy. *Acta Neurol Scand* 1988, 78:81–84.
53. Miranda-Pfeilsticker B, Figarella-Branger D, Pellissier JF, Serratrice G. Le syndrome postpoliomyelitique: 29 cas. *Rev Neurol (Paris)* 1992, 148:355–361.
54. Apostolski S, Dozic S, Bugarski C, Vukanic D. Clinical heterogeneity of inclusion body myositis (IBM). In: *Proceedings of the 9th International Meeting on Neuromuscular Diseases* (abstract). 1988, p. 108.
55. Arahata K, Engel AG. Monoclonal antibody analysis of mononuclear cells in myopathies. III. Immunoelectron microscopy aspects of cell-mediated muscle fiber injury. *Ann Neurol* 1986, 19:112.
56. Arahata K, Engel AG. Monoclonal antibody analysis of mononuclear cells in myopathies. IV. Cell-mediated cytotoxicity and muscle fiber necrosis. *Ann Neurol* 1988, 23:168.
57. Arahata K, Engel AG. Monoclonal antibody analysis of mononuclear cells in myopathies: IV. Identification and quantitation of T8+ suppressor cells. *Ann Neurol* 1988, 23:493.
58. Engel AG, Arahata K. Monoclonal antibody analysis of mononuclear cells in myopathies. II. Phenotypes of autoinvasive cells in polymyositis and inclusion body myositis. *Ann Neurol* 1984, 16:209.
59. Lindberg C, Oldfors A, Tarkowski A. Restricted use of T cell receptor V genes in endomysial infiltrates of patients with inflammatory myopathies. *Eur J Immunol* 1994, 24:2659–2663.
60. Mendell JR, Sahenk Z, Paul L. Amyloid filaments in inclusion body myositis: novel findings provide new insights into nature of filaments. *Arch Neurol* 1991, 48:1229.
61. Askanas V, Engel WK, Alvarez RB. Enhanced detection of Congo-red positive amyloid deposits in muscle fibers of inclusion body myositis. *Neurology* 1993, 43:1265.

62. Askanas V, Engel WK, Alvarez RB. Light and electron microscopic localization of β-amyloid protein in muscle biopsies in patients with inclusion body myositis. *Am J Pathol* 1992, 141:31.

63. Askanas V, Serdaroglu P, Engel WK, et al. Immunolocalization of ubiquitin in muscle biopsies of patients with inclusion body myositis and oculopharyngeal dystrophy. *Neurosci Lett* 1991, 130:73.

64. Askanas V, Alvarez RB, Engel WK. β-amyloid precursor epitopes in muscle fibers of inclusion body myositis. *Ann Neurol* 1993, 34:551.

65. Sarkosi B, Askanas V, Engel WK. Abnormal accumulation of prion protein mRNA in muscle fibers of patients with sporadic inclusion body myositis and hereditary inclusion body myositis. *Am J Pathol* 1994, 145:1280–1284.

66. Carpenter S, Karpati G. The pathological diagnosis of specific inflammatory myopathies. *Brain Pathology* 1992, 2:13–19.

67. Nalbantoglu J, Karpati G, Carpenter S. Conspicuous accumulation of a single-stranded DNA binding protein in skeletal muscle fibers in inclusion body myositis. *Am J Pathol* 1994, 144:874–882.

68. Argov Z, Yarom R. "Rimmed vacuole myopathy" sparing the quadriceps: a unique disorder in Iranian Jews. *J Neurol* 1984, 65:33.

69. Massa R, Weller B, Karpati G, et al. Familial inclusion body myositis among Kurdish-Iranian Jews. *Arch Neurol* 1991, 48:519–522.

70. Sadeh M, Gadoth N. Vacuolar myopathy sparing the quadriceps. *Neurology (suppl 1)* 1991, 41:275.

71. Hentati F, Ben Hamida C, Tomé FMS, et al. Familial inclusion body myositis sparing the quadriceps with asymptomatic leukoencephalopathy in a Tunisian kindred. *Neurology (suppl 1)* 1991, 41:422.

72. Neville HE, Ringel SP, Baumbach LL. Familial inclusion body myositis. *Neurology (suppl 1)* 1990, 40:120.

73. Fardeau M, Askanas V, Tomé FMS, et al. Hereditary neuromuscular disorder with inclusion body myositis-like filamentous inclusions. Clinical, pathological and tissue culture studies. *Neurology (suppl 1)* 1990, 40:120.

74. Klingman JG, Gibbs MA, Creek W. Familial inclusion body myositis. *Neurology (suppl 1)* 1991, 41:275.

75. Cole AJ, Kuzniecky R, Karpati G, et al. Familial myopathy with changes resembling inclusion body myositis and periventricular leucoencephalopathy: a new syndrome. *Brain* 1988, 11:1025.

76. Welander L. Myopathia distalis tarda hereditaria: 249 examined cases in 72 pedigrees. *Acta Med Scand* 1951:141–1.

77. Thornell LE, Edström L, Billeter R, et al. Muscle fibre type composition in distal myopathy (Welander). An analysis with enzyme and immuno-histochemical, gel electrophoretic and ultra-structural techniques. *J Neurol Sci* 1984, 65:269–292.

78. Borg K, Tomé FMS, Edström L. Intranuclear and intracytoplasmic filamentous inclusions in distal myopathy (Welander). *Acta Neuropathol* 1991, 82:102.

79. Lindberg C, Borg K, Edström L, et al. Inclusion body myositis and Welander distal myopathy: a clinical, neurophysiological and morphological comparison. *J Neuro Sci* 1991, 103:76.

80. Murone I, Sato T, Shirakawa K, et al. Distal myopathy: a case of nonhereditary distal myopathy. *Clin Neurol (Tokyo)* 1963, 3:387–393.

81. Sasaki K, Mori H, Takahashi K, Nakamura H. Distal myopathy: report of four cases. *Clin Neurol (Tokyo)* 1969, 9:627–637.

82. Miyoshi S, Santa T, Ohta M, Araki S. A case report of sporadic distal myopathy, with special reference to vacuolar degeneration and rod-like body in muscle fibers. *Clin Neurol (Tokyo)* 1970, 10:111–120.

83. Ideta T, Shikai T, Uchino M, et al. Distal myopathy: report of four cases in two families. *Clin Neurol (Tokyo)* 1973, 13:579–586.

84. Fukuhara N, Kumamoto T, Tsubaki T. Rimmed vacuoles. *Acta Neuropathol (Berlin)* 1980, 51:229–235.

85. Nonaka I, Sunohara N, Ishiura S, Satoyoshi E. Familial distal myopathy with rimmed vacuoles and lamellar (myeloid) body formation. *J Neurol Sci* 1981, 51:141.

86. Mizusawa H, Kurisaki H, Takatsu M, et al. Rimmed vacuolar distal myopathy. A clinical, electrophysiological, histopathological and computed tomographic study of 7 cases. *J Neurol* 1987, 234:129.

87. Sunohara N, Nonaka I, Kamei N, Satoyoshi E. Distal myopathy with rimmed vacuole formation. A follow-up study. *Brain* 1989, 112:65.

88. Nonaka I, Sunohara N, Satoyoshi E, Terasawa K, Yonemoto K. Autosomal recessive distal muscular dystrophy: a comparative study with distal myopathy with rimmed vacuoles formation. *Ann Neurol* 1985, 17:51–59.

89. Markesbery WR, Griggs RC, Leach RP, Lapham LW. Late onset hereditary distal myopathy. *Neurology* 1974, 23:127.

90. Udd B, Partanen J, Halonen P, et al. Tibial muscular dystrophy – late adult onset distal myopathy in 66 Finnish patients. *Arch Neurol* 1993, 50:604–608.

91. Gowers WR. A lecture on myopathy and a distal form. *Lancet* 1902, 11:89–92.

92. Milhorat AT, Wolff HG. Progressive muscular dystrophy of distal type; report on a family; report of autopsy. *Arch Neurol Psych* 1943, 49:655–664.

93. Summer D, Crawford M, Harriman DGF. Distal muscular dystrophy in an English family. *Brain* 1971, 94:51–60.

94. Oldfors A, Larsson N, Lindberg C, Holme E. Mitochondrial DNA deletions in inclusion body myositis. *Brain* 1993, 116:325–336.

95. Santorelli FM, Sciacco M, Shanske S, Griggs RC, et al. Mitochondrial DNA deletions in patients with inclusion body myositis (abstract). *Neurology (suppl 2)* 1994, 44:A131.

96. Dalakas MC. Polymyositis, dermatomyositis and inclusion body myositis. *N Engl J Med* 1991, 325:1487–1498.

Part III

Sporadic Inclusion-Body Myositis: Clinical
and Diagnostic Considerations

3

Sporadic Inclusion-Body Myositis: Clinical and Laboratory Features and Diagnostic Criteria

JERRY R. MENDELL

Sporadic inclusion-body myositis belongs to the group of idiopathic inflammatory myopathies. The term "inclusion-body myositis" was coined in 1971 by Yunis and Samaha (1). Controversy concerning the specificity of its histopathology delayed its general acceptance as a distinct disorder, but it is now unequivocally established as a well-defined entity separate from dermatomyositis and polymyositis (2–4).

Before describing the clinical and laboratory features, it is extremely important to clarify the distinction between sporadic inclusion-body myositis (s-IBM) and hereditary inclusion-body myopathy (h-IBM). s-IBM, the principal topic of this chapter, is by definition a form of myositis (where "myositis" refers to an inflammatory condition). s-IBM must be differentiated from the two forms of h-IBM that have been well characterized: the autosomal-recessive disorder of Persian Jews with quadriceps sparing (5–7) and the autosomal-dominant disorder with weakness in a limb-girdle distribution (8). From a historical perspective, these inherited conditions were originally considered to be variants of inclusion-body myositis (IBM); however, neither involves inflammation, and for that reason, a sharp distinction must be made between the inflammatory condition s-IBM and the inherited disorders known as h-IBM. Table 3.1 lists these conditions and distinguishes s-IBM and h-IBM from the other disorders that feature rimmed vacuoles.

Sporadic IBM Inclusion-Body Myopathy

Clinical Features

s-IBM is the second most common idiopathic inflammatory myopathy and the most common among patients over the age of 50 years. Childhood-onset cases of IBM have been reported, but these fit more appropriately into the h-IBM group (9–11). Lotz et al. (4) placed the mean

107

Table 3.1. *Myopathies with rimmed vacuoles*

Sporadic inclusion-body myositis (s-IBM)
Hereditary inclusion-body myopathies (h-IBMs)
  Autosomal-recessive, affecting Persian Jews (quadriceps-sparing)
  Autosomal-dominant (limb-girdle distribution)
Other inherited rimmed-vacuole myopathies
  Oculopharyngeal muscular dystrophy
  Oculopharyngodistal myopathy
  Welander distal myopathy
  Markesbery distal myopathy
  Finnish tibial dystrophy
  Nonaka distal myopathy
  Marinesco-Sjögren syndrome
  X-linked myopathy with excessive autophagia
  Acid-maltase deficiency
  Lysomal storage disease with normal acid maltase

age of onset of symptoms at 56.1 years; in their cohort of 40 patients, only 7 were younger than 50 years. There is an unequivocal male preponderance, with men affected at least three times more often than women (M : F = 3 : 1) (1,2,4).

s-IBM involves a distinctive pattern of muscle weakness, allowing a clear distinction from the other inflammatory myopathies. In most cases, weakness begins in the lower extremities and progresses slowly to involve the arms. At the time of diagnosis, both proximal and distal muscles are affected in the majority of patients, and typical findings include weakness of the wrist flexors and finger flexors, with relative preservation of strength in wrist and finger extensors. Atrophy of the volar forearm muscles is characteristic. In the lower extremities, prominent weakness and atrophy of the quadriceps muscles, combined with proximal and distal weakness, provide a characteristic picture. In some cases we have studied, quadriceps weakness and atrophy have been the predominant features, simulating a disorder diagnosed as quadriceps myopathy in earlier eras (12). Asymmetry in the degrees of weakness is commonly observed in s-IBM.

Dysphagia occurs in about one-third of patients with s-IBM. Rarely, dysphagia can be the presenting manifestation (13), and it can be a debilitating feature leading to aspiration, in which case the patient may benefit from cricopharyngeal myotomy (13,14). Findings on barium x-rays indicate that the major dysfunction resides in the upper esophageal

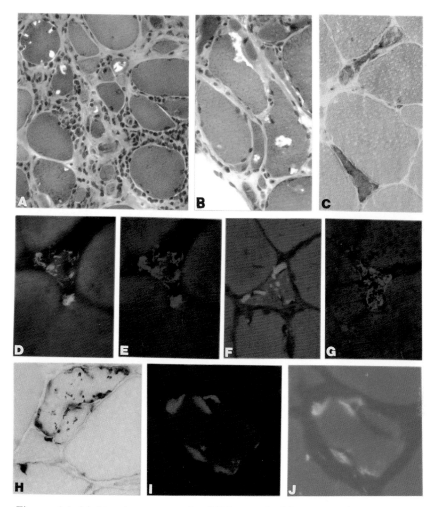

Figure 1.1 Light microscopy of s-IBM muscle biopsy specimens. A and
B: Engel-Gomori trichrome staining. There is mononuclear-cell inflammation in
A. Several vacuolated muscle fibers are shown in A and B (A, ×600; B, ×1,320).
C: Pan-esterase staining demonstrates small, angular, darkly stained muscle
fibers indicative of denervation (×1,320). E–G: Examples of Congo-red positivity visualized through Texas-red filters. D: The same fiber as in E is visualized
through green fluorescence (FITC) filters; Congo-red positivity appears orange
through FITC filters (D–G, ×1,200). H: Peroxidase-antiperoxidase (PAP) staining of abnormal muscle fibers using SMI-31 antibody; SMI-31 positivity appears
in the form of squiggly or dotty inclusions (×1,320). Co-localization of Congo-red
positivity (I) and SMI-310 immunoreactivity (J) using double staining on the
same section (×1,600). There is close co-localization between Congo-red-positive deposits and SMI-310-immunoreactive deposits (indicative of phosphorylated tau)

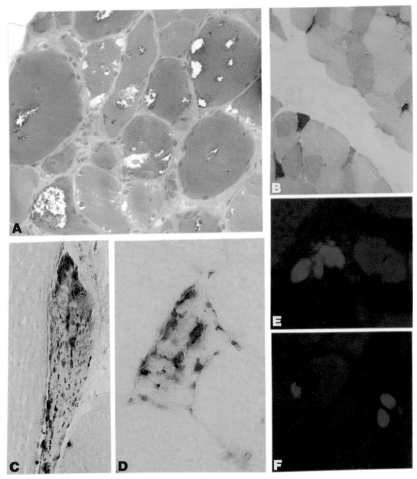

Figure 1.6. h-IBM, light-microscopy of muscle biopsy. A: Engel-Gomori trichrome staining illustrating many vacuolated muscle fibers in autosomal-recessive h-IBM. Only a few of the vacuoles are rimmed; most appear empty; and some are filled with a purple-grayish material ($\times$1,320). B: Pan-estarase reaction demonstrates several darkly-stained, small angular muscle fibers indicative of denervation ($\times$450). C and D: PAP reaction in autosomal-recessive h-IBM, illustrating SMI-31 immunoreactivity in vacuolated muscle fibers ($\times$1,320). E and F: Examples of Congo-red positivity in autosomal-dominant IBM ($\times$1,320). In contrast to s-IBM, in which Congo-red positivity occurs in the form of squiggly or rod-like inclusions, Congo-red positivity in autosomal-dominant IBM occurs in the form of round inclusions.

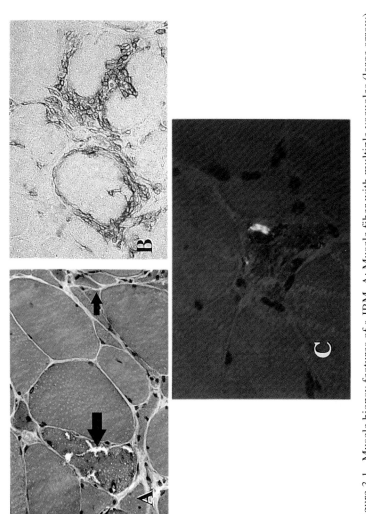

Figure 3.1. Muscle biopsy features of s-IBM. A: Muscle fiber with multiple vacuoles (large arrow) and several small angular fibers (small arrow) in the same field in a section stained with Engel-Gomori trichrome. B: Two non-necrotic muscle fibers invaded by CD8+ mononuclear cells. C: Muscle fiber showing apple-green birefringence of amyloid in Congo-red stain viewed with polarized light.

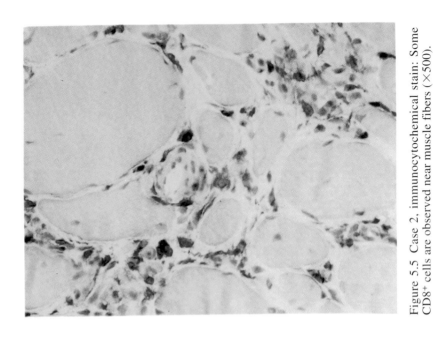

Figure 5.5 Case 2, immunocytochemical stain: Some CD8+ cells are observed near muscle fibers (×500).

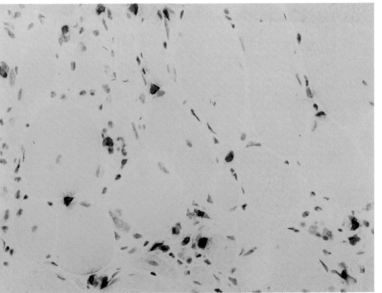

Figure 5.4. Case 2, immunocytochemical stain: Numerous CD4+ cells are present in endomysium near muscle fibers (×400).

muscles (2,4). Facial-muscle weakness (particularly of the orbicularis oculi) is present in approximately one-third of patients. Respiratory muscles are usually spared in patients with s-IBM. Muscle stretch reflexes typically are normal, although loss of quadriceps reflexes may accompany significant atrophy of this muscle (4).

Heart involvement has not been documented as a manifestation of s-IBM. However, given that s-IBM affects an older population of patients, cardiovascular abnormalities are commonly encountered but are independent of the underlying disorder (4). There is an increased incidence of peripheral neuropathy in s-IBM patients (9). There is no documented association with malignancy.

Of particular interest are the relationships between s-IBM and various immune-mediated diseases, including idiopathic thrombocytopenic purpura, interstitial lung disease, diabetes mellitus, systemic lupus erythematosus, and Sjögren syndrome (4,15). We have observed s-IBM in the setting of common variable immunodeficiency disease, and similar cases have been reported by Dalakas and Illa (16). An association of s-IBM with autoimmune diseases is supported by an overrepresentation of the major histocompatibility alleles B8 and DR3 (17).

Laboratory Features

The serum concentration of creatine kinase is usually elevated twofold to fivefold in s-IBM patients. In exceptional cases, concentrations may reach 12 times normal. Autoantibodies defining subsets of myositis (17,18) are not observed in s-IBM. Erythrocyte sedimentation rates usually are normal or only mildly elevated. Multiple mitochondrial-DNA deletions are common in s-IBM (19,20) (as discussed elsewhere in this text) but have no role in diagnosis.

In s-IBM, electromyography will demonstrate increased insertional activity, often with fibrillations accompanied by short-duration, polyphasic, early recruited motor-unit potentials. The incidence of long-duration potentials is also increased, and a mixed pattern of short- and long-duration potentials supports a diagnosis of IBM (9).

An unequivocal diagnosis of s-IBM rests on the muscle biopsy picture. Four features are characteristic (Figure 3.1, following page 104): (i) Single or multiple rimmed vacuoles lined with granular material are present in fresh-frozen sections stained with hematoxylin and eosin or Engel-Gomori trichrome. (ii) A cardinal feature is the presence of endomysial inflammation, particularly invasion of non-necrotic muscle fibers by

CD8+ T cells (21). Macrophages may also be present, but are less specific. The pattern of inflammation is similar to that of polymyositis, although perimysial and perivascular inflammatory infiltrations occur less often in s-IBM. (iii) Intracellular amyloid deposits are found within muscle fibers (22). The deposits demonstrate apple-green birefringence using polarized light. Congo-red positivity can be enhanced using a fluorescence technique described by Askanas et al. (23). (iv) Electron-microscopic examination of s-IBM muscle demonstrates nonbranching filaments, also referred to as tubulofilaments (Figure 3.2). The tubulofilaments measure 15–18 nm in diameter and vary in length from 1 to 5 nm. These filaments can occur in compact or loose bundles and in parallel or random orientations, most often in close association with rimmed vacuoles. Tubulofilaments also occur within the nucleus, usually surrounded by a thin rim of marginated chromatin.

The rimmed vacuoles in s-IBM are composed of whorls of membranous material and myelin figures, as well as amorphous debris, when viewed by electron microscopy (Figure 3.2). Small groups of atrophic fibers are also commonly observed in this disorder, raising the possibility of a superimposed neurogenic component (9).

Family History

In two families studied at The Ohio State University, siblings were affected by a condition meeting all the proposed criteria (Table 3.2) for s-IBM. Similar familial occurrences of this disorder have been observed by Dalakas et al. (personal communication). These do not represent multigeneration families; only siblings have been affected. Current thinking suggests that these familial cases occur as a result of a predisposition based on genetic factors (such as sharing major histocompatibility alleles). The presence of inflammation is revealed by muscle biopsy, distinguishing these familial cases from h-IBM.

Diagnostic Criteria

Diagnostic criteria for s-IBM have been recommended (20), as listed in Table 3.2. A definite diagnosis of s-IBM remains a histologic diagnosis, established in any individual showing the cardinal muscle biopsy features described. It is worthy of note that the histologic criteria permit a definite diagnosis of s-IBM if either amyloid deposits (shown by light microscopy) or tubulofilaments (shown by electron microscopy) are found. That can

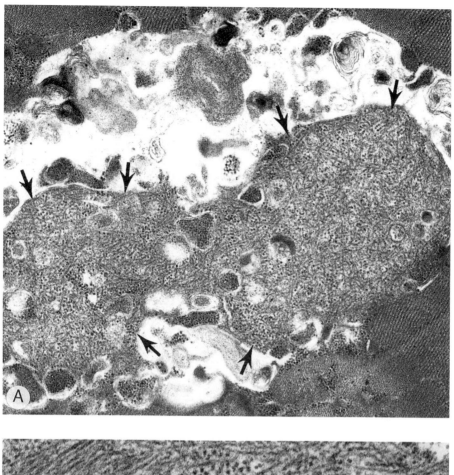

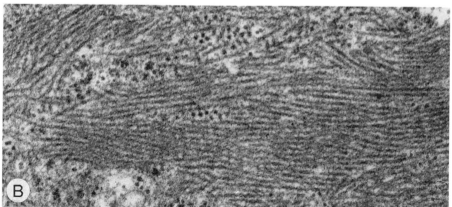

Figure 3.2. Electron micrographs of s-IBM. A: Clusters of closely packed, poorly aligned tubulofilaments (arrows) are seen within a typical vacuole containing membranous debris; among the filaments, free and membrane-bound glycogen granules can be seen. B: Closely aligned 15–18-nm tubulofilaments are seen.

Table 3.2. *Diagnostic criteria for s-IBM*

I. Characteristic features
    A. Clinical
        1. Duration of illness: more than 6 months
        2. Age of onset: more than 30 years old
        3. Muscle weakness must affect the proximal and distal muscles of
            arms and legs, *and*
            the patient must exhibit at least one of the following features:
            (a) Finger-flexor weakness
            (b) Wrist-flexor weakness greater than wrist-extensor weakness
            (c) Quadriceps-muscle weakness (grade 4 MRC)
    B. Laboratory
        1. Serum creatine kinase less than 12 times normal
        2. Muscle biopsy
            (a) Inflammatory myopathy characterized by mononuclear-cell in
                 vasion of non-necrotic muscle fibers
            (b) Vacuolated muscle fibers
            (c) Either
                 (i)   Intracellular amyloid deposits (must use fluorescence
                       method of identification before excluding the presence of
                       amyloid) *or*
                 (ii) 15–18-nm tubulofilaments shown by electron microscopy
        3. Electromyography findings must be consistent with the features of
            an inflammatory myopathy (i.e., irritable myopathy); long-duration
            potentials are commonly observed and do not
            exclude a diagnosis of s-IBM
    C. Family history
        Rarely, s-IBM can be observed in families. This condition is
        different from h-IBM without inflammation. Familial cases of s-IBM
        require documentation of the inflammatory component by
        muscle biopsy, in addition to vacuolated muscle fibers, intracellular
        (within muscle fibers) amyloid, and 15–18-nm tubulofilaments.
    D. Associated disorders
        IBM can occur with a variety of other disorders, especially immune-
        mediated conditions. The presence of an associated condition does not
        preclude a diagnosis of s-IBM if the following diagnostic criteria are
        met.
II. Diagnostic criteria for s-IBM
    A. *Definite* s-IBM
        Patients must exhibit all muscle biopsy features, including invasion of
        non-necrotic fibers by
        mononuclear cells, vacuolated muscle fibers, and intracellular (within
        muscle fibers) amyloid deposits or 15–18-nm tubulofilaments. None of
        the other clinical or laboratory features are mandatory if the muscle
        biopsy features are diagnostic.
    B. *Possible* s-IBM
        If the muscle shows only inflammation (invasion of non-necrotic muscle
        fibers by mononuclear cells) *without* other muscle biopsy features of
        IBM, *then* a diagnosis of "possible s-IBM" can be made if the patient
        exhibits the characteristic clinical (I.A.1,2,3) and laboratory (I.B.1,3)
        features. Neither I.C nor I.D should exclude a diagnosis of s-IBM.

avoid the delay and expense of carrying out electron microscopy for all patients suspected of having s-IBM.

Most s-IBM patients will show the characteristic clinical and laboratory features described earlier and listed in Table 3.2. Exceptions, however, do occur, especially early in the evolution of the disorder. The diagnostic criteria have been drafted (20) in recognition of the fact that there are patients who do not meet all of the histologic criteria at the time of initial encounter. Such patients are placed in the group designated as "possible s-IBM." The "possible s-IBM" category includes those who have the clinical and laboratory features of s-IBM, in association with inflammation seen at muscle biopsy (non-necrotic muscle fibers invaded by mononuclear cells), but who lack rimmed vacuoles, intracellular amyloid deposits, and 15–18-nm tubulofilaments. The precise number of these patients has not been determined, but it may reach as high as 15% of the total cohort who will eventually develop all the features of s-IBM. The importance of the category of "possible s-IBM" to future clinical trials cannot be underestimated.

As previously mentioned, neither familial occurrences nor associated disorders preclude a diagnosis of s-IBM as outlined in Table 3.2.

Hereditary Inclusion-Body Myopathies

The inherited forms of IBM (i.e., the h-IBMs) are discussed elsewhere in this volume. Here, only the features and diagnostic criteria for s-IBM have been defined. It is important to again emphasize that although s-IBM and h-IBM have certain overlapping features, they are distinct nosologic entities. The link between s-IBM and h-IBM concerns the presence of rimmed vacuoles, intracellular amyloid deposits, and 15–18-nm tubulofilaments (24). These histologic findings are present in both the autosomal-recessive form of h-IBM among Persian Jews and the autosomal-dominant form of h-IBM with a limb-girdle distribution of muscle weakness. Neither of these inherited conditions demonstrates mononuclear inflammatory-cell invasion of non-necrotic muscle fibers. A brief summary of the clinical features of the h-IBMs (5–9) is given in Table 3.3.

Additional rimmed-vacuole myopathies, each with distinct clinical features, and all lacking inflammation of muscle biopsy specimens, are listed in Table 3.1. Some of these conditions are discussed further elsewhere in this volume. Perhaps adding to the chaos and blurring the distinctions based on morphology is the observation that some of these rimmed-vacuole myopathies (Welander and Nonaka distal myopathies, Finnish tibial

Table 3.3. *Hereditary inclusion-body myopathies (h-IBMs)*

I. Autosomal-recessive disorder (5–8)
   A. Affects Persian Jews (Kurdish Iranians) and may affect Egyptians and Afghans
   B. Onset before 35 years of age
   C. Affects proximal and distal muscles, with sparing of quadriceps muscles in the majority
   D. Muscle biopsy shows rimmed vacuoles, amyloid deposits, and 15–18-nm tubulofilaments, but no inflammation
II. Autosomal-dominant disorder (9)
   A. Onset before 30 years of age
   B. Affects proximal and distal muscles, including quadriceps muscles
   C. Dysphagia common
   D. Muscle biopsy shows rimmed vacuoles, amyloid deposits, and 15–18-nm tubulofilaments, but no inflammation

dystrophy, and oculopharyngeal muscular dystrophy, as discussed in other chapters of this volume) may also feature amyloid deposits and 15–18-nm tubulofilaments. The significance of these findings is under study and should be clarified by further research.

Conclusions

The objective of this chapter has been to describe the clinical and laboratory features and the histologic profile for s-IBM. Delineating these features and defining the diagnostic criteria (Table 3.2) for s-IBM are important steps in the clinical management of patients, in addition laying the foundation for future prospective studies of s-IBM. The hereditary forms of IBM are discussed in other chapters of this volume.

References

1. Yunis EJ, Samaha FJ. Inclusion body myositis. *Lab Invest* 1971, 25:240–248.
2. Carpenter S, Karpati G, Heller I, Eisen A. Inclusion body myositis: a distinct variety of idiopathic inflammatory myopathy. *Neurology* 1978, 28:8–17.
3. Ringel SP, Kenney CE, Neville HE, Giorno R, Carry MR. Spectrum of inclusion body myositis. *Arch Neurol* 1978, 44:1154–1157.
4. Lotz BP, Engel AG, Nishino H, Stevens JC, Litchy WJ. Inclusion body myositis: observations in 40 patients. *Brain* 1989, 112:727–747.
5. Argov Z, Yarom R. "Rimmed vacuole myopathy" sparing the quadriceps. *J Neurol Sci* 1984, 64:33–43.

6. Cole AJ, Kuzniecky R, Karpati G, Carpenter S, Andermann E, Andermann F. Familial myopathy with changes resembling inclusion body myositis and periventricular leukoencephalopathy: a new syndrome. *Brain* 1988, 111:1025–1037.

7. Sadeh M, Gadoth N, Hadar H, Ben-David E. Vacuolar myopathy sparing the quadriceps. *Brain* 1993, 116:217–232.

8. Neville HE, Baumbach LL, Ringel SP, Russo LS Jr, Sujansky E, Garcia CA. Familial inclusion body myositis: evidence for autosomal dominant inheritance. *Neurology* 1992, 42:897–902.

9. Eisen A, Berry K, Gibson S. Inclusion body myositis (IBM): myopathy or neuropathy? *Neurology* 1983, 33:1109–1114.

10. Riggs JE, Schochat SS, Gutmann L, Lerfald SC. Childhood onset inclusion body myositis mimicking limb-girdle muscular dystrophy. *J Child Neurol* 1989, 4:283–285.

11. Danon MJ, Reyes MG, Perurena OH, Masdea JC, Manaligod JR. Inclusion body myositis: a corticosteroid-resistant idiopathic inflammatory myopathy. *Arch Neurol* 1982, 39:760–764.

12. Walton JN. Two cases of myopathy limited to the quadriceps. *J Neurol Neurosurg Psychiatry* 1956, 19:106.

13. Riminton DS, Chambers ST, Parkin PJ, Pollock M, Donaldson IM. Inclusion body myositis presenting solely as dysphagia. *Neurology* 1993, 43:1241–1243.

14. Danon MJ, Friedman M. Inclusion body myositis associated with progressive dysphagia: treatment with cricopharyngeal myotomy. *Can J Neurol Sci* 1989, 16:436–438.

15. Chad D, Good P, Adelman L, Bradley WG, Mills J. Inclusion body myositis associated with Sjögren's syndrome. *Arch Neurol* 1982, 39:186–188.

16. Dalakas MC, Illa I. Common variable immuodeficiency and inclusion body myositis: a distinct myopathy mediated by natural killer cells. *Ann Neurol* 1995, 37:806–810.

17. Plotz PH, Rider LG, Targoff IN, Raben N, O'Hanlon TP, Miller FW. NIH Conference. Myositis: immunologic contributions to understanding cause, pathogenesis and therapy [review]. *Ann Intern Med* 1995, 122:715–724.

18. Tan EM. Autoantibodies to nuclear antigens (ANA): their immunobiology and medicine. *Adv Immunol* 1982, 33:167–240.

19. Oldfors A, Larsson NG, Lindberg C, Holme E. Mitochondrial deletions in inclusion body myositis. *Brain* 1993, 116:325–336.

20. Griggs RC, Askanas V, DiMauro S, Engel A, Karpati G, Mendell JR, Rowland LP. Inclusion body myositis and myopathies. *Ann Neurol* 1995, 38:705–713.

21. Arahata K, Engel AG. Monoclonal antibody analysis of mononuclear cells in myopathies. I: Quantitation of subsets according to diagnosis and sites of accumulation and demonstration and counts of muscle fibers invaded by T cells. *Ann Neurol* 1994, 16:193–208.

22. Mendell JR, Sahenk Z, Gales T, Paul L. Amyloid filaments in inclusion body myositis. *Arch Neurol* 1991, 48:1229–1234.

23. Askanas V, Engel WK, Alvarez RB. Enhanced detection of Congo-red positive amyloid deposits in muscle fibers of inclusion body myositis and brain of Alzheimer's disease using fluorescence technique. *Neurology* 1993, 43:1265–1267.

24. Mendell JR, Sahenk Z. Inclusion body myositis. *Neurology* 1992, 42:2231–2232.

4

Inclusion-Body Myositis: Natural History

FRANÇOISE BILLÉ-TURC

Inclusion-body myositis (IBM) is a disease of unknown cause, and its natural history is largely unknown, with only few available reports. Determining the natural history of IBM is of major interest for characterizing the course of the disease and its response to therapeutic trials. Natural-history knowledge will provide information concerning the age of onset of the disease, the prediagnosis period, and the course of the disease following muscle biopsy (linear or remitting). Moreover, there are many differences in the course of sporadic (s-IBM) and hereditary (h-IBM) cases.

For the past few years we have been observing 18 patients with s-IBM, more than 80% of them men. The age at onset of the disease varied from 17 to 70 years (mean age 46.22 ± 17). The disease reached a peak around 60 years (Figure 4.1). The latency period before diagnosis varied from 1 to 20 years, with a peak in the early period and a mean latency of 5.4 ± 4.8 years. Table 4.1 shows the age of the patients at time of diagnosis and the follow-up. The progression of functional disability is described in Table 4.2. In the follow-up, despite steroid treatment, there was no improvement in 11 cases. One case showed stabilization. In two cases, myalgias disappeared following steroid treatment, and in one case, following treatment with intravenous immunoglobulin (IVIG). In some cases with associated mitochondrial abnormalities, coenzyme Q did not produce improvement.

Approach to a Natural History of s-IBM

The incidence of s-IBM varies from 15% to 28% among the idiopathic inflammatory myopathies (1). s-IBM is the most frequent myopathy among patients referred for "steroid-resistant" polymyositis. There is no really effective treatment, and there have been no prospective studies of the natural history of IBM. So many questions remain, with few answers. Is IBM a benign or severe disease? Is IBM a chronic, progressive, or relapsing disease? According to the recent IBM literature, combined

116

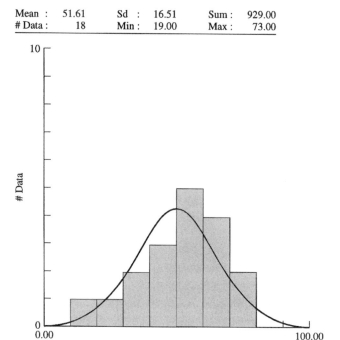

| Mean : | 51.61 | Sd : | 16.51 | Sum : | 929.00 |
| # Data : | 18 | Min : | 19.00 | Max : | 73.00 |

Figure 4.1. Age at time of diagnosis: horizontal scale, age of patients; vertical scale, number of patients.

with our own cases, there have been about 250 sporadic cases (155 male and 76 female in the literature).

Onset

IBM is most often a disease affecting old men, but there have been some cases during childhood, and one-third of cases occur in women, with one report during pregnancy. Eisen et al. (2) and Chou (3) described a bimodal disease that most often occurs during the second and sixth decades. Others have seen IBM as a one-peak disease occurring after 50 years (4–6). The age at onset of symptoms varies from 16 to 81 years (average 53.7). In most cases (50%) the disease starts between 50 and 70 years, but in 20% of cases it begins between 10 and 30 years. However, h-IBM has an earlier onset. It could be due to a hormonal or infectious factor.

Table 4.1. *Disease duration and age at diagnosis (vertical scale, number of cases; horizontal scale, age of patients; in black, time from first symptoms to diagnosis; in white, time from diagnosis to last follow-up)*

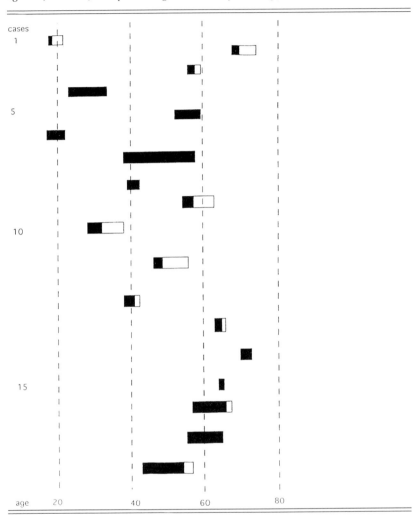

Prediagnosis Period

There tends to be a long latency before diagnosis. The duration of symptoms before biopsy diagnosis has varied from 4 months to 36 years, with an average of 6 years. In the study by Sayers et al. (7), the disease duration before diagnosis was less than 37 months, and initially 40% were incorrectly diagnosed. Granted, 3 years is still a long time, but it is clearly an improvement over earlier studies.

Table 4.2. *Progression of functional disability in 18 patients*

	1 - 4	5 - 9	10 - 14	15 - 19	20 ⟶
5					
4	++++	++	+		+
3	++	+++	+	+	+
2	+				
1	+				

Note: + represents 1 patient. Vertical axis: 1 represents a bedridden or wheel-chair-bound patient; 5 is an ambulatory patient with minimal disability. Horizontal axis: years of disease evolution, from 1 year to more than 20 years.

There are some partial explanations: The disease is often slow to develop, and there are some misleadings forms, with dysphagia, myalgia, tiredness, or pseudoneurogenic involvement. There have been some cases in which the diagnosis was delayed because the disease was unknown to general practitioners. It seems important to have an early diagnosis, because it is logical that treatment will be more effective if initiated earlier. Even the partially effective treatments that are known will not work after the disease has progressed to a certain point or reached a plateau.

At Time of Diagnosis

At this time, the developmental pattern appears to include focal asymmetrical forms, rapidly progressive forms, and some cases associated with immune disorders. Often there is proximal weakness of the lower limbs (quadriceps) severe in that progresses slowly to the arms and then the distal musculature, but deep finger-flexor muscles are often involved at early stages of the disease. At the time of diagnosis, distal weakness is detected in about half of patients, but it is greater than or equal to the degree of proximal weakness in only 35% of patients. Weakness is asymmetrical in one-third of cases. Mild facial, cervical, or scapular weakness occurs in 20% of patients, and facial involvement was mentioned in one-third of the Sekul and Dalakas cases (1). Dysphagia is frequent, affecting about 27% of the IBM population, but in one study it was reported to occur in 4 of 40 patients at onset of the disease and in 16 of 40 at the time of diagnosis (8). Sekul and Dalakas (1) found that 43% of patients had difficulty with swallowing, and more than 90% had abnormal swallowing studies. Knee reflexes were decreased, even without severe quadriceps weakness. They typically disappeared about 10 years after diagnosis. There is no sensory deficit, except in patients who also have a peripheral neuropathy. Some diseases can be associated with IBM, such as cardiovascular abnormality (18%, and only 2 cases of cardiomyopathy), diabetes mellitus, carcinoma. Those diseases seem rather to be induced by old age or to be iatrogenic (steroids), rather than having any direct relationship to IBM. However, an association with an immune disorder (dermatomyositis, scleroderma, systemic lupus erythematosus, thrombocytopenia) can cause a different course to the disease.

Ambulatory Period

A patient's prognosis will depend on the form of the disease. There are some slowly developing chronic forms with selective muscle involvement and, on the other hand, some rapidly progressive forms. The variability in the patient's state during the ambulatory period should be assessed quantitatively as a guide to the prognosis.

Progression of the Disease

There have been few reports of improvement among IBM patients. Levin et al. (9) described a 60-year-old woman who experienced spontaneous recovery. However, most patients deteriorate, and the disease rarely stabilizes, despite treatment. Death is not frequent and most often occurs because of cardiorespiratory deficiency. So IBM is not really a fatal disease, but despite the fact that there are some moderate forms involving little disability, patients often need help with their daily activities.

Is IBM a severe or benign disease? Very little has been written about this topic. Sekul and Dalakas (1) studied 14 patients for more than 5 years; 10 required a cane or support for ambulation by the fifth year after the onset of disease, and 3 of 5 patients with symptoms for 10 years or more were essentially wheelchair-bound. Usually there is a slow progression of IBM, but the degree of disability in relation to the duration of the disease had not been adequately studied until the work of Lotz et al. (8). They assessed functional disability on a scale graduated from 1 (wheelchair-bound) to 5 (minimal involvement).

Course in Treated Patients

In most cases, the course of IBM in treated patients is relentless. With steroid treatment, rare patients have experienced transient improvement, and some have had longer benefit (5,10). Immunosuppressive drugs seem not to work, despite some reports that the combination of oral azathioprine plus oral methotrexate or intravenous methotrexate (11) has led to stabilization. Soueidan and Dalakas (12) reported improvement with high-dosage IVIG. Other treatment such as leukocytopheresis, plasmapheresis, cyclosporin, and total-body irradiation have been ineffective.

Sayers et al. (7) reviewed the cases of 32 patients; 68% of those treated experienced decrements in functioning and muscle strength or stabilization of function. There were only 3 cases of long-term improvement. All untreated patients deteriorated clinically.

Leff et al. (11) examined responses to immunosuppressive treatment in a retrospective study. Prednisone appeared to have been of some modest clinical benefit in 10 of 25 patients (40%). Immunosuppressive drugs such as azathioprine and methotrexate halted the progression of weakness in 8 of 35 trials (23%). In a prospective study, the combination of oral azathioprine and methotrexate and a biweekly infusion of high-dosage intravenous methotrexate with leucovorin rescue appeared to stabilize or even slightly improve strength and functional abilities in some patients.

Improvement occurred rarely and often when other diseases such as collagen vascular disease (10) or systemic lupus erythematosus (13) were associated.

Moderate clinical responses to administration of steroids have been described in some cases (5,14,15).

Soueidan and Dalakas (12) reported, in an open study, that 3 of 4 patients had improved after monthly infusions of high-dosage IVIG. In a further randomized crossover study conducted in 19 patients, Dalakas et al. (16) reported objective signs of improvement in one-third of the patients. However, in an open study, Amato et al. (17) reported worsening, despite IVIG, in all 9 patients treated. Griggs et al. (18) reported similar declines in quantitative myometry and in muscle mass for 7 patients during the natural progression and IVIG treatment (a 6-month period without treatment, compared with a subsequent 6 months of monthly IVIG).

In summary, steroids, IVIG, and immunosuppressive drugs have produced only slight improvements in a minority of patients, and most studies have shown side effects from the treatments, without improvement for the patients. Now it will be important to determine if immunosuppressive drugs can be of predictable benefit and, because of their cost, to determine if IVIG will be more efficient in some subset of patients.

Natural History of h-IBM

There have been few reports on the natural history of h-IBM. Some authors (19–21) have described h-IBM occurring in patients of Iranian Jewish origin, with onset in childhood, a slow progression, and quadriceps sparing. In that group, some patients become wheelchair-bound at an early stage. Most of the patients can still walk after 15–20 years of disease. Other forms without sparing of the quadriceps have been reported: 5 families with juvenile or adult onset (22–24), 5 cases in one family with onset after birth, highly progressive forms with leukoencephalopathy, and one Tunisian family with relative sparing of the quadriceps. Clarification of the relationship between s-IBM and h-IBM awaits discovery of a mutant gene in h-IBM.

Is It Possible to Determine Prognostic Criteria?

Age at Onset

In s-IBM, the age at onset is not predictive of major disability. There are severe cases in young patients and benign courses in some old patients. h-IBM begins in childhood or young adulthood, frequently spares the quadriceps muscles, and can involve the brain with an asymptomatic leukoencephalopathy (25). Incapacity most often occurs a decade after the onset.

Type of Disease

The forms that feature asymmetrical and multifocal atrophy usually involve slow progression (e.g., weakness affecting biceps, brachioradialis, wrist extensors, peroneal or pelvic-girdle muscles on one side). Usually such cases progress slowly, with asymmetrical and multifocal weakness and wasting (2,26–28).

Pseudopolymyositic forms have the features of chronic corticosteroid-resistant polymyositis, with dysphagia, myalgias, and weakness. The prognosis seems poor.

Pseudodegenerative forms mimic muscular dystrophies or progressive spinal atrophies. The duration of the disease before diagnosis tends to be lengthy. The progression seems slower than for the other type of the disease (2,29).

Significance of Laboratory Data

Normal erythrocyte sedimentation rates and serum creatine kinase (CK) concentrations seem to have no prognostic value, but an increased CK concentration may initially indicate a better prognosis, with the response to steroids depending on the inflammatory status of the disease. According to Barohn et al. (30), despite decreased serum CK concentrations, muscle strength declined after prednisone treatment.

CT Scan

Neuroimaging of IBM muscle may be of some use for follow-up purposes. However, there is no criterion to indicate the prognosis for the disease.

Histopathology

Barohn et al. (30) treated 8 IBM patients with steroids and performed muscle biopsies before and after treatment. Inflammation had decreased in the muscle biopsy specimens, but the number of vacuolated and amyloid-positive fibers had increased after oral prednisone treatment. They suggested that inflammatory lesions may play a secondary role and that IBM may represent a degenerative muscle disorder.

Conclusion

Prospective studies will be necessary to determine the natural history of IBM and to guide the decision whether or not to treat. Future research will be needed to develop a nontoxic, economically realistic treatment that can produce improvement or sustained long-term maintenance of strength and function.

References

1. Sekul EA, Dalakas MC. Inclusion body myositis: new concepts. *Semin Neurol* 1993, 13:256–263.
2. Eisen A, Berry K, Gibson G. Inclusion body myositis (IBM): myopathy or neuropathy? *Neurology* 1983 33:1109–1114.
3. Chou SM. Inclusion body myositis: a chronic persistent mumps myositis? *Human Pathol*, 1986, 17:765–777.
4. Danon MJ, Reyes MG, Peruena OH, et al. Inclusion body myositis. A corticosteroid-resistant idiopathic inflammatory myopathy. *Arch Neurol* 1982, 39:760–764.
5. Julien J, Vital CL, Vallat JM, Lagueny A, Sapina D. Inclusion body myositis. Clinical, biological and ultrastructural study. *J Neurol Sci* 1982, 55:15–24.
6. Ringel SP, Kenny CE, Neville HE, Giorno R, Carry MR. Spectrum of inclusion body myositis. *Arch Neurol* 1987, 44:1154–1157.
7. Sayers MA, Chou SM, Calabrese LH. Inclusion body myositis: analysis of 32 cases. *J Rheumatol* 1992, 19:1385–1389.
8. Lotz BP, Engel AG, Nishino H, et al. Inclusion body myositis: observations of 40 patients. *Brain* 1989, 112:727.
9. Levin K, Mitsumoto H, Agamanolis O. Steroid-responsiveness and clinical variability in inclusion body myositis. *Muscle Nerve* 1986, 9:217.
10. Lane RJM, Fulthorpe JJ, Hudgson P. Inclusion body myositis: a case with associated collagen vascular disease responding to treatment. *J Neurol Neurosurg Psychiatry* 1985, 48:270–273.
11. Leff RL, Miller FW, Hicks J, Fraser DD, Plotz PH. The treatment of inclusion body myositis: a retrospective review and a randomized, prospective trial of immunosuppressive therapy. *Medicine*, 1993, 72:225–235.
12. Soueidan SA, Dalakas MC. Treatment of inclusion-body myositis with high-dose intravenous immunoglobulin. *Neurology* 1993, 43:876–879.
13. Yood RA, Smith TW. Inclusion body myositis and systemic lupus erythematosus. *J Rheumatol* 1985, 12:568–570.
14. Hughes JT, Esiri MM. Ultrastructural studies in human polymyositis. *J Neurol Sci* 1975, 25:347.
15. Mikol J, Felten-Papaiconomou A, Ferchal F, et al. Inclusion body myositis: clinicopathological studies and isolation of an adenovirus type II from muscle biopsy specimen. *Ann Neurol* 1982, 11:576.
16. Dalakas MC, Dambrosia JM, Sekul EA, et al. The efficacy of high-dose intravenous immunoglobulin in patients with inclusion-body-myositis. *Neurology* 1995, 45(S):208 (abstract).
17. Amato AA, Barohn RJ, Sahenk Z, et al. Inclusion body myositis: treatment with intravenous immunoglobulin. *Neurology* 1994, 44:1516–1518.
18. Griggs RC, Askanas V, DiMauro S, Engel A, Karpati G, Mendell JR, Rowland LP. Inclusion body myositis and myopathies. *Ann Neurol* 1995, 38:705–713.
19. Argov Z, Yarom R. "Rimmed vacuole myopathy" sparing the quadriceps: a unique disorder in Iranian Jews. *J Neurol* 1984, 64:33.

20. Massa R, Weller B, Karpati G, Schoubridge E, Carpenter S. Familial inclusion body myositis among Kurdish-Iranian Jews. *Arch Neurol* 1991, 48:519–522.

21. Sadeh M, Gadoth N. Vacuolar myopathy sparing the quadriceps. *Neurology (suppl 1)* 1991, 41:275.

22. Neville HE, Baumach LL, Ringel SP, Russo LS, Sujansky E, Garcia CA. Familial inclusion body myositis: evidence for autosomal dominant inheritance. *Neurology* 1992, 42:897–902.

23. Fardeau M, Askanas V, Tomé F, et al. Hereditary neuromuscular disorder with inclusion body myositis-like filamentous inclusions: clinical, pathological and tissue culture studies. *Neurology (suppl 1)* 1990, 40:120.

24. Klingman JG, Gibbs MA, Creek W. Familial inclusion body myositis. *Neurology (suppl 1)* 1991, 41:275.

25. Hentati F, Ben Hamida C, Tomé F, et al. "Familial inclusion body myositis" sparing the quadriceps with asymptomatic leukoencephalopathy in a Tunisian kindred. *Neurology (suppl 1)* 1991, 41:422.

26. Jerusalem F, Baumgartner G, Wyler R. Virus-ähnliche Einschlüsse bei chronischen neuro-muskulären Prozessen. Elecktronenmikroskopische Biopsiebefunde von 2 Fällen. *Arch Psychiatr Nervenkr* 1972, 215:148–166.

27. Lisson G, Pongratz D, Hübner G, Wallesch C. Klinik und Morphologie der sog. "Einschlusskörpermyositis." *Fortschr Neurol Psychiat* 1980, 48:121–127.

28. Tomé FMS, Fardeau M, Lebon P, Chevallay M. Inclusion body myositis. *Acta Neuropathol*, 1981, 287–291.

29. Ketelsen UP, Beckmann R, Zimmermann H, Sauer M. Inclusion body myositis: a "slow-virus" infection of skeletal musculature? *Klin Wochen* 1977, 23:1063–1066.

30. Barohn RJ, Amato AA, Sahenk Z. Inclusion body myositis: explanation for poor response to immunosuppressive therapy. *Neurology* 1995, 45:1302–1304.

5

Uncommon Clinicopathologic Forms of Sporadic Inclusion-Body Myositis: Report of 4 Cases

MICHÈLE COQUET, OLIVIER COQUET, XAVIER FERRER, JEAN JULIEN AND CLAUDE VITAL

We have had the opportunity to study 30 cases of sporadic inclusion-body myositis (s-IBM). Most of them met the classic criteria for diagnosis the disease (3,6,15,21,27), though 4 cases had uncommon clinical or pathologic features: One case started as an isolated severe dysphagia for 5 years, another featured atypical inflammatory infiltrates and a clinical pattern mimicking distal myopathy with rimmed-vacuole formation, and 2 cases were associated with sarcoid myopathy.

Methods

Muscle biopsy specimens were obtained from the deltoid (case 1), the gastrocnemius (case 2), and the quadriceps (cases 3 and 4). In all patients, conventional techniques were used, and histochemical and ultrastructural studies were performed. In cases 2 and 4 immunocytochemistry was performed using either the peroxidase or alkaline phosphatase system with diaminobenzidine or new fuschin as substrate.

Case Reports

Case 1

A 72-year-old man was referred to the hospital for severe dysphagia with significant weight loss. He also suffered from myocardial ischemia and temporal arteritis. Esophagoscopy revealed cricopharyngeal dysfunction, but no tumor. Neurologic examination and electromyographic (EMG) findings were normal. Three years later, limb weakness and gait difficulty appeared. A diagnosis of polymyositis was then made at muscle biopsy. Steroid treatment was begun, but the patient did not improve. At age 78 he could be fed only by gastric tube. A second biopsy performed on the right deltoid revealed the usual IBM lesions: angulated fibers, rimmed vacuoles, and lymphocyte infiltrates surrounding non-necrotic fibers. Electron microscopy showed filaments 16–18 nm in diameter in the cytoplasm (Figure 5.1). The patient died 6 months later from cardiac infarction.

Case 2

A 20-year-old woman without family antecedents complained of a 2-year history of progressive leg weakness with bilateral foot-drop. The first symptom was peroneal atrophy, and gastrocnemius-muscle atrophy developed later. Slight bilateral atrophy and weakness were noted in the finger muscles. The serum creatine kinase concentration was 450 U/L, and EMG study disclosed a myopathic pattern.

Muscle biopsy showed a vacuolar myopathy with inflammatory exudates. In cryostat sections, clusters of atrophic angulated fibers with numerous rimmed vacuoles were observed (Figure 5.2). Immunocytochemical studies showed clusters of B lymphocytes (Figure 5.3) near the vessels, often surrounded by T lymphocytes. CD4+ cells (Becton) were more numerous (Figure 5.4, following page 104) than CD8+ cells (Becton) (Figure 5.5, following page 104). The margins of the rimmed vacuoles reacted with dystrophin antibody (Novocastra); ubiquitin (Sigma)

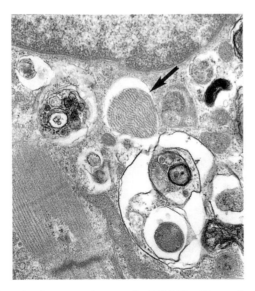

Figure 5.1. Case 1, electron micrograph: IBM-like filaments (arrow) near a nucleus and membranous debris (×15,000).

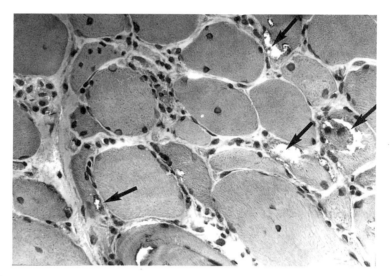

Figure 5.2. Case 2, frozen section, H&E stain: Angulated fibers, fibers with rimmed vacuoles (arrows), and inflammatory infiltrates are observed (×350).

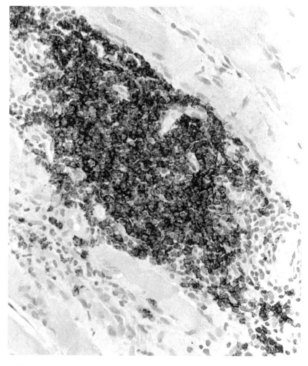

Figure 5.3. Case 2, immunocytochemical stain L26: Numerous B lymphocytes are seen around vessels.

was positive in the vacuoles, and β-amyloid protein (Dako) and τ protein (Dako) were negative. HLA class I (Immunotech) was not clearly expressed. Semithin sections showed numerous rimmed vacuoles, often located at the periphery of the fibers. By electron microscopy, collections of tubular filaments about 18 nm in diameter (Figure 5.6), partly membrane-bound, were sometimes observed near membranous whorls. No filaments were found in the nuclei. Mitochondrial abnormalities were not observed.

The patient was treated with steroids, but showed no improvement. Three years later, her condition had worsened considerably, and walking was increasingly difficult.

Cases 3 and 4

In these two cases the clinical features were similar. Both were women, ages 64 and 63. They had complained of walking difficulties for several years. Quadriceps atrophy followed later in both. EMG showed both myopathic and neurogenic changes. The first patient also had a Sjögren syndrome. The second patient died 1 year later of cardiac infarction. In

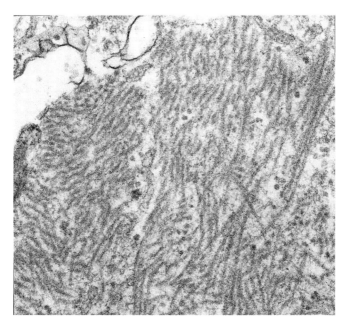

Figure 5.6. Case 2, electron micrograph: Twisted filaments in cytoplasm of a muscle fiber (×45,000).

both cases, despite cutaneous anergy for tuberculin, no systemic sarcoidosis could be found.

Muscle biopsies showed, in both cases, atrophic angulated fibers, rimmed vacuoles, and non-necrotic fibers surrounded or infiltrated by T lymphocytes. In case 4, CD8+ cells were numerous around non-necrotic cells. By ultrastructural study, filaments 16 to 18 nm in diameter were observed both in the cytoplasm and in nuclei (Figures 5.7 and 5.8). Furthermore, in both cases there were several circumscribed granulomatous nodules without necrosis that were composed of histiocytes, epithelioid cells, and lymphocytes (Figure 5.9). In case 4, Langhans giant cells (Figure 5.10), sometimes with asteroid bodies, were observed and were CD68 (Dako). Numerous granulomas were observed on semithin sections. Ultrastructural study showed epithelioid cells and giant cells (Figure 5.11), as already reported in sarcoidosis (19,30).

Discussion

Dysphagia in patients with s-IBM has been reported in several series. Lotz et al. (18) reported that 30–40% of patients complained of varying degrees of dysphagia. Cases with involvement of cricopharyngeal muscle and severe dysphagia were reported by Danon and Friedman (8) and

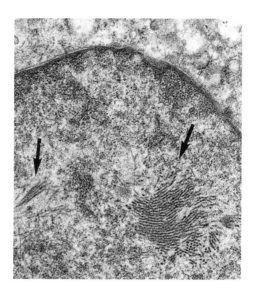

Figure 5.7.   Case 3, electron micrograph: Filaments 16–18 nm in diameter within a myonucleus (×15,000).

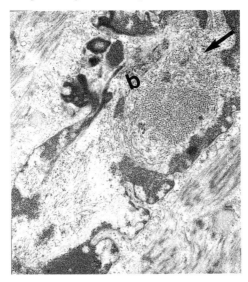

Figure 5.8. Case 4, electron micrograph: Transverse section of filaments about 16 nm in diameter within a degenerate myonucleus (×7,500).

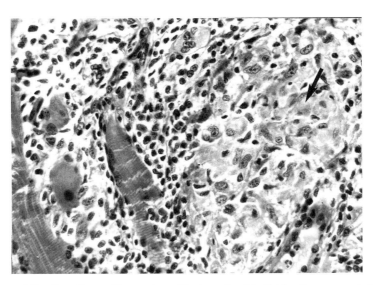

Figure 5.9. Case 3, paraffin section: Cluster of epithelioid cells surrounded by lymphocytes is seen near fragments of muscle fibers (×350).

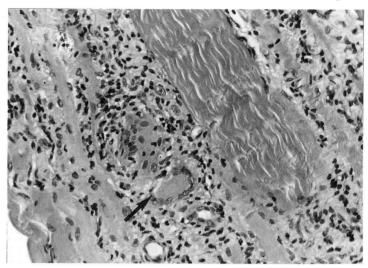

Figure 5.10. Case 4, paraffin section: Inflammatory infiltrate with a Langhans-type giant cell (arrow) in endomysium (×350).

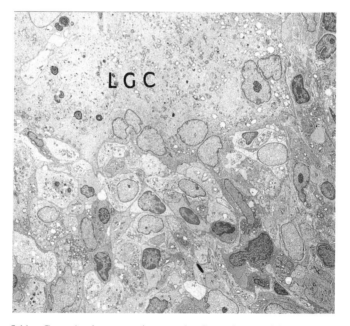

Figure 5.11. Case 4, electron micrograph: Granuloma with a Langhans-type giant cell (LGC) (×1,050).

Verma et al. (29). However, IBM presenting solely with dysphagia, as in our case 1, is rare; only 3 cases were reported by Wintzen et al. (31), and 2 by Riminton et al. (26). The interval between dysphagia and limb weakness can be as long as 7 years, as in one the cases reported by Wintzen et al. (31). Cricopharyngeal muscle biopsy performed in 3 cases (26,29) showed the typical changes of s-IBM. Dysphagia should always be considered in the presence of an isolated dysphagia. Patients treated with cricopharyngeal myotomy (26,29) showed marked improvement.

In s-IBM the cell infiltrates are composed mainly of CD8+ cytotoxic T cells (1,14,16), whereas B lymphocytes are rare (10,11). In our case 2, CD4+ cells were more numerous than CD8+ cells, and there were numerous B lymphocytes around vessels, as in dermatomyositis. The association with dermatomyositis is improbable, because there was no cutaneous rash nor any tubuloreticular inclusions in the endothelial cells, and there was no response to steroid treatment. This case also illustrates the possible linkage between s-IBM and distal myopathy with rimmed-vacuole formation (DMRV). This myopathy was described by Nonaka et al. (23) in 1981. It is characterized by female predominance and autosomal-recessive inheritance, but sporadic cases have been reported. The initial and preferential peroneal-muscle involvement appears in the second or third decade of life (22,24). The disease leads progressively to a non-ambulant state within 10 years after onset. Muscle biopsy shows myopathic changes and rimmed vacuoles, and filaments 16–18 nm in diameter in the cytoplasm and sometimes in the nuclei are revealed by electron microscopy. Inflammatory exudates are always absent. Our case is clinically and pathologically similar to DMRV, except for the presence of inflammatory exudates; therefore our case resembles both s-IBM and DMRV. Two hypotheses can be suggested: s-IBM and DMRV may be different forms of the same entity (so that our case could be an intermediate form); s-IBM and DMRV may be two distinct entities (so that our case could be considered an atypical form of s-IBM).

The association of s-IBM and sarcoidosis has rarely been reported. Carpenter and Karpati (2) and Mhiri and Gherardi (20) described typical s-IBM occurring in patients with systemic sarcoidosis without sarcoid myopathy. Nevertheless, muscle sarcoidosis could exist without the presence of granulomatous lesions in the biopsy specimen, as they are irregularly distributed within the muscle. It appears that the first report of IBM with muscle sarcoidosis came in 1980 from Matsubara (19), who described intranuclear IBM-like inclusions in 2 cases of sarcoidosis with granulomatous myopathy and changes similar to those of polymyositis.

Since then, only the case reported by Danon et al. (7) has shown, at autopsy, the association of the two typical lesions in the muscle, as in our cases 3 and 4. The question arises whether or not the sarcoidosis is confined solely to the skeletal muscles. In a series of 25 cases of muscular granulomatous sarcoidosis, Vital et al. (30) observed 13 cases in which the sarcoidosis was present only in the muscle. Those authors assumed that in the course of sarcoidosis, muscle involvement might precede the other localizations. In addition, there have been cases in which autopsy, performed in patients with apparently isolated muscle sarcoidosis, has shown sarcoid involvement of other organs (5,9,12). The patient in our case 3 also suffered from Sjögren syndrome. Association of s-IBM with this immunologic disorder has already been reported (4,13).

These 4 cases of uncommon clinicopathologic forms of s-IBM raise the question of the nosologic status of s-IBM. Our review points toward it being either an autoimmune disease or an authentic dystrophy with inflammatory reaction, as suggested by Pellissier et al. (25).

Acknowledgments

We would like to thank Dr. D. Henin for kindly reviewing the manuscript, R. Cooke for linguistic help, Miss Naya, Miss Nehaye, Mrs. Coadou, Mrs. Herfaut, and Mrs. Raso for their technical assistance, and Mr. Castaniera for his photographic expertise.

References

1. Askanas V, Engel WK. New advances in inclusion body myositis. *Curr Opin Rheumatol* 1993, 5:732–741.
2. Carpenter S, Karpati G. Inflammatory myopathies. In *Pathology of Skeletal Muscle*, Carpenter S, Karpati G(eds). New York, Churchill-Livingstone, 1984, p. 567.
3. Carpenter S, Karpati G. The pathological diagnosis of specific inflammatory myopathies. *Brain Pathol* 1992, 2:13–19.
4. Chad D, Good P, Adelman L, Bradley WG, Mills J. Inclusion body myositis associated with Sjögren's syndrome. *Arch Neurol* 1982, 39:186–188.
5. Crompton MR, McDermot V. Sarcoidosis associated with progressive muscular wasting and weakness. *Brain* 1961, 84:62–74.
6. Dalakas MC. Polymyositis, dermatomyositis and inclusion-body myositis. *N Engl J Med* 1991, 325:1487–1498.
7. Danon MJ, Perurena OH, Ronan S, Manaligod JR. Inclusion body myositis associated with systemic sarcoidosis. *Can J Neurol Sci* 1986, 13:334–336.
8. Danon MJ, Friedman M. Inclusion body myositis associated with progressive dysphagia. Treatment with cricopharyngeal myotomy. *Can J Neurol Sci* 1989, 16:436–438.

9. Douglas AC, McLeod JG, Matthews JD. Symptomatic sarcoidosis of skeletal muscle. *J Neurol Neurosurg Psychiatry* 1973, 36:1034–1040.
10. Engel AG, Arahata K. Monoclonal antibody analysis of mononuclear cells in myopathies: II. Phenotypes of autoinvasive cells in polymyositis and inclusion body myositis. *Ann Neurol* 1984, 16:209–215.
11. Figarella-Branger D, Pellissier JF, Bianco N, DeVictor B, Toga M. Inflammatory and non-inflammatory inclusion body myositis. Characterization of the mononuclear cells and expression of the immunoreactive class I major histocompatibility complex product. *Acta Neuropathol* 1990, 79:528–536.
12. Gardner-Thorpe L. Muscle weakness due to sarcoid myopathy (six case reports and an evaluation of steroid therapy). *Neurology* 1972, 22:917–928.
13. Gutmann L, Govindan S, Riggs JE, Schochet S. Inclusion body myositis and Sjögren's syndrome. *Arch Neurol* 1985, 42:1021–1022.
14. Hohlfeld R, Engel AG. Coculture with autologous myotubes of cytotoxic T cells isolated from muscle in inflammatory myopathies. *Ann Neurol* 1984, 4:809–816.
15. Julien J, Vital C, Vallat JM, Lagueny A, Sapina D. Inclusion body myositis: clinical, biological and ultrastructural study. *J Neurol Sci* 1982, 55:2415–2416.
16. Kalovidouris AE. Immune aspects of myositis. *Curr Opin Rheumatol* 1992, 4:809–814.
17. Khraishi MM, Jay V, Keystone EC. Inclusion body myositis in association with vitamin B_{12} deficiency and Sjögren's syndrome. *J Rheumatol* 1992, 19:306–309.
18. Lotz BP, Engel AG, Nishino H, Stevens JC, Litchy WJ. Inclusion body myositis: observation in 40 patients. *Brain* 1989, 112:427–447.
19. Matsubara S. Ultrastructural changes in granulomatous myopathy. *Acta Neuropathol* 1980, 50:91–96.
20. Mhiri C, Gherardi R. Inclusion body myositis in French patients. A clinicopathological evaluation. *Neuropathol Appl Neurobiol* 1990, 16:333–344.
21. Mikol J, Engel AG. Inclusion body myositis. In *Myology*, Engel AG, Franzini-Armstrong C (eds). New York, McGraw-Hill, 1994, pp. 1384–1398.
22. Murakami N, Ihara Y, Nonaka I. Muscle fiber degeneration in distal myopathy with rimmed vacuole formation. *Acta Neuropathol* 1995, 89:29–34.
23. Nonaka I, Sunohara N, Ishiura S, Satoyoshi E. Familial distal myopathy with rimmed vacuole and lamellar (myeloid) body formation. *J Neurol Sci* 1981, 51:141–155.
24. Nonaka I, Sunohara N, Satoyoshi E, Terasawa K, Yonemoto K. Autosomal recessive distal muscular dystrophy: a comparative study with distal myopathy with rimmed vacuole formation. *Ann Neurol* 1985, 17:51–59.
25. Pellissier JF, Figarella-Branger D, Pouget J, Serratrice G. Myosite à inclusions et maladies neuromusculaires à vacuoles bordées. In *Nervous System, Muscles and Systemic Diseases*, Serratrice G (ed). Paris, Expansion Scientifique Française, 1993, pp. 99–108.
26. Riminton DS, Chambers ST, Parkin PJ, Pollock M, Donalson IM. Inclusion body myositis presenting solely as dysphagia. *Neurology* 1993, 43:1241–1243.

27. Serratrice G, Pellissier JF, Pouget J, Figarella-Branger D. Formes cliniques des myosites à inclusions: 12 cas. *Rev Neurol (Paris)* 1989, 145:781–788.
28. Sunohara N, Nonaka I, Kamei N, Satoyoshi E. Distal myopathy with rimmed vacuole formation. A follow-up study. *Brain* 1989, 112:65–83.
29. Verma A, Bradley WG, Adesina AM, Sofferman R, Pendlebury WW. Inclusion body myositis with cricopharyngeus muscle involvement and severe dysphagia. *Muscle Nerve* 1991, 14:470–473.
30. Vital C, Vallat JM, Gruyer G, Coquet M, Rivel J. Etude anatomoclinique de 25 cas de sarcoidose musculaire. Examen ultra structural de 2 biopsies. *Arch Anat Cytol Path* 1980, 28:214–221.
31. Wintzen AR, Bots GTAM, de Bakker HM, Hulshof JH, Padberg GW. Dysphagia in inclusion body myositis. *J Neurol Neurosurg Psychiatry* 1988, 51:1542–1545.

6

Inclusion-Body Myositis: Pathologic Changes

DOMINIQUE FIGARELLA-BRANGER, ALEX
BAETA-MACHADO, GIOVANNI PUTZU, AND
JEAN FRANÇOIS PELLISSIER

Inclusion-body myositis (IBM) is a term coined (1) to describe a form of myopathy that clinically resembles chronic polymyositis and pathologically is characterized by the presence of inflammatory exudates and vacuoles containing eosinophilic inclusions and 16–18-nm tubulofilamentous inclusions, as first reported by Chou (2).

At the beginning of the IBM story, these inclusions were thought to be specific, and efforts have been made to characterize them. Their exact nature has not yet been determined, however, and their specificity seems questionable, because they also occur in other conditions, namely, familial IBM and neuromuscular disorders associated with rimmed vacuoles and tubulofilamentous inclusions. The latter group includes various neuromuscular disorders. In some of them, those that are well-defined sporadic or genetically linked diseases, rimmed vacuoles are not consistently observed, whereas in others, rimmed vacuoles containing tubulofilamentous inclusions constitute one of the most salient pathologic features (Table 6.1).

Inflammation usually does not occur, either in familial IBM [although it has been observed in the cases of two families (3,4)] or in the various neuromuscular disorders associated with rimmed vacuoles.

Thus far, more than 240 sporadic cases of IBM have been cited in the literature (review: 5). The clinical picture of sporadic IBM is heterogeneous, and three main clinical features have been observed (6): (i) asymmetrical muscle involvement, (ii) a polymyositis-like syndrome unresponsive to corticosteroid treatment, and (iii) forms mimicking chronic spinal muscular atrophy. The diagnosis has always been based on the characteristic muscle biopsy findings.

In addition, up to 60 cases of so-called familial IBM have been reported. Whether these cases should be called familial IBM or inclusion-body myopathies is a matter of some debate. These patients always have

Table 6.1. *Heterogeneous group of neuromuscular disorders in which rimmed vacuoles and tubulofilamentous inclusions occur*

I. Diseases characterized by numerous rimmed vacuoles:
  A. Distal myopathies with rimmed vacuoles: familial IBM or inclusion-body myopathies?
     Japanese type (autosomal-recessive)
     Welander type (autosomal-dominant)
  B. Oculopharyngeal muscular dystrophy (OPMD)

II. Diseases occasionally associated with rimmed vacuoles:
  A. Genetically linked muscle diseases
     Desminopathy
     Glycogenosis (adult type II, type III, and McArdle disease)
     Ceroid lipofuscinosis
     Facioscapulohumeral myopathy with rimmed vacuoles
     Steinert disease
     Adrenoleukodystrophy
  B. Sporadic neuromuscular disorders
     Distal myopathy with rimmed vacuoles
     Limb-girdle myopathy
     Chronic denervation syndromes (ALS, chronic spinal muscular atrophy, post-poliomyelitis syndrome, paraneoplastic neuropathy)

distal involvement. This term includes the familial "rimmed-vacuole myopathy" that spares the quadriceps, as first described by Argov and Yarom (7) in 1984, which has now been reported in 9 families (8,9). In these patients of Iranian Jewish origin, the disease begins in childhood or in early adulthood and progresses slowly, involving many limb and axial muscles, but sparing the quadriceps. Familial IBM not sparing the quadriceps has been reported in 5 families of various origins (10–12,34). Here again, the disease can have a juvenile or adult onset. It is associated in some families with a leukoencephalopathy (4,10).

Taken as a whole, these findings show that the tubulofilamentous inclusions are not specific to IBM and raise a question about the nosology of IBM: Is IBM an inflammatory myopathy, or a muscle dystrophy with occasional inflammatory exudates? Are sporadic IBM and familial IBM the same, or distinct entities? Nowadays, IBM can be defined as a particular neuromuscular disorder that is unresponsive to corticosteroid treatment and is characterized by a constellation of clinical, morphologic, and electromyographic features, none of which is specific to IBM.

In this chapter we propose to describe the morphologic hallmarks of IBM, to discuss their potential utility as diagnostic tools, and, when possible, to assess their contribution the pathogenesis of IBM. The morphologic hallmarks of IBM (sporadic and familial) are as follows:

Rimmed (lined) vacuoles
Endomysial inflammatory exudates (present only in sporadic IBM)
Small groups of round or angulated atrophic fibers
Eosinophilic cytoplasmic inclusions
Small amyloid deposits within or near vacuoles and within nuclei
Abnormal nuclear and cytoplasmic filaments 16–18 nm in diameter
Nuclear-membrane abnormalities and nuclear breakdown
Other findings (necrotic regenerative fibers, fibrosis, and ragged red fibers)

Rimmed Vacuoles

Vacuoles rimmed with basophilic material have been observed in IBM muscle fibers. The number of fibers showing rimmed vacuoles varies from one case to another, but at least 1% of fibers with rimmed vacuoles is a quite common finding (13). The sizes and shapes of the rimmed vacuoles are quite variable (Figure 6.1A).

These vacuoles contain lysosomal markers such as cathepsin B and D (14), and some are strongly reactive with acid phosphatase (Figure 6.1E). Under electron microscopy, myelinated bodies can be observed. These cytoplasmic degradation products correspond to the vacuoles observed under light microscopy (Figure 6.1B-E). The vacuoles are assumed to be autophagic, but many are not completely surrounded by membrane (Figure 6.1F).

The presence of rimmed vacuoles is an absolute requisite for the diagnosis of IBM. These vacuoles are not specific, however, and can be associated with various neuromuscular disorders (Table 6.1). On the other hand, the occurrence of rimmed vacuoles in the context of an inflammatory myopathy is highly suggestive of IBM, although IBM can be associated with systemic autoimmune or connective-tissue diseases in up to 20% of the patients (15).

Endomysial Inflammatory Exudates

Slight to conspicuous endomysial inflammation is almost consistently observed in sporadic IBM, although it is usually absent from familial IBM and inclusion-body myopathies (Figure 6.2A,B).

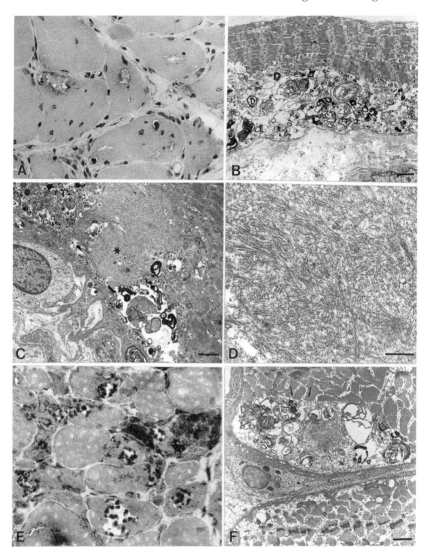

Figure 6.1. A: Rimmed vacuoles of various sizes in muscle fibers (hematoxylin and eosin, ×315). B and C: Ultrastructural feature of a rimmed vacuole: accumulation of membranous structures, myeloid bodies, and tubulofilamentous inclusions (*) (bar = 2 mm). D: Intracytoplasmic filaments at higher magnification. Filaments are oriented in different directions, and some may each contain a central lumen (bar = 500 mm). E: Rimmed vacuoles strongly stained by acid phosphatase (×195). F: Rimmed vacuole partially surrounded by membrane (arrow)(bar = 1 mm).

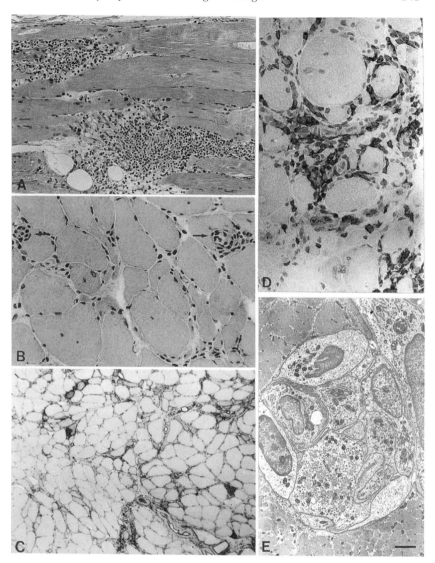

Figure 6.2. Endomysial inflammatory exudates. Profuse (A) and scarce (B) endomysial inflammation in sporadic IBM. Note the partial invasion (arrow) (A, ×145; B, ×315; hematoxylin and eosin). C: Fibers, usually located near inflammatory exudates, express MHC class I antigen on their surface membranes (×80). D: Inflammatory cells are mainly cytotoxic CD8+ lymphocytes (×195). E: Ultrastructural feature of partial invasion (bar = 1 mm).

As occurs in polymyositis, mononuclear cells surround and partly invade non-necrotic muscle fibers (partial invasion, Figure 6.2E). The cells are rather cytotoxic CD8+ cells and macrophages (Figure 6.2D). B cells and natural-killer cells are mainly absent (16,17). Near CD8+ cells, muscle fibers abnormally express class I antigens of the major histocompatibility complex (MHC) (18,19) (Figure 6.2C).

The inflammatory cells in IBM are activated, because they express MHC class I and II antigens and ICAM-1. ICAM-1 is also expressed on the surfaces of non-necrotic muscle fibers invaded by autoaggressive cells and serves as a ligand for these cells (15,20). These findings strongly suggest that an antigen-directed cytotoxicity mediated by cytotoxic T cells occurs in IBM. Unlike what occurs in patients with polymyositis, however, IBM patients are unresponsive to corticosteroid treatment. If inflammation plays a pathogenic role in IBM, it is therefore not the only factor involved. In our opinion, inflammation must be present for the diagnosis of sporadic IBM to be made.

Small Groups of Round or Angulated Atrophic Fibers

Groups of atrophic fibers are always observed in IBM. This typical feature was first described by Eisen et al. (21) and then by Lotz et al. (13), who observed it in 96% of the IBM cases investigated. The atrophic fibers are of both types. They are strongly stained when treated with NADH diaphorase. The mechanism underlying the formation of small groups of atrophic fibers in IBM has not yet been elucidated. At least four hypotheses can be put forward: These groups may consist of split fibers, such as those observed after necrosis and regeneration, but necrotic fibers are scarce in familial IBM (whereas numerous angulated fibers are common). The fibers may be apoptotic or denervated fibers. Lastly, the fibers may be atrophic, as a result of nuclear damage.

Although the electron-microscopic features have rarely included any of the typical apoptotic changes, some muscle fibers in IBM have been found to express the oncoprotein Bcl-2, which is an inhibitor of apoptosis (22) (Figure 6.3D). Bcl-2 expression by some atrophic fibers may be an attempt to escape programmed cell death. Less than 5% of the atrophic fibers express Bcl-2, but, interestingly, muscle fibers do not express Bcl-2 in any of the other idiopathic inflammatory myopathies.

On the other hand, the atrophic fibers may in fact be denervated fibers. The NCAM expression on the cell-surface membrane, together with the lack of polysialylated NCAM (Figure 6.3A,B) expression, argues in favor

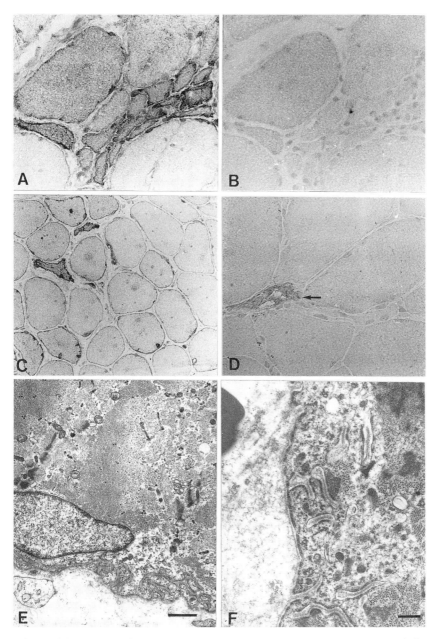

Figure 6.3. Denervation and apoptosis in IBM. Strong NCAM expression (A),
but lack of polysialylated NCAM expression (B), in atrophic fibers (×315). C:
Fibers with sub-sarcolemmal rimmed vacuoles also express NCAM (×195). D:
Atrophic fiber expressing Bcl-2 oncoprotein (arrow) (×195). E and F: Denervated endplates demonstrated by electron microscopy (E, bar = 1 mm; F, bar =
500 nm).

of this hypothesis (23). In addition, type grouping has sometimes been observed in IBM [3 of 21 patients in our series, 3 of 48 patients in the series of Lotz et al. (13)], and we detected some denervated endplates in 3 patients under electron microscopy (Figure 6.3E,F). These findings, together with the frequent occurrences of mixed EMG potentials, suggest that neurogenic impairment may occur in IBM. In addition, peripheral neuropathy has been reported by some authors to be associated with IBM (24,25). Not only atrophic fibers but also vacuolated fibers strongly express NCAM throughout their cell membranes (Figure 6.3C), as previously described (8,23).

Lastly, muscle fibers may become atrophic in IBM because they gradually lose their myonuclei (26). It is likely that a combination of these mechanisms may occur in IBM.

Although they are less numerous, small atrophic fibers can also be observed in various neuromuscular disorders characterized by rimmed vacuoles. Here again, the pathogenesis remains to be elucidated.

Eosinophilic Inclusions

Eosinophilic inclusions were always observed in our series of patients, but they were present in only 58.3% of the series investigated by Lotz et al. (13). The inclusions are located in the cytoplasm, usually in the vicinity of vacuoles. Eosinophilic inclusions should not be confused with cytoplasmic bodies, which are frequently observed in IBM. Eosinophilic inclusions are composed of abnormal filaments. They can also be encountered in the various neuromuscular disorders in which rimmed vacuoles occurs, where they are less numerous, however. In some IBM muscles, large nuclei containing homogeneous eosinophilic or amphophilic material can be observed (1,27; D. Figarella-Branger et al., unpublished data).

Small Amyloid Deposits within or near Vacuoles and within Nuclei

In 1991, Mendell et al. (28) established that the inclusions typical of IBM, or some of the materials associated with these inclusions, have a congophilic green birefringent appearance in polarized light and are therefore indicative of amyloidosis (Figure 6.4A,B,D,E). We have observed very few congophilic green birefringent inclusions in our IBM muscle biopsies, however. This is probably because true amyloid fibrils (measuring 7–10 nm in diameter) are rarely located near IBM filaments, on the basis of the electron-microscopic findings (Figure 6.4G,H). Interestingly, as re-

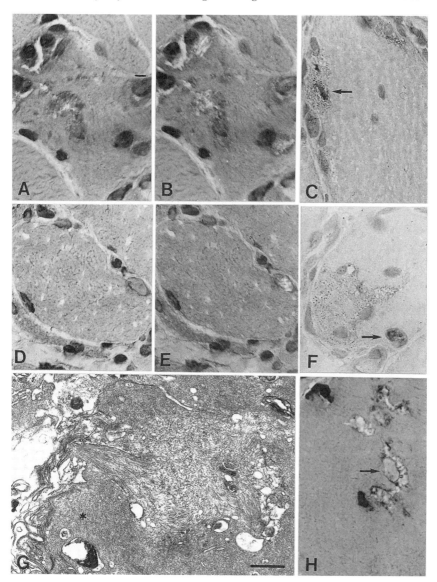

Figure 6.4.   Amyloid deposits. Congophilic (A and D) and green birefringent (B and E) intracytoplasmic (A and B) and intranuclear (D and E) amyloid deposits (all, ×500). Rimmed vacuole (C) and nucleus (F, arrow) strongly stained with anti-ubiquitin antibody (both, ×315). G: True amyloid fibrils (*) located near IBM filaments (bar = 1 mm). H: Only some rimmed vacuoles contain congophilic deposits (arrow) (Congo red, ×700).

ported by Askanas et al. (29), congophilia is easiest to detect by examining sections stained with Congo red under fluorescence illumination using fluorescein isothiocyanate (TITC) or Texas-red filters. (However, because it is not possible with that technique to explore the β-sheet configuration of the deposits, which shows up only after exposure to polarized light, it cannot be definitely stated whether or not the fluorescent deposits are actually due to amyloidosis.)

The cytoplasmic and nuclear inclusions immunoreact with ubiquitin (30–33) (Figure 6.4C-F). In addition, in studies performed mainly by V. Askanas and co-workers, β-amyloid protein (Aβ), β-amyloid precursor protein (βAPP), τ protein, abnormally phosphorylated τ (Alz-50), prion, and apolipoprotein E (ApoE) immunoreactivities were detected in IBM (14,30–40) (Table 6.2). In addition, Sarkozi et al. (35) reported that the expression of βAPP mRNA was increased in IBM. Suprisingly, in attempting to assess, using a cDNA probe, whether or not IBM was asso-

Table 6.2. *Amyloid and amyloid-related proteins in IBM and inclusion-body myopathies*

Protein	IBM	Neuromuscular disorders with rimmed vacuoles
Ubiquitin	Askanas et al. (30), Albrecht and Bilbao (31), Leclerc et al. (32), Pellissier et al. (33)	Villanova et al. (14),[a] Leclerc et al. (32),[a] Pellissier et al. (33),[b] Murakami et al. (40)[c]
βAPP	Askanas et al. (34), Sarkozi et al. (35), Villanova et al. (14), Pellissier et al. (33)	Pellissier et al. (33), Murakami et al. (40)
Aβ	Askanas et al. (36), Villanova et al. (14), Leclerc et al. (32)	Murakami et al. (40)
τ protein and Alz-50	Pellissier et al. (33), Askanas et al. (37)	Pellissier et al. (33), Murakami et al. (40)
Prion protein	Askanas et al. (38)	
ApoE	Askanas et al. (39)	

Notes: βAPP, β-amyloid precursor protein; Aβ, β-amyloid protein; Alz-50, abnormally phosphorylated τ protein; ApoE, apolipoprotein E.
[a] Results from patients with oculopharyngeal muscular dystrophy (OPMD).
[b][c] Japanese autosomal-recessive distal myopathy with rimmed-vacuole formation.
[b] OPMD, types II and III glycogenosis, and McArdle disease, also observed in desmin myopathy (D. Figarella-Branger et al., unpublished data).

ciated with an increase in βAPP mRNA, Nalbantoglu et al. (41) noted a conspicuous accumulation of a single-strand-DNA-binding protein in skeletal-muscle fibers.

The DNA-binding protein involved in IBM has not yet been identified. Because the most common nuclear protein that binds single-strand DNA is replicating protein A (RP-A), a multi-subunit chromosomal protein with 70-, 34,- and 13-kDa polypeptides, we searched for an increase in RP-A expression in IBM using a monoclonal antibody directed against the 34-kDa subunit (generously provided by J. Hurwitz, New York). We observed that a diffuse increase in RP-A expression occurred in IBM myonuclei. Occasionally, accumulation in some cytoplasmic inclusions is seen (Figure 6.5E). However, because the pattern of expression was different from that of the single-strand-DNA-binding protein, RP-A may not have been responsible for the binding (42).

In IBM we have observed anti-βAPP immunoreactivity, τ immunoreactivity, a high level of abnormally phosphorylated τ immunoreactivity (Figure 6.5A-D). Aβ immunoreactivity was observed only in muscle from one IBM patient and one OPMD patient (33). The discrepancies between the levels of Aβ expression are difficult to explain. Besides, it should be noted that none of the findings described are unique or specific to IBM. Amyloid deposits also occur in OPMD, in distal myopathies with rimmed vacuoles, and occasionally in acid maltase deficiency, limb-girdle dystrophy, and Becker dystrophy (14,43). Ubiquitin deposits and βAPP occur in OPMD. We have observed amyloid deposits, βAPP, ubiquitin, τ, and abnormally phosphorylated τ in cases of OPMD, muscle glycogenosis, and desmin myopathy (Table 6.2).

Whether the ectopic expression of these multiple proteins in muscle actually plays a role in the pathogenesis of IBM and neuromuscular disorders in which rimmed vacuoles occur or whether, on the contrary, the ectopic expression results from the formation of rimmed vacuoles is still an open question.

Abnormal Nuclear and Cytoplasmic Filaments 16–18 nm in Diameter

Abnormal filaments such as those first described by Chou (2) can be seen in some of the muscle fibers in all IBM biopsy specimens. They have been extensively studied (review: 5). Briefly, using conventional electron-microscopic techniques (after glutaraldehyde fixation and resin embedding), they have a tubulo-filamentous appearance and measure 16–20 mm in diameter (Figure 6.1A-C). They are composed of ubiquitinated

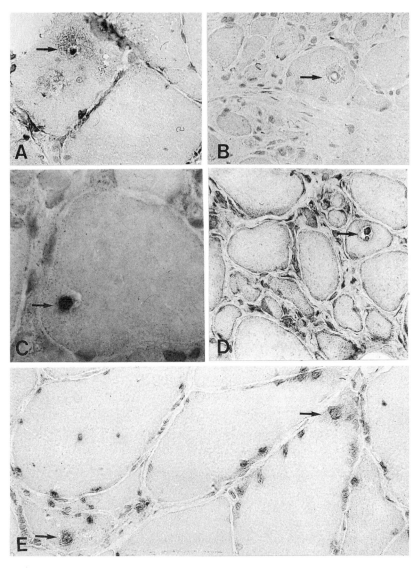

Figure 6.5.   Abnormal protein accumulation. βAPP accumulation in cytoplasmic inclusions (A, arrow), but lack of Aβ accumulation in some (B, arrow); τ (C) and abnormally phosphorylated τ (D) in cytoplasmic inclusions. E: RP-A 34-kDa accumulation in nuclei and in some inclusions (arrows) (all, $\times$315).

material, as shown by immuno-electron microscopy (30), but their exact composition is not yet known. They are located within the cytoplasm, usually in the vicinity of autophagic vacuoles, but sometimes also within nuclei, although the intranuclear filaments can be difficult to detect. Abnormal intranuclear filaments have been detected in only about 40% of all the cases studied, but abnormal intracytoplasmic filaments in 100%. These filaments are not specific to IBM, because they have been reported to occur in a large number of inclusion-body myopathies (Table 6.1). The occurrence of intranuclear filaments in the latter group of diseases appears to be extremely rare, however (44–46).

Nuclear-Membrane Abnormalities and Nuclear Breakdown

Enlarged nuclei filled with eosinophilic or amphophilic material that pushes the chromatin material up against the nuclear envelope have been observed under conventional microscopy in some cases of IBM. However, the number of abnormal nuclei turns out to be much higher at electron-microscopic examination. Nuclei can be filled by abnormal filaments, and in some cases the nuclear envelope is perforated, with filaments extruding into the adjacent cytoplasm (Figure 6.6F). The nuclear membrane can be abnormal and is sometimes absent (Figure 6.6E). In many nuclei the nuclear matrix is abnormally highly condensed (Figure 6.6D). These features appear to be highly characteristic of IBM, and so far as we know they have not been reported in any of the various neuromuscular disorders involving rimmed vacuoles. The contribution of myonuclei to the pathogenesis of IBM will be discussed later in this volume.

Other Findings

Various degenerative phenomena, such as necrosis and regenerative fibers, have been observed in IBM, but of course they are not specific to the disease. One interesting observation is that mitochondrial abnormalities are frequently encountered in IBM. Ragged red fibers have often been noted in IBM muscles, and numerous cytochrome-c-oxidase-negative fibers have been observed. One frequent electron-microscopic feature is an accumulation of mitochondria showing a high matrix density and numerous paracrystalline inclusions. Moreover, deficiencies in various complexes of the respiratory chain, as well as mitochondrial-DNA deletions, have been reported to occur in IBM (47). The exact reason for

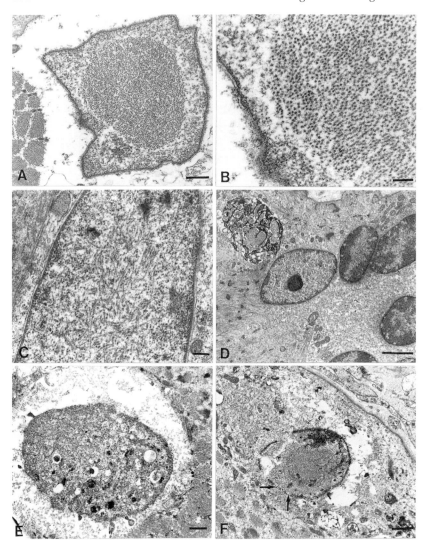

Figure 6.6. Nuclear abnormalities. Accumulation of tubulofilamentous inclusions in nuclei (A, bar = 500 nm; B and C, bar = 200 nm). Abnormal condensation of nuclear matrix in some nuclei (D) and lack of nuclear membrane (E). F:
Perforation of the nuclear envelope and extrusion of filaments in adjacent cytoplasm (arrows)(bar = 1 mm).

the mitochondrial abnormalities in IBM has not been determined, but they may be due to a combination of some or all of the following mechanisms: Various conditions such as viruses, aging, and inflammation are known to generate mitochondrial abnormalities (48). Aging and inflammation are features commonly associated with sporadic IBM. Interestingly, mitochondrial abnormalities are less numerous in familial IBM occurring in younger patients, whose muscle biopsy specimens are devoid of inflammation. Besides, the mitochondrial changes occurring in IBM are highly suggestive of nuclear DNA abnormalities. It is likely, although not yet proven, that the various nuclear abnormalities occurring in IBM may alter some of the nuclear genes involved in mitochondrial functions.

Conclusions and Unanswered Questions

As we have seen, IBM is characterized by several hallmarks, but none of them is specific to the disease. In our opinion, sporadic IBM can definitely be diagnosed if the clinical history and electromyographic data point in this direction and if the muscle biopsies show rimmed vacuoles, tubulofilamentous inclusions with or without amyloidosis, and endomysial inflammatory exudates. If inflammatory exudates are lacking, IBM may be responsible, but some neuromuscular disorders can also lead to rimmed vacuoles and tubulofilamentous inclusions.

It is questionable, however, that inflammatory exudates constitute a suitable criterion on which to base the diagnosis of a disease in which the pathogenic role of inflammation is unknown and the patients are unresponsive to corticosteroid treatment. Moreover, if familial IBM and sporadic IBM are really the same entity, it is difficult to understand why inflammation is always lacking in the familial cases.

As mentioned earlier, the tubulofilamentous inclusions always observed in both cytoplasm and nuclei in cases of IBM are not characteristic of IBM. The exact nature of the tubulofilamentous inclusions in unknown. They are composed of ubiquitinated material and may be associated with amyloidosis; this disease is characterized by accumulations of various proteins, as often occurs in Alzheimer disease and prion disease. Whether or not IBM is triggered by an excess of Aβ in the muscle, leading to loss of muscle fibers, remains to be determined. In addition, it seems unlikely that other well-defined disease, such as OPMD, in which Aβ is also accumulated, would have the same pathogenesis as IBM.

On the other hand, some myonuclear abnormalities that occur almost exclusively in IBM (sporadic and familial) may be the initial pathologic phenomena and may play major roles in the pathogenesis of IBM, as suggested by Karpati and Carpenter (26). If the nuclear hypothesis is true, however, and if this means that rimmed vacuoles are secondary to nuclear breakdown, how are we explain the formation of rimmed vacuoles in spite the absence of nuclear abnormalities in the various neuromuscular disorders in which rimmed vacuoles occur?

Some final questions arise: Are familial IBM and sporadic IBM the same, or distinct entities? What is the link between familial IBM and inclusion-body myopathies, such as distal myopathies and OPMD? It seems likely that only discovery of the gene responsible for familial IBM will make it possible to answer such questions.

References

1. Yunis EJ, Samaha FJ. Inclusion body myositis. *Lab Invest* 25:240–248, 1971.
2. Chou SM. Myxovirus-like structures and accompanying nuclear changes in chronic polymyositis. *Arch Pathol* 86:649–658, 1968.
3. Neville HE, Ringel SP, Baumbach LL. Familial inclusion body myositis. *Neurology (Suppl 1)* 40:120, 1990.
4. Hentati F, Ben Hamida C, Tomé F, Oueslati S, Fardeau M. "Familial inclusion body myositis" sparing the quadriceps with asymptomatic leukoencephalopathy in a Tunisian kindred. *Neurology (suppl 1)* 41:422, 1991.
5. Mikol J, Engel AG, Franzini-Amstrong C. Inclusion body myositis. In *Myology*, Engel AG, Franzini-Amstrong C (eds). New York, McGraw-Hill, 1994.
6. Serratrice G, Pellissier JF, Pouget J, Figarella-Branger D. Formes cliniques des myosites à inclusions: 12 cas. *Rev Neurol* 145(11):781–788, 1989.
7. Argov Z, Yarom R. "Rimmed vacuole myopathy" sparing the quadriceps. A unique disorder in Iranian Jews. *J Neurol Sci* 64:33–43, 1984.
8. Massa R, Weller B, Karpati G, Shoudbridge E, Carpenter S. Familial inclusion body myositis among Kurdish-Iranian Jews. *Arch Neurol* 48:519–522, 1991.
9. Sadeh M, Gadoth N, Hadar H, Ben-David E. Vacuolar myopathy sparing the quadriceps. *Brain* 116:217–232, 1993.
10. Cole AJ, Kuzniecky R, Karpati G, Carpenter S, Andermann E, Andermann F. Familial myopathy with changes resembling inclusion body myositis and periventricular leucoencephalopathy: a new syndrome. *Brain* 11:1025–1037, 1988.
11. Fardeau M, Askanas V, Tomé FMS, Engel KW, Alvarez RB, Chavallay M. Hereditary neuromuscular disorder with inclusion body myositis-like filamentous inclusions: clinical, pathological, and tissue culture studies. *Neurology (suppl 1)* 40:120, 1990.
12. Klingman JG, Gibbs MA, Creek W. Familial inclusion body myositis. *Neurology (suppl 1)* 41:275, 1991.

13. Lotz BP, Engel AC, Nishino H, Stevens JC, Litchy WJ. Inclusion body myositis: observations of 40 patients. *Brain* 112:727–747, 1989.
14. Villanova M, Kawai M, Lübke U, Oh SJ, Perry G, Six J, Ceuterick C, Martin JJ, Cras P. Rimmed vacuoles of inclusion body myositis and oculopharyngeal muscular dystrophy contain amyloid precursor protein and lysosomal markers. *Brain Res* 603:343–347, 1993.
15. Dalakas MC. Immunopathogenesis of inflammatory myopathies. *Ann Neurol (Suppl 1)* 37: 574–586, 1995.
16. Arahata K, Engel AG. Monoclonal antibody analysis of mononuclear cells in myopathies: I. Quantitation of subsets according to diagnosis and sites of accumulation and demonstration and counts of muscle fibers invaded by T cells. *Ann Neurol* 16:193–208, 1984.
17. Engel AG, Arahata K. Mononuclear cells in myopathies: quantitation of functionally distinct subsets, recognition of antigen-specific cell-mediated cytotoxicity in some diseases, and implications for the pathogenesis of the different inflammatory myopathies. *Hum Pathol* 17:704–721, 1986.
18. Karpati G, Pouliot Y, Carpenter S. Expression of immunoreactive major histocompatibility complex products in human skeletal muscles. *Ann Neurol* 23:64–72, 1988.
19. Figarella-Branger D, Pellissier JF, Bianco N, DeVictor B, Toga M. Inflammatory and noninflammatory inclusion body myositis. Characterization of the mononuclear cells and expression of the immunoreactive class I major histocompatibility complex product. *Acta Neuropathol* 79:528–536, 1990.
20. De Bleecker JL, Engel AG. Expression of cell adhesion molecules in inflammatory myopathies and Duchenne dystrophy. *J Neuropathol Exp Neurol* 53:369–376; 1994.
21. Eisen A, Berry K, Gibson G. Inclusion body myositis (IBM) myopathy or neuropathy? *Neurology* 33:1109–1114, 1983.
22. Hockenbery D, Nunez G, Milliman C, Schreiber RD, Korsmeyer SJ. Bcl-2 is an inner mitochondrial membrane protein that blocks programmed cell death. *Nature* 348:334–336, 1990.
23. Figarella-Branger D, Nedelec J, Pellissier JF, Boucrau J, Bianco N, Rougon G. Expression of various isoforms of neural cell adhesive molecules and their highly polysialylated counterparts in diseased human muscle. *J Neurol Sci* 98:21–36, 1990.
24. Lindberg C, Oldfors A, Edtröm A. Inclusion body myositis. Peripheral nerve involvement, combined morphological and electrophysiological studies on peripheral nerves. *J Neurol Sci* 99:327, 1990.
25. Schröder JM, Neudecker S. Peripheral neuropathy associated with inclusion body myositis: proof by sural nerve biopsy. *J Neuropathol Appl Neurobiol* 21:449, 1995.
26. Karpati G, Carpenter S. Evolving concepts about inclusion body myositis. In Serratrice G, Pellissier JF, Pouget J, et al. (eds), *Système nerveux, muscles et maladies systémiques: acquisitions récentes.* Paris, Expansion Scientifique Française, 1993, pp. 93–98.
27. Carpenter S, Karpati G, Heller I, Eisen A. Inclusion body myositis: a distinct variety of idiopathic inflammatory myopathy. *Neurology* 28:8–17, 1978.
28. Mendell JR, Sahenk Z, Paul L. Amyloid filaments in inclusion body myositis: novel findings provide new insights into nature of filaments. *Arch Neurol* 48:1229–1234, 1991.

29. Askanas V, Engel WK, Alvarez RB. Enhanced detection of Congo-red positive amyloid deposits in muscle fibers of inclusion body myositis. *Neurology* 43:1265–1266, 1993.

30. Askanas V, Serdaroglu P, Engel WK, Alvarez RB. Immunolocalization of ubiquitin in muscle biopsies of patients with inclusion body myositis and oculopharyngeal dystrophy. *Neurosci Lett* 130:73–76, 1991.

31. Albrecht S, Bilbao M. Ubiquitin expression in inclusion body myositis: an immunohistochemical study. *Arch Pathol Lab Med* 117:789–793, 1993.

32. Leclerc A, Tomé FMS, Fardeau M. Ubiquitin and β-amyloid-protein in inclusion body myositis (IBM), familial IBM-like disorder and oculopharyngeal muscular dystrophy: an immunocytochemical study. *Neuromuscular Disord* 3(4):283–291, 1993.

33. Pellissier JF, Figarella-Branger D, Pouget J, Serratrice G. Myosites à inclusions et maladies neuromusculaires avec vacuoles bordées. In Serratrice G, Pellissier JF, Pouget J, et al. (eds), *Système nerveux, muscles et maladies systémiques: acquisitions récentes.* Paris, Expansion Scientifique Française, 1993, pp. 99–108.

34. Askanas V, Alvarez RB, Engel WK. β-amyloid precursor epitopes in muscle fibers of inclusion body myositis. *Ann Neurol* 34:551–560, 1993.

35. Sarkozi E, Askanas V, Johnson SA, Engel WK, Alvarez RB. β-amyloid precursor protein mRNA is increased in inclusion body myositis muscle. *Neuroreport* 4:815–818, 1993.

36. Askanas V, Engel WK, Alvarez RB. Light and electron microscopic localization of β-amyloid protein in muscle biopsies in patients with inclusion body myositis. *Am J Pathol* 141:31–36, 1992.

37. Askanas V, Engel WK, Bilak M, Alvarez RB, Selkoe DJ. Twisted tubulofilaments of inclusion body myositis muscle resemble paired helical filaments of Alzheimer brain and contain hyperphosphorylated. *Am J Pathol* 144(1):177, 1994.

38. Askanas V, Bilak K, Engel WK, Alvarez RB, Tomé F, Leclerc A. Prion protein is abnormally accumulated in inclusion body myosites. *Neuroreport* 5:25–28, 1993.

39. Askanas V, Mirabella M, Engel WK, Alvarez RB, Weisgraber KH. Apoprotein E immunoreactive deposits in inclusion-body diseases. *Lancet* 343:364, 1994.

40. Murakami N, Ihara Y, Nonaka I. Muscle fiber degeneration in distal myopathy with rimmed vacuoles formation. *Acta Neuropathol* 89:29–34, 1995.

41. Nalbantoglu J, Karpati G, Carpenter S. Conspicuous accumulation of a single stranded DNA binding protein in skeletal muscle fibers in inclusion body myositis. *Am J Pathol* 144:874–882, 1994.

42. Figarella-Branger D, Karpati G, Carpenter S, Nalbantoglu J. Replication protein A (RP-A) is a candidate single stranded DNA binding protein in inclusion body myositis (IBM). *Muscle Nerve (suppl 1)* p. S117, 1994.

43. Satoyoshi E, Murakami N, Takemitu M, Nonaka I. Significance of rimmed vacuoles in various neuromuscular disorders. In Serratrice G, Pellissier JF, Pouget J, et al. (eds), *Système nerveux, muscles et maladies systémiques: aquisitions récentes.* Paris, Expansion Scientifique Française, pp. 83–92, 1993.

44. Nonaka I, Sunohara N, Ishiura S, Satoyoshi E. Familial distal myopathy with rimmed vacuole and lamellar (myeloid) body formation. *J Neurol Sci* 51:141–155, 1981.

45. Smith T, Chad D. Intranuclear inclusions in oculopharyngeal dystrophy. *Muscle Nerve* 7:339–341, 1984.
46. Borg K, Tomé FMS, Edström L. Intranuclear and cytoplasmic filamentous inclusions in distal myopathy (Welander). *Acta Neuropathol* 82:102–106, 1991.
47. Oldfors A, Larsson N, Lindberg C, Home E. Mitochondrial DNA deletions in inclusion body myositis. *Brain* 116:325–336, 1993.
48. Di Mauro S, Moraes CT. Mitochondrial encephalomyopathies. *Arch Neurol* 50:1197–1208, 1993.

7

Unusual Pathologic Forms of Inclusion-Body Myositis and Neuromuscular Disorders with IBM-like Changes

JEAN FRANÇOIS PELLISSIER, ALEX
BAETA-MACHADO, GIOVANNI PUTZU, AND
DOMINIQUE FIGARELLA-BRANGER

There are unusual pathologic forms of inclusion-body myositis (IBM) that can be related to various other conditions, but their actual existence as distinct entities is open to question. If all the morphologic hallmarks of IBM are considered together, none of those changes is specific for the disease. Diagnostic criteria (Table 7.1) have been proposed by several authors (1–11).

The associations and numbers of lesions are the most important factors for histopathologic diagnosis. In most cases, if rimmed vacuoles, atrophic fibers, inflammatory exudates, and cytoplasmic and nuclear 18-nm filaments are present simultaneously, the diagnosis of IBM becomes more likely. If, in addition, eosinophilic inclusions and intravacuolar amyloid deposits are found, the diagnosis is virtually certain.

Morphologic Variants of IBM

On the basis of the pathologic hallmarks of IBM it should be possible to recognize three conditions as morphologic variants of IBM: the noninflammatory forms, forms with absence of amyloid deposits, and forms with absence of eosinophilic cytoplasmic inclusions.

The definitions of the noninflammatory forms are indeed controversial, and whether they are variant types of IBM or non-IBM diseases has yet to be determined (12). Most of them correspond to so-called familial IBM (13–18). In studies of this condition, only two families were found to have inflammatory exudates at muscle biopsy (19,20). The other patients in whom there is familial expression belong in the category of

Table 7.1 *Histopathologic criteria for IBM*

Abnormal nuclear and cytoplasmic 18-nm-diameter filaments
Rimmed (lined) vacuoles
Endomysial inflammatory exudates, with partial invasion of non-necrotic fibers
Small groups of round or angulated atrophic fibers
Eosinophilic cytoplasmic inclusions (different from cytoplasmic bodies)
Small amyloid deposits within or near vacuoles and within nuclei
Nuclear-membrane abnormalities and nuclear breakdown
Necrotic and regenerative fibers
Ragged red fibers
Fibrosis

so-called rimmed-vacuole myopathy, also known nowadays as inclusion-body myopathy.

Amyloid material, when present, is normally observed in or near the rimmed vacuoles (9,21). It corresponds to 8–10-nm fibrils in these areas, coexisting with abnormal tubulofilamentous material 18 nm in diameter. Amyloid material can also be observed as intranuclear deposits. Nevertheless, the presence of amyloid material has variously been reported in 50% to 90% of cases (22).

Eosinophilic cytoplasmic inclusions are frequently found in rimmed vacuoles or near vacuoles. These inclusions must not be confused with cytoplasmic bodies (12), which are quite numerous in some cases and are observed at the same locations. Moreover, as seen by electron microscopy, eosinophilic inclusions correspond to 18-nm tubulofilamentous material, not to cytoplasmic bodies nor to amyloid material. In our experience, we have seen no IBM without cytoplasmic inclusions. They have been detected less frequently in other series (6).

We contend that the other suggested variant forms, such as IBM without rimmed vacuoles, or IBM without atrophic fibers, do not exist. Reports of IBM without typical filaments probably resulted from inadequate ultrastructural studies of insufficient muscle specimens.

Neurosmuscular Disorders with IBM Pathologic Changes

Many neuromuscular disorders show several of the morphologic features of IBM, but obviously are not IBM (23). All of them are noninflammatory conditions, corresponding either to diseases with a genetic transmission pattern or to sporadic or acquired disorders (Table 7.2).

Table 7.2. *Neuromuscular disorders with rimmed vacuoles and IBM-type filaments*

Hereditary diseases
  Oculopharyngeal muscular dystrophy (OPMD)
  Desminopathies
  Glycogenosis
    Adult type II
    Type III
    McArdle disease
  Steinert disease
  Ceroid lipofuscinosis
  Inclusion-body myopathies
    Familial distal myopathies with rimmed vacuoles
    Facioscapulohumeral myopathy with rimmed vacuoles
    Leukoencephalopathy associated with IBM-like myopathy
    Rimmed-vacuole myopathy sparing the quadriceps

Sporadic and acquired diseases
  Inclusion-body myopathies
    Limb-girdle myopathy
    Distal myopathy with rimmed vacuoles
  Chronic denervation syndromes
    Amyotrophic lateral sclerosis
    Chronic spinal muscular atrophy
    Post-poliomyelitis syndrome
    Paraneoplastic neuropathy
    Polyglucosan-body disease

Hereditary Muscle Diseases with IBM Pathologic Changes

In the group of hereditary diseases, oculopharyngeal muscular dystrophy (OPMD) is the most important, because light microscopy consistently reveals a high incidence of rimmed vacuoles in atrophic fibers in OPMD patients. Some of these muscle fibers contain amyloid deposits (Figure 7.1a). Membranous whorls and IBM-like filaments (24,25) are observed in most cases (Figure 7.2a,b). By immunohistochemistry, ubiquitin (Ub)

Figure 7.1. OPMD, cryostat sections. (a) Atrophic muscle fiber with rimmed vacuoles, showing the presence of green birefringence material (arrows) (Congo-red staining and polarized light, ×900). (b and c) Serial sections of a vacuolated muscle fiber showing Aβ and ubiquitin (Ub) accumulation (immunoperoxidase; b, Aβ monoclonal antibody; c, anti-Ub monoclonal antibody; ×470). (d) Immunoreactivity of abnormally phosphorylated τ protein in rimmed vacuoles (immunoperoxidase, monoclonal Alz-50 antibody; ×900).

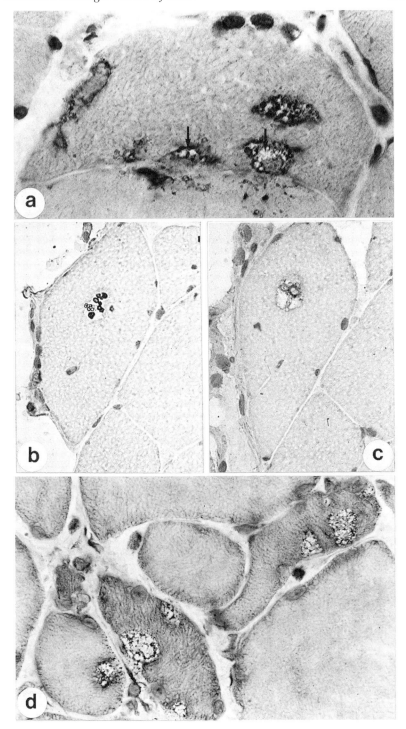

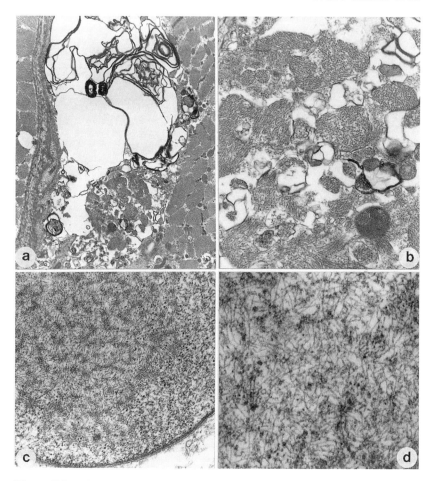

Figure 7.2. Electron microscopy in OPMD. (a) Ultrastructure of a rimmed vacuole in muscle fiber containing membranous whorls and focal aggregates of abnormal filaments (×8,000). (b) Cluster of intracytoplasmic tubular filaments 18 nm in diameter (×30,000). (c) Intranuclear palisading filamentous inclusion, marker of the disease (×40,000). (d) Higher magnification of intranuclear inclusion consisting of filaments 8 nm in diameter (×80,000).

is seen to be immunoreactive in these vacuoles, as are also τ protein and abnormally phosphorylated τ protein (Figure 7.1d), β-tubulin, and β-amyloid precursor protein (βAPP) (23,26,28). In only one patient in our series were both β-amyloid protein (Aβ) and Ub immunoreactive in a vacuole of a single fiber at serial section (Figure 7.1b,c). On the other hand, intranuclear 8-nm inclusions (29) are the specific markers of OPMD

(Figure 7.2c,d). IBM-like intranuclear filaments have been reported only once in an OPDM patient (30).

Muscle biopsy specimens in type III glycogenosis and in McArdle disease show vacuolar myopathy. Numerous sub-sarcolemmal and inter-myofibrillar vacuoles contain PAS-positive material. Besides glycogen accumulation, some atrophic muscle fibers contain rimmed vacuoles and amyloid deposits (Figure 7.3a-d) (23,31). Electron-microscopic studies will confirm the 18-nm tubulofilamentous inclusions (Figures 7.4a,b and 7.5e). Moreover, these abnormal inclusions can also be observed in blebs of glycogen particles in stored fibers (Figures 7.4c,d and 7.5d). Strong immunoreactivity for Ub is found in rimmed-vacuole inclusions (Figures 7.3f and 7.5a), and ubiquitinous material is also visible in blebs of glyco-gen storage (23) (Figures 7.3e and 7.5c). Aβ immunoreactivity is not observed, but anti-βAPP immunoreactivity is present in rimmed vacuoles (Figure 7.3g). Ubiquitinated material can be detected in rare nuclei in type III glycogenosis (Figure 7.5b). In only one case of type III glyco-genosis did one abnormal nucleus show disintegrative changes and con-tain 18-nm tubulofilamentous aggregates at electron microscopy.

In two studies of familial desminopathies with a "rubbed-out" appear-ance of muscle fibers, rimmed vacuoles were always observed in some atrophic fibers (32,33). Those vacuoles were immunoreactive with Ub antibodies. IBM-like filaments were visible in vacuoles by electron mi-croscopy (Figure 7.6a-c). No intranuclear inclusions were observed.

Finally, rimmed vacuoles and 18-nm tubulofilamentous inclusions can be observed in other diseases, such as ceroid lipofuscinosis of a pro-tracted late-infantile type (J.F. Pellissier et al., personal observation). Membranous whorls and abnormal filaments sometimes coexist with enlarged lysosomes showing characteristic accumulations of curvilinear bodies (Figure 7.7a,b).

Familial distal myopathies of dominant (34–38) or recessive (39–45) autosomal inheritance can feature prominent vacuoles with membranous bodies and tubulofilamentous inclusions. They were initially considered to be in the category of rimmed-vacuole distal myopathy (46,47), and nowadays they could be included in the category of inclusion-body myopathy, along with other conditions clinically expressed as familial facioscapulohumeral myopathy (J.F. Pellissier et al., personal observa-tion), myopathy sparing the quadriceps (13), and leukoencephalopathy with IBM-like myopathy (14). Some authors have classified these last two diseases in the group of familial IBM. Whether or not familial distal myopathy of dominant or recessive inheritance is also familial IBM is a

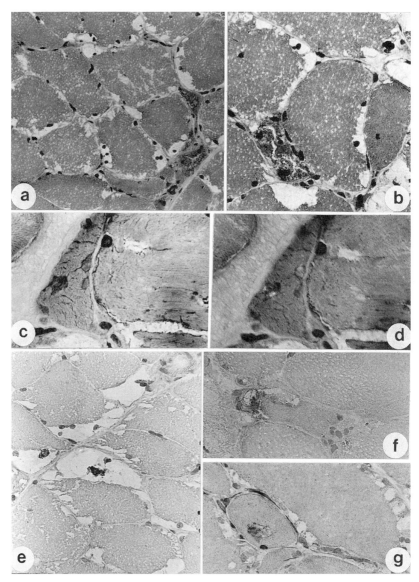

Figure 7.3. McArdle disease, cryostat sections. (a and b) Rimmed vacuoles in atrophic fibers among numerous fibers containing multiple storage vacuoles (H & E; a, ×200; b, ×325). (c and d) Amyloid deposits with green birefringence (arrows) in a rimmed vacuole (c, Congo red; d, polarized light; ×810). (e) Ub-positive material in sub-sarcolemmal blebs of glycogen (immunoperoxidase, anti-Ub monoclonal antibody; ×325). (f) Atrophic muscle fiber with rimmed vacuole immunoreactive for (immunoperoxidase, anti-Ub monoconal antibody; ×325). (g) Immunoreactivity for APP of inclusions in a rimmed vacuole (immunoperoxidase, anti-APP monoclonal antibody; ×325).

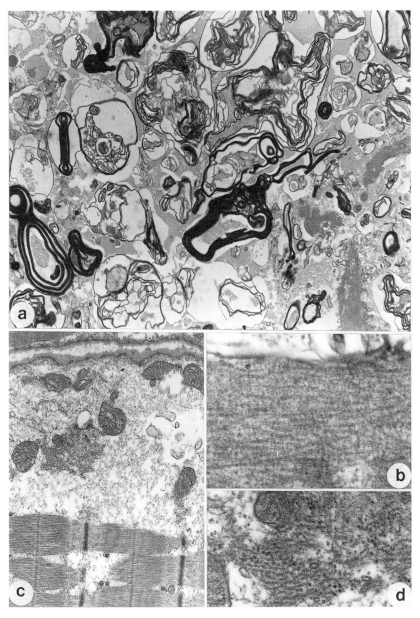

Figure 7.4. Electron microscopy in McArdle disease. (a) Large amounts of myeloid bodies and membrane fragments in a rimmed vacuole associated with fascicles of abnormal filamentous inclusions (right side) (×8,000). (b) Detail of tubulofilamentous inclusion in longitudinal section (×100,000). (c) Tubulofilamentous material in a sub-sarcolemmal vacuole containing glycogen particles and mitochondria (×20,000). (d) Higher magnification of tubulofilamentous inclusion in glycogen vacuole (×80,000).

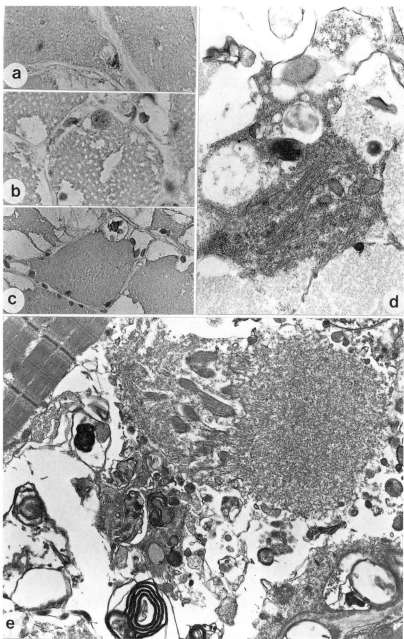

Figure 7.5. Cryostat sections and electron microscopy in type III glycogenosis. (a) Rimmed vacuoles immunoreactive for Ub (immunoperoxidase, anti-Ub monoclonal antibody; ×600). (b) Enlarged nucleus immunoreactive for Ub (immunoperoxidase, anti-Ub monoclonal antibody; ×600). (c) Ub-positive material

matter of nosologic debate. Only genetic studies will be able to solve this conceptual problem.

Sporadic or Acquired Neuromuscular Diseases with IBM Hallmarks

In sporadic forms of distal myopathy, numerous muscle fibers can be involved with rimmed vacuoles that occasionally contain large cytoplasmic inclusions and cytoplasmic or spheroid bodies (48,49). Membranous whorls and abnormal filamentous aggregates are observed at electron microscopy. The same findings can be seen in patients with a progressive limb-girdle myopathy (J.F. Pellissier et al., personal observation). These two last conditions can be included in the subgroup of inclusion-body myopathy.

Finally, variable numbers of muscle fibers with rimmed vacuoles (Figure 7.8a-c) and tubulofilamentous aggregates (Figure 7.8d) can be found in post-poliomyelitis syndrome (50,51) and in other subacute or chronic denervation processes (3,51,52), as well as in chronic spinal muscular atrophy (7).

Histopathologic diagnosis of IBM remains difficult, as compared with diagnoses of other inflammatory myopathies, such as polymyositis and dermatomyositis, for which criteria have been adequately defined. The existence of morphologic variants of IBM has to be questioned, but what is important is that there are neuromuscular disorders of well-defined nosography that share some of the pathologic hallmarks of IBM. Further investigations will be essential to determine the exact significance of the inflammatory cells and the type of this corticosteroid-resistant autoimmunity, even if the inflammatory response is not the main mechanism. Another important consideration will be to determine whether or not there really is a specific marker for this puzzling disease. Each structural change seen in IBM can be found in almost any neuromuscular disorder; therefore, in IBM the numbers and associations of lesions are higher than in other diseases, and nuclear changes are particularly apparent in IBM. Nevertheless, whether or not the same deleterious processes, from affected nuclei to rimmed-vacuoles formation with 18-nm filaments, occur in IBM and other non-IBM diseases, is a matter of some debate.

---

in sub-sarcolemmal bleb of glycogen (immunoperoxidase, anti-Ub monoclonal antibody; ×325). (d) Aggregate of tubulofilamentous material in sub-sarcolemmal glycogen vacuole (×24,000). (e) Ultrastructural feature of a rimmed vacuole with myeloid bodies, membranous formations, granular material, and a large cluster of abnormal tubular filaments (×10,000).

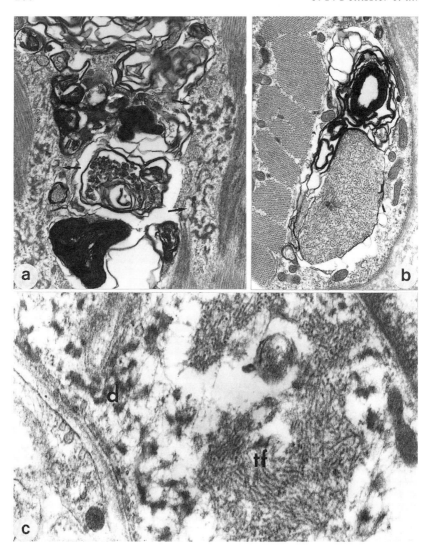

Figure 7.6. Electron microscopy in desminopathy. (a) Large mass of membranous bodies and membranovesicular inclusions between two aggregates of desmin deposits (arrows) (×20,000). (b) Cluster of abnormal tubular filaments associated with myeloid bodies and other membranous fragments beneath the sarcolemma (×76,000). (c) Sub-sarcolemmal area containing both tubulofilamentous inclusions (tf) and desmin aggregates (d) (×60,000).

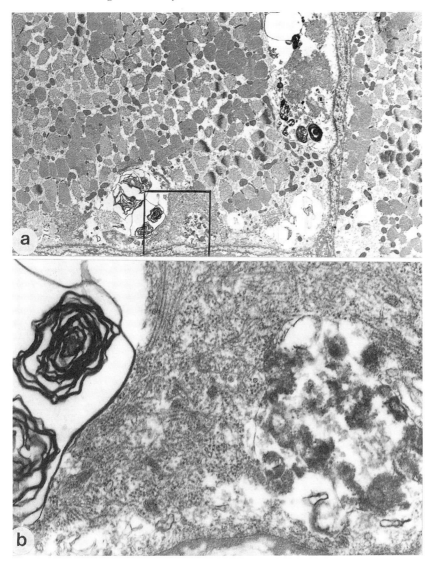

Figure 7.7. Electron microscopy in neuronal ceroid lipofuscinosis. (a) Muscle fiber with lysosomal storage material associated with myeloid bodies and membranous whorls (×6,000). (b) Small cluster of intracytoplasmic tubular filaments between membranous whorls (left) and abnormal lysosome (right); enlargement of part a (×40,000).

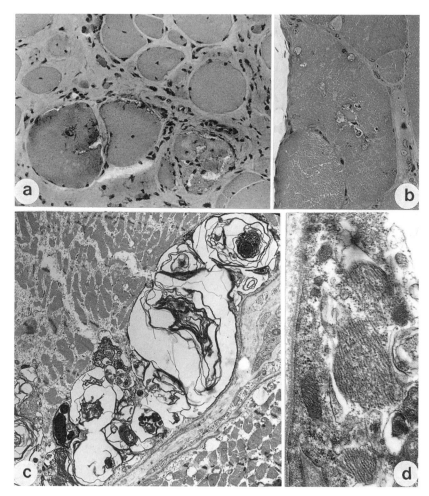

Figure 7.8.   Light and electron microscopy in post-poliomyelitis syndrome. (a) Muscle fibers with rimmed vacuoles. (cryostat section; H&E; ×200). (b) Rimmed vacuole with round inclusion material adjacent to membranous whorls (resin section, toluidine blue; ×325). (c) Myeloid bodies and other membranous formations in a sub-sarcolemmal rimmed vacuole (×5,000). (d) Small clusters of cytoplasmic tubulofilamentous inclusions beneath the sarcolemma (×40,000).

References

1. Carpenter S, Karpati G, Heller I, Eisen A. Inclusion body myositis: a distinct variety of idiopathic inflammatory myopathy. *Neurology* 1978, 28:8–17.

2. Julien J, Vital C, Vallat JM, Lagueny A, Sapina D. Inclusion body myositis: clinical, biological and ultrastructural study. *J Neurol Sci* 1982, 55:15–24.
3. Eisen A, Berry K, Gibson G. Inclusion body myositis (IBM): myopathy or neuropathy? *Neurology* 1983, 33:1109–1114.
4. Engel AG, Arahata K. Mononuclear cells in myopathies: quantitation of functionally distinct subsets, recognition of antigen-specific cell mediated cytotoxicity in some diseases, and implications for the pathogenesis of the different inflammatory myopathies. *Hum Pathol* 1986, 17:704–721.
5. Ringel SP, Kenny CE, Neville HE, Giorno R, Carry MR. Spectrum of inclusion body myositis. *Arch Neurol* 1987, 44:1154–1157.
6. Lotz BP, Engel AG, Nishino H, Stevens JC, Litchy WJ. Inclusion body myositis: observations in 40 patients. *Brain* 1989, 112:727–747.
7. Serratrice G, Pellissier JF, Pouget J, Figarella-Branger D. Formes cliniques des myosites à inclusions: 12 cas. *Rev Neurol* 1989, 11:781–788.
8. Figarella-Branger D, Pellissier JF, Bianco N, DeVictor B, Toga M. Inflammatory and non-inflammatory inclusion body myositis. Characterization of the mononuclear cells and expression of the immunoreactive class I major histocompatibility complex product. *Acta Neuropathol* 1990, 79:528–536.
9. Mendell JR, Samenk Z, Gales T, Paul L. Amyloid filaments in inclusion body myositis. *Arch Neurol* 1991, 48:1229–1234.
10. Oldfors A, Larsson NG, Lindberg G, Holme E. Mitochondrial DNA deletions in inclusion body myositis. *Brain* 1993, 116:325–336.
11. Mikol J, Engel AG. Inclusion body myositis. In *Myology*, 2nd ed., Engel AG, Franzini-Armstrong C (eds.). New York, McGraw-Hill, 1994, pp. 1384–1398.
12. Karpati G, Carpenter S. Evolving concepts about inclusion body myositis. In *Advances in Neuromuscular Diseases: Nervous System, Muscles and Systemic Diseases*, Serratrice G, Pellissier JF, Pouget J (eds). Paris, Expansion Scientifique Française, 1993, pp. 93–98.
13. Argov Z, Yarom R. "Rimmed vacuole myopathy" sparing the quadriceps. *J Neurol Sci* 1984, 64:33–43.
14. Cole AJ, Kuzniecky R, Karpati G, Carpenter S, Andermann E, Andermann F. Familial myopathy with changes resembling inclusion body myositis and periventricular leucoencephalopathy. *Brain* 1988, 111:1025–1037.
15. Fardeau M, Askanas V, Tomé FMS, Engel WK, Alvarez RB, Chevallay M. Hereditary neuromuscular disorder with inclusion body myositis-like filamentous inclusion: clinical, pathological and tissue culture studies. *Neurology (suppl 1)* 1990, 40:120.
16. Massa R, Weller B, Karpati G, Shoubridge E, Carpenter S. Familial inclusion body myositis among Kurdish-Iranian Jews. *Arch Neurol* 1991, 48:519–522.
17. Klingman JG, Gibbs MA, Creek W. Familial inclusion body myositis. *Neurology (suppl 1)* 1991, 41:275.
18. Sadeh M, Gadoth N, Hadar H, Ben-David E. Vacuolar myopathy sparing the quadriceps. *Brain* 1993, 116:217–232.
19. Hentati F, Ben Hamida C, Tomé FMS, Oueslati S, Fardeau M, Ben Hamida M. "Familial inclusion body myositis" sparing the quadriceps with asymptomatic leucoencephalopathy in a Tunisian kindred. *Neurology* 1991, 41:422.

20. Neville HE, Baumbach LL, Ringel SP, Russo LS, Sujansky E, Garcia CA. Familial inclusion body myositis: evidence for autosomal dominant inheritance. *Neurology* 1992, 42:897–902.
21. Askanas V, Engel WK, Alvarez RB. Enhanced detection of Congo red-positive amyloid deposits in muscle fibers of inclusion body myositis and brain of Alzheimer's disease using fluorescence technique. *Neurology* 1993, 43:1265–1267.
22. Dalakas MC. Immunopathogenesis of inflammatory myopathies. *Ann Neurol (suppl 1)* 1995, 37:S74–S86.
23. Pellissier JF, Figarella-Branger D, Pouget J, Serratrice G. Myosite à inclusions et maladies neuromusculaires à vacuoles bordées. In *Advances in Neuromuscular Diseases. Nervous System, Muscles and Systemic Diseases*, Serratrice G, Pellissier JF, Pouget J (eds). Paris, Expansion Scientifique Française, 1993, pp. 99–108.
24. Serratrice G, Pellissier JF. Myopathies oculaires. *S Presse Med* 1987, 16:1969–1974.
25. Coquet O, Vital C, Julien J. Presence of inclusion body myositis-like filaments in oculopharyngeal muscular dystrophy. Ultrastructural study of 10 cases. *Neuropathol Appl Neurobiol* 1990, 16:393–400.
26. Tomé FMS, Leclerc A. Differential features of the skeletal muscle fiber involvement in oculopharyngeal muscular dystrophy and inclusion body myositis. In *Advances in Neuromuscular Diseases. Nervous System, Muscles and Systemic Diseases*, Serratrice G, Pellissier JF, Pouget J (eds). Paris, Expansion Scientifique Française, 1993, pp. 109–115.
27. Leclerc A, Tomé FMS, Fardeau M. Ubiquitin and β-amyloid protein in inclusion body myositis (IBM), familial IBM-like disorder and oculopharyngeal muscular dystrophy: an immunocytochemical study. *Neuromusc Disord* 1993, 3:283–291.
28. Villanova M, Kawai M, Lübke U, Oh SJ, Perry G, Six J, Ceuterick C, Martin JJ, Cras P. Rimmed vacuoles of inclusion body myositis and oculopharyngeal muscular dystrophy contain amyloid precursor protein and lysosomal markers. *Brain Res* 1993, 603:343–347.
29. Tomé FMS, Fardeau M. Nuclear inclusions in oculopharyngeal muscular dystrophy. *Acta Neuropathol* 1980, 49:85–87.
30. Smith T, Chad D. Intranuclear inclusions in oculopharyngeal dystrophy. *Muscle Nerve* 1984, 7:339–341.
31. Figarella-Branger D, Pellissier JF, Pouget J, Calore EE, Azulay JP, Desnuelle C, Serratrice G. Myosites à inclusions et maladies neuromusculaires avec vacuoles bordées. *Rev Neurol* 1992, 118:281–290.
32. Pellissier JF, Pouget J, Charpin C, Figarella-Branger D. Myopathy associated with desmin type intermediate filaments. An immunoelectron microscopic study. *J Neurol Sci* 1989, 89:49–61.
33. Telermann-Topet N, Bauherz G, Noel S. Auriculo ventricular block and distal myopathy with rimmed vacuoles and desmin storage. *Clin Pathol* 1991, 10:61–64.
34. Markesbery WR, Griggs C, Leach RP, Lowell WL. Late onset hereditary distal myopathy. *Neurology* 1974, 24:124–134.
35. Matsubara S, Tanabe H. Hereditary distal myopathy with filamentous inclusions. *Acta Neurol Scand* 1982, 65:363–368.
36. Borg K, Solders G, Borg J, Edström L, Kristensson K. Neurogenic involvement in distal myopathy (Welander). *J Neurol Sci* 1989, 91:53–70.

37. Borg K. Tomé FMS, Edström L. Intranuclear and cytoplasmic filamentous inclusion in distal myopathy (Welander) *Acta Neuropathol* 1991, 82:102–106.

38. Lindberg C, Borg K, Edström L, Hedström A, Oldfors A. Inclusion body myositis and Welander distal myopathy: a clinical, neurophysiological and morphological comparison. *J Neurol Sci* 1991, 103:76–81.

39. Fukuhara N, Kumamoto T, Subaki T. Rimmed vacuoles. *Acta Neuropathol* 1980, 51:229–235.

40. Nonaka I, Sunohara N, Ishiura S, Satoyoshi E. Familial distal myopathy with rimmed vacuole and lamellar myeloid body formation. *J Neurol Sci* 1981, 51:141–155.

41. Nonaka I, Sunohara N, Satoyoshi E, Terasawa K, Yonemoto K. Autosomal recessive distal muscular dystrophy: a comparative study with distal myopathy with rimmed vacuole formation. *Ann Neurol* 1985, 17:51–59.

42. Sunohara N, Nonaka I, Kamei N, Satoyoshi E. Distal myopathy with rimmed vacuole formation. A follow up study. *Brain* 1989, 112:65–83.

43. Udd B, Partanen J, Halonen P, Falck B, Hakamies L, Heikkilä H, Ingo S, Kalimo H, Kääriänen H, Laulumaa V, Paljärvi L, Rapola J, Reumanen M, Sonninen V, Somer H. Tibial muscular dystrophy. Late adult-onset distal myopathy in 66 Finnish patients. *Arch Neurol* 1993, 50:604–608.

44. Partanen J, Laulumaa V, Paljärvi L, Partanen K, Naukkarinen A. Late onset foot-drops muscular dystrophy with rimmed vacuoles. *J Neurol Sci* 1994, 125:158–167.

45. Murakami N, Ihara Y, Nonaka I. Muscle fiber degeneration in distal myopathy with rimmed vacuole formation. *Acta Neuropathol* 1995, 89:29–34.

46. Misuzawa H, Kurisaki H, Takatsu H, Inoue K, Mannen T, Toyokura V, Nakanishi T. Rimmed vacuolar distal myopathy: a clinical, electrophysiological, histopathological and computed tomographic study of seven cases. *J Neurol* 1987, 234:129–136.

47. Misuzawa H, Kurisaki H, Takatsu H, Inoue K, Mannen T, Toyokura Y, Nakanishi T. Rimmed vacuolar distal myopathy: an ultrastructural study. *J Neurol* 1987, 234:137–145.

48. Markesbery WR, Griggs RC, Herr B. Distal myopathy: electron microscopic and histochemical studies. *Neurology* 1977, 27:727–735.

49. Miller RG, Blank NK, Layzer RB. Sporadic distal myopathy with early adult onset. *Ann Neurol* 1979, 5:220–227.

50. Abarbanel JM, Lichtenfeld Y, Zirkin H, Louzon Z, Osimani A, Farkash P, Herishan U. Inclusion body myositis in post-poliomyelitis muscular atrophy. *Acta Neurol Scand* 1988, 78:81–84.

51. Miranda-Pfeifsticker B, Figarella-Branger D, Pellissier JF, Serratrice G. Le syndrome post-poliomyelitique: à propos de 29 nouvelles observations. *Rev Neurol* 1992, 148:355–361.

52. Ketelsen UP, Beckmann R, Zimmermann H, Sauer M. Inclusion body myositis: a "slow virus" infection of skeletal musculature. *Klin Wochenschr* 1977, 55:1063–1066.

53. Mhiri C, Gherardi R. Inclusion body myositis in French patients. A clinicopathological evaluation. *Neuropathol Appl Neurobiol* 1992, 148:355–361.

8

Electrophysiologic Findings in Inclusion-Body Myositis

JEAN-PHILLIPPE AZULAY, JEAN POUGET, AND
GEORGES SERRATRICE

The definition of inclusion-body myositis (IBM) is based on characteristic histopathologic features that are fully described in other chapters of this volume. It is not clearly established that this myopathy can be distinguished from other inflammatory muscle diseases on the basis of a combination of clinical and electrophysiologic features. Moreover, the electrophysiologic findings are controversial in regard to the hypothesis of an associated neurogenic component or a concomitant neuropathy. We will review these different aspects as reflected in 14 IBM patients in order to delineate the electrophysiologic characteristics of this syndrome.

Patients and Methods

We studied 14 consecutive patients with IBM, as proved by muscle biopsy: 11 males and 3 females, with a mean age of 53.4 years. Nerve conduction velocities (NCVs) for motor and sensory nerves were determined following conventional methods. The nerves tested included the median, ulnar, peroneal, tibial, and sural. Needle electromyography (EMG) was carried out in at least eight muscles. The distal and proximal parts of upper and lower limbs were explored, including affected and spared muscles. Motor-unit-potential (MUP) analysis was carried out using the Dorfman or Andreassen technique (1,2), and 20–40 MUPs were analyzed in each muscle.

Results

NCV studies demonstrated reduced compound muscle action potential (CMAP) amplitudes in 7 cases and reduced sensory nerve action potential (SNAP) amplitudes in 3 cases in lower limbs; velocities were slow in lower limbs in 5 cases. All the electrophysiologic parameters were normal in upper limbs. Needle examination demonstrated abnormalities in all cases. Abnormal spontaneous muscle-fiber activity (fibrillations, positive sharp waves) was observed in all patients. It was associated with early recruitment, polyphasic MUPs of reduced amplitude and duration consistent with myopathic changes in 8 cases. That pattern was designated the "myositic pattern." In only one case was the spontaneous activity associated with neurogenic changes characterized by an increased recruitment frequency of long-duration high-amplitude potentials, called the "neurogenic pattern." An association of neurogenic and myogenic changes in different parts of a given muscle (mixed pattern) was seen in the last 5 patients. MUP analysis was performed in 7 patients and demonstrated myogenic or normal parameters in 5 cases (Table 8.1).

Concerning the histopathologic features of denervation, our studies never showed target fibers. Necrotic fibers, which were present in almost all the cases (12 of 14), probably constituted the major cause of the spontaneous activity. Type grouping was seen in 5 cases, and small groups of atrophic fibers in 8 cases. The combination of both abnormalities was seen in 4 cases, all with a mixed EMG pattern.

Discussion

The arguments for a coexisting neurogenic component in IBM are based on clinical, biologic, morphologic, and EMG features. Distal weakness, loss of tendon reflexes, a normal or mildly elevated serum creatine kinase concentration, and the presence of small groups of angulated atrophic fibers, type grouping, and target fibers seen at muscle biopsy are suggestive of a neurogenic disorder. Several electrophysiologic studies of IBM patients have confirmed such neurogenic abnormalities, showing typical neurogenic changes (3) or a mixed pattern of neurogenic and myogenic features, considered as highly suggestive (4). Other studies have reported abnormalities of NCVs that may support the concept of peripheral-nerve involvement in IBM (5).

Table 8.1 *MUP analysis (7 patients)*

Parameter	Elevated	Reduced	Normal
Amplitude	1	5	1
Duration	3	3	1
Polyphasism	2		5
MU mean firing rate	2		4

A pattern of associated neurogenic and myogenic changes with spontaneous activity in single muscles, the so-called mixed pattern, is considered by some authors as most suggestive of IBM (4), but it has the same incidence in long-standing polymyositis (6–8), probably reflecting disease chronicity rather than a cause. The most frequent changes observed in our study, as in previous reports, consisted in an association of spontaneous activity and myopathic MUPs, identical with the pattern commonly seen in other inflammatory myopathies (9–11).

The occurrences of isolated neurogenic changes reported by some authors (12,13) are very rare, as was the case in our study, where we found only one such isolated neurogenic pattern. Considering that conventional EMG techniques have failed to clearly delineate the neurogenic and myogenic components of this myopathy, some authors have used more specific techniques to evaluate denervation. Our quantitative study of MUP parameters confirmed the high incidence of myopathic changes. Single-fiber EMG (SFEMG) reports were provided by Eisen et al. (3) for 7 cases. They found a high fiber density (mean, 6.3; $N < 2$) and abnormal jitter (83 μsec; $N < 60$). Those findings led them to believe that IBM had a major neurogenic component, but Joy et al. (4) were unable to confirm those findings, reporting only mildly abnormal jitter (mean, 46.5 μsec) and a modestly increased fiber density (2.6), which they considered compatible with a myopathic process. Because SFEMG is performed in distal muscles, the differences between the two studies may have resulted from the occurrence of prominent distal involvement in the patients of Eisen et al. (3), compared with proximal weakness in those of Joy et al. (4). Another investigation, macro-EMG, was used in 1987 by Pouget et al. (13), who reported on a patient with a normal fiber density an abnormally high amplitude of the macro-MUP, suggesting a larger size for the motor units, probably due to compensatory and regeneration mechanisms. In 1995, Luciano and Dalakas (14) carried out macro-EMG in 11 patients and found myogenic or normal macro-EMG potentials. We can conclude from these different studies that it may not be possible to define a specific EMG pattern, whatever the technique used, and that denervation is not a main feature in IBM. The different atypical electrophysiologic findings reported for IBM patients probably result from chronic compensatory processes.

Concerning the NCV abnormalities, the most frequent feature is a mild neuropathy of axonal type (4,5,8,15). The incidence of this neuropathy was as high as 50% in the study by Hartlage et al. (16) and in our study, although NCV findings were normal in all patients studied by Luciano and Dalakas (14). When present, the neuropathy is characterized by a loss of amplitude of the CMAP with normal or subnormal velocities, affecting only the lower limbs. The hypothesis of a concomitant neuropathy in IBM is supported by these findings, but the role of the neuropathy does not seem to be essential or important.

Conclusions

It was not possible, on the basis of our findings, to correlate histologic abnormalities and an EMG pattern. Considering the different findings in the various electrophysiologic studies of IBM, we can conclude that isolated neurogenic abnormalities are infrequent and that mixed potentials are not specific and are found in other inflammatory myopathies, reflecting disease chronicity, and probably are due to separation of muscle fibers from their endplates by segmental myonecrosis (17,18).

A mild neuropathy is frequent in IBM patients. It is not contributive to the weakness, but may explain areflexia and some neurogenic features. The question of a specific nerve involvement in IBM is not yet settled, and an associated dysimmune neuropathy may be considered as far as an autoimmune process is implicated in IBM.

References

1. Dorfman LJ, McGill KC. Automatic decomposition electromyography (ADEMG): validation and normative data in brachial biceps. *Electroencephalogr Clin Neurophysiol* 1985, 61:453–461.
2. Andreassen S. Computerized analysis of motor unit firing. *Prog Clin Neurophysiol* 1983, 10:150–163.
3. Eisen A, Berry K, Gibson G. Inclusion body myositis (IBM): myopathy or neuropathy? *Neurology* 1983, 33:1109–1114.
4. Joy JL, Oh SJ, Baysal AI. Electrophysiological spectrum of inclusion body myositis. *Muscle Nerve* 1990, 13:949–951.
5. Lindberg C, Person LI, Björkander J, Oldfors A. Inclusion body myositis: clinical, morphological, physiological and laboratory findings in 18 cases. *Acta Neurol Scand* 1994, 89:123–131.
6. Mechler F. Changing electromyographic findings during the chronic course of polymyositis. *J Neurol Sci* 1974, 23:237–242.
7. Uncini A, Lange DJ, Hayes AP, Lovelace RE. Long-duration polyphasic potentials in myopathies: a pathologic correlation. *Neurology* (*suppl 1*) 1987, 37:115.
8. Lotz BP, Engel AG, Nishino H, Stevens JC, Litchy WJ. Inclusion body myositis, observations in 40 patients. *Brain* 1989, 112:727–747.
9. Sawchak JA, Kula RW, Sher JH, Shafiq SA, Clark LM. Clinicopathologic investigations in patients with inclusion body myositis (IBM). *Neurology* (*suppl 2*) 1983, 33:237.

10. Gutman L, Govindan S, Riggs JE, Schochet SS. Inclusion body myositis and Sjögren syndrome. *Arch Neurol* 1985, 42:1021–1022.
11. Calabrese LH, Mitsumoto H, Chou SM. Inclusion body myositis presenting as a treatment-resistant polymyositis. *Arthritis Rheum* 1987, 39:397–403.
12. Mikol J, Felten-Papaiconomou A, Ferchal F, Perol Y, Gautier B, Haguenau B, Pepin B. Inclusion-body myositis: clinicopathological studies and isolation of an adenosvirus type 2 from muscle biopsy specimen. *Ann Neurol* 1981, 11:576–581.
13. Pouget J, Pellissier JF, Serratrice G. Aspects électromyographiques des myosites à inclusions. Etude en macroélectromyographie. *Rev EEG Neurophysiol* 1987, 17:319–328.
14. Luciano CA, Dalakas MC. A macro-EMG study of inclusion-body myositis: no evidence for a neurogenic component. *Neurology (suppl)* 1995, 45:227.
15. Dalakas MC. Polymyositis, dermatomyositis and inclusion body myositis. *N Engl J Med* 1991, 325:1487–1498.
16. Hartlage P, Rivner M, Henning W, Levy R. Electrophysiologic and prognostic factors in inclusion body myositis. *Muscle Nerve* 1988, 11:984.
17. Sekul EA, Dalakas MC. Inclusion body myositis: new concepts. *Semin Neurol* 1993, 13:256–263.
18. Shields RW, Shymansky S, Estes M. EMG–muscle biopsy correlations in inclusion body myositis. *Neurology (suppl 1)* 1991, 41:422.

9

Genetic Factors in Sporadic Inclusion-Body Myositis

MICHAEL J. GARLEPP, LORI BLECHYNDEN,
HYACINTH TABARIAS, CASSANDRA LAWSON,
FRANK VAN BOCKXMEER, AND FRANK L.
MASTAGLIA

Inclusion-body myositis (IBM) is one of a group of diseases that are referred to as the inflammatory muscle diseases (1). As discussed in detail in other chapters in this volume, IBM is characterized by the presence of distinctive rimmed vacuoles that contain a characteristic array of proteins (2). Clinically, IBM can be distinguished from polymyositis and dermatomyositis by its characteristic distribution of affected muscles, its absence of skin involvement, and its relative resistance to treatment with corticosteroids and other immunosuppressive agents (3). IBM has generally been considered to be an autoimmune muscle disease (1). That classification has been based on the predominance of CD8[+]T cells among the mononuclear cells in the inflammatory lesions of affected muscles (4,5), the demonstration that non-necrotic muscle fibers are invaded by T lymphocytes (4,5), a limited amount of evidence showing *in vitro* lymphocyte reactivity to muscle cells (6), and the co-occurrence of other autoimmune diseases in around 15% of these patients (7).

Genetic factors that may predispose to the development of inflammatory muscle diseases have been sought for many years (review: 8). In polymyositis and dermatomyositis the most commonly examined markers have been those in the major histocompatibility complex (MHC). Weak associations with class II or class I HLA antigens in these subgroups of inflammatory muscle disease have been reported by several groups (8). Genetic analyses of IBM have been less frequent (9,10). It is clear from the occurrence of familial IBM that genetic factors can play roles in the development of certain forms of IBM, although the histologic features of these patients may differ from those of patients with sporadic IBM (2,11). When considering genetic factors that are most likely to be involved in the predisposition to the development of IBM, two groups of genes are obvious candidates. The first comprises genes that previously have been associated with autoimmune diseases, particularly autoimmune muscle diseases, and that may play roles in the immune response. Foremost among these are the genes within the MHC, but the T-cell-receptor loci, and perhaps genes encoding certain cytokines, may also be relevant. The other set of genes to be considered includes those that encode the proteins that are commonly found in the inclusions of IBM.

MHC Genes

The MHC on the short arm of chromosome 6 in humans encompasses 4,000 kb and encodes a variety of different types of genes (Figure 9.1), many of which are intimately involved in both specific and non-specific immune responses (12). Many of the genes in this complex display a high degree of genetic polymorphism, which manifests at the amino acid level as

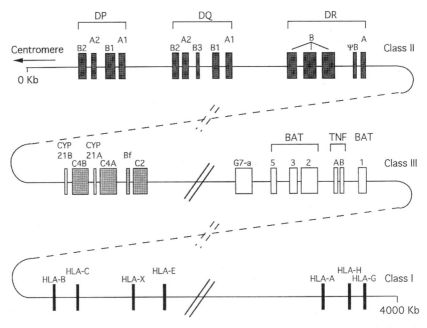

Figure 9.1. A simplified map of the human MHC, adopted from Campbell and Trowsdale (12), illustrating the diversity of the genes present in this complex, the multiplicity of genes of each type, and their diversity of functions. Genes whose products are functionally similar (i.e., class I, class II, or complement genes) have been shaded similarly. The unshaded genes represent only a fraction of the other genes located within the MHC. Some encode products whose functions are unknown (e.g., BAT genes), and some encode cytokines (e.g., TNF-α and -β [From Garlepp (8), with permission.]

antigenic differences and which often results in differences in functions between alleles. The class I and II genes encode the HLA antigens that are primarily involved in the presentation of antigenic peptides to the T-cell receptors (TCRs) on antigen-specific T lymphocytes. Class I MHC molecules present peptides to $CD8^+$ T cells, whereas the peptides presented by class II molecules are recognized by $CD4^+$ T cells (13). Also included in this complex are numbers of genes encoding components of the complement system, genes encoding enzymes such as 21-hydroxylase (CYP21), genes encoding the tumor-necrosis-factor (TNF) cytokines TNF-α and TNF-β, and several other genes of known and unknown functions (12).

We have carried out a detailed analysis of the class I, II, and III MHC genes in our group of patients with IBM (10). The alleles at each of these loci in our patient group are shown in Table 9.1. There was a striking increase in the frequency of DR3 (Table 9.2), as well as increases in the frequencies of B8, DR1, and null alleles at the C4A locus.

Certain combinations of alleles at various loci within the MHC exhibit very strong linkage disequilibrium; that is, they occur together on a given

Table 9.1. *HLA and complement typing in IBM*

Subject	HLA			Complement		
	A	B	DR	C4A	C4B	Bf
1	2, 11	7, 8	2, 3	Q0	1	S
2	1, 3	8, 35	1, 3	2, 3	1	S, F
3	1, 28	5, 8	3, 13	Q0, 3	1	S
4	2, 19	40	3, 13	3	1	S, F
5	1, 23	8, 44	3	3	1	S, F1
6	2, 28	7, 21	1, 3	Q0, 3	1	S, F
7	1, 11	8, 15	3, 6	ND[a]	ND	ND
8	1, 11	8, 35	1, 3	Q0, 3	1	S
9	ND	ND	3, 15	ND	ND	ND
10	2	7, 18	2, 3	3	Q0, 1	S, F1
11	2	8, 44	3, 13	Q0, 3	1	S, F
12	1, 11	5, 8	1, 13	ND	ND	S, F
13	1, 3	8, 40	3, 4	Q0, 3	1	S
14	2, 9	18, 27	3	3	Q0, 1	S, F1
15	1, 28	8, 44	1, 3	ND	ND	ND

Note: Class I typing by serology; class II typing by serology and allele-specific oligonucleotide typing; complement typing by gel electrophoresis and immunofixation.
[a]ND, not done.

Table 9.2. *Selected MHC allele frequencies in IBM*

Allele	IBM (%)	Controls[a] (%)	p[b]
B8	71	28	<.01
DR3	93	25	<.005
DR1	33	15	ns
DR6 (13)	33	20	ns
DR52	100	80	ns
C4A*Q0[c]	77	30	<.005
C4B*Q0	35	34	ns

[a]Control frequencies for DR and B8 from Garlepp et al. (10).
[b]p values determined by chi-square analysis; ns, not significant (p > .05).
[c]Figures for C4A*Q0 and C4B*Q0 in IBM patients were derived from complement allotyping and C4 restriction-fragment polymorphism data. Control frequencies from Christiansen et al. (27).

haplotype more often than would be expected by chance. Detailed analysis of such haplotypes from many unrelated individuals has suggested that the DNA sequences between the marker genes for each haplotype probably are identical (14). The class II MHC antigen DR3 is represented on two such ancestral haplotypes (Table 9.3). The first, marked by B8 and DR3, contains a deletion in the class III region that results in a null allele at the C4A locus and deletion of the CYP21A gene (15). The second is marked by B18 and DR3 and also carries a deletion in the class III region, although this results in a null allele at the C4B locus and deletion of the CYP21A gene (14,15). Southern-blot analysis using probes for C4 and for CYP21 allows assessment of the presence of these characteristic deletions (15). The B8/DR3 haplotype is marked by a unique 6.4-kb C4-hybridizing DNA fragment after Taq I digestion and the absence of a 3.2-kb

Table 9.3. *DR3-bearing ancestral haplotypes in IBM*

Haplotype	Other disease associations
B8 C4A*Q0 C4B BfS DR3	Myasthenia gravis
	Systemic lupus erythematosus
	Insulin-dependent diabetes mellitus
	Autoimmune liver disease
B18 C4A3 C4B*Q0 BfF1 DR3	Insulin-dependent diabetes mellitus

CYP21 hybridizing fragment (15). The B18/DR3 haplotype is characterized by the absence of the 3.2-kb CYP21-hybridizing fragment as well as the absence of fragments characteristic of C4B (6.0 or 5.4 kb) after digestion with the same enzyme (10,15). DNA from 10 of the 13 patients we subjected to this analysis showed the 6.4-kb C4 fragment characteristic of the null allele of C4A on the B8/DR3 haplotype. Two patients had evidence of a deletion at the C4B locus, along with the CYP21A gene (Figure 9.2). Two of the patients for whom DNA analysis was not carried out possessed B18, a null allele at the C4B locus, and BfF1, indicating that the DR3 was likely to be carried on the B18/DR3 haplotype. These data suggest that the DR3 in these patients with IBM is present on the two well-recognized ancestral haplotypes.

Each of these haplotypes has been associated with other autoimmune diseases (Table 9.3). The frequency of the B8/DR3 haplotype is increased in patients with myasthenia gravis, insulin-dependent diabetes mellitus (IDDM), sytemic lupus erythematosus (SLE), autoimmune thyroid disease, polymyositis, and dermatomyositis (8,16,17). In polymyositis the most striking association is found in that subgroup of patients with antibodies to histidyl-tRNA synthetase (Jo-1) and interstitial lung disease (18). None of the patients in our group had antibodies to Jo-1, and pulmonary involvement was not a clinical feature. The B18/DR3 haplotype has been associated with IDDM (19).

The B8/DR3 haplotype has also been associated with selective IgA deficiency (20), as well as common variable immunodeficiency (21–23). Two recent reports have described patients with IBM and common variable immunodeficiency (24,25). We assayed serum concentrations of IgG, IgA, and IgM in our patients with IBM, and all fell within the normal range (M. Garlepp, unpublished data). It is possible that the association of immunoglobulin deficiency and IBM in those patients (24,25) relates to the presence of the B8/DR3 haplotype, although the HLA types were not reported. This haplotype presumably carries genes that predispose to both conditions, and manifestation of either or both of these diseases may depend on the actions of other factors, either genetic or environmental.

Because of the strong linkage disequilibrium between genes in the class II and class III regions of the MHC, and particularly in the DR/DQ region, it is difficult to ascribe the primary association to a particular locus. The presence of DR3 in 14 of 15 patients and its presence on two distinct haplotypes support a direct role for DR3 or an MHC class II gene in strong linkage disequilibrium with DRB1*0301 (26). The T-cell infiltrate in IBM is composed primarily of CD8+ cells, which are believed

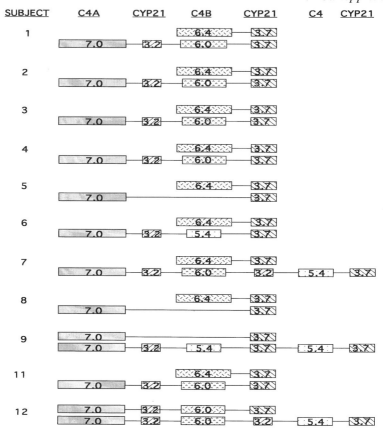

Figure 9.2. Probable class III arrangements in some of our patients with IBM derived from analyses of C4 and CYP21 restriction-fragment length polymorphisms (RFLPs), complement typing, and previous knowledge of extended haplotypes and C4 and CYP21 combinations. The genes are labeled according to the size of the corresponding Taq I RFLP. Data from patients 10, 13, 14, and 15 (Table 9.1) are not shown. [From Garlepp et al. (10), with permission.]

to invade the muscle fibers. Because these cells recognize antigen presented by class I MHC, any direct role for DR3 in antigen presentation must be at the level of the CD4+ T helper cells that are required to initiate, and perhaps maintain, the CD8+ T-cell response (13).

Alternatively, other genes that form part of these ancestral haplotypes might play roles. Fourteen of our 15 patients had deletions of either the C4A or C4B locus, and at least 19 of the 30 haplotypes exhibited some genetic aberration (deletion or duplication) of the class III region. The high frequency of C4 null alleles might suggest a role for partial C4 deficiency in this disease. This has been suggested in the case of SLE, where it has been proposed that the mechanism is related to a defect in immune-complex clearance (27). It is difficult to envisage such a mechanism in IBM. Other genes that form parts of these haplotypes have the potential to play a role. For example, the genes for TNF are encoded in the class III region (Figure 9.1). These molecules have the capacity to mediate cell damage, and aberrant production of TNF-α has been associated with the B8/DR3 haplotype (28). Several other genes whose functions have yet to be determined have also been located in the MHC. One recently described gene with preferential expression in skeletal muscle (29) may be worthy of further investigation.

Genes Encoding the Proteins Associated with the Rimmed Vacuoles in IBM

Several proteins and their mRNAs have been localized to the inclusion bodies in IBM (2). Mutations or polymorphisms of at least three of these proteins have been associated with their deposition in other diseases. Mutations in the gene encoding β-amyloid, the amyloid precursor-protein (APP) gene, have been associated with increased deposition of βA4 in Alzheimer disease (AD) and in Dutch-type hereditary cerebral hemorrhage (30). These mutations occur in DNA sequences within or flanking the βA4 fragment of APP and seem to promote aberrant processing of the APP and increased production and deposition of βA4. We have sequenced exons 16 and 17 of the APP gene, which encode the βA4 fragment, in our group of patients with IBM and have found no evidence of sequence abnormalities (M. Garlepp et al., unpublished data).

Mutations in the prion-protein gene are also associated with increased deposition of this protein in diseases such as Gerstmann-Sträussler-Scheinker disease and Creutzfeldt-Jakob disease (CJD) (31). Two common alleles of the prion gene can be distinguished by a polymorphism at codon 129 that results in an amino acid change from methionine to valine. Patients with iatrogenic and sporadic CJD have increased frequencies of homozygosity at codon 129, as compared with controls (31,32). We have sequenced the entire coding region of the prion gene in each of our patients with IBM and have found no evidence of a mutation. Furthermore, the frequencies of the allelic variants at codon 129 were similar to those reported in the healthy population (Table 9.4).

Table 9.4. *Frequencies of prion-gene codon-129 polymorphisms in IBM*

Genotype	IBM[a] (%)	Control frequency[b] (%)
Homozygous Val/Val	15	12
Heterozygous Val/Met	46	37
Homozygous Met/Met	38	51

Note: Approximately 95% of patients with sporadic CJD are homozygous for either Met or Val at codon 129 (31).
[a]DNA from 14 patients with IBM was sequenced.
[b]Control frequencies from DeArmond and Prusiner (31).

The ε4 variant of apolipoprotein E (ApoE) has been associated with late-onset familial and sporadic AD (33,34). Because several of the proteins found in the inclusions of IBM patients, including βA4, prion, and ApoE itself, are also associated with the characteristic plaques of AD, we and others have analyzed the distribution of the alleles of ApoE in IBM (35,36). In our patient group, the gene frequency of the ε4 allele was 0.29, compared with a frequency of 0.13 in healthy controls ($p < .05$). This frequency approaches that reported for AD (0.32–0.42). In a separate study (36), a slight increase in the frequency of the ε4 allele was reported in IBM, but that was not statistically significant. Because the numbers of patients in both studies were small, this point requires clarification.

APO E4 has been demonstrated to have a higher binding affinity for βA4 and lower affinity for the tau protein than the other ApoE alleles (37,38). These properties have been suggested to contribute to its role in AD and to the accelerated formation of the plaques characteristic of that disease (38). These properties may also contribute to the deposition of βA4 in IBM (in the presence of increased APP production) and the accumulation of hyperphosphorylated tau. APOE plays a major role in the redistribution of lipid between and within tissues (39) and is implicated in the process of nerve regeneration and repair, as well as smooth-muscle proliferation and regeneration (39). Whether or not ApoE plays a role in skeletal-muscle metabolism is unknown. Of interest in the context of inflammatory muscle disease, however, are the reports that ApoE is capable of modulating T-lymphocyte activation by mitogens and antigens (40,41). Because IBM is characterized by the accumulation of T lymphocytes and macrophages, which are potent producers of ApoE, a role in an immune response to skeletal muscle should be considered. The various allelic forms may differ in their efficiencies for each of these functions.

Conclusion

To date we have demonstrated a very strong association between the HLA antigen DR3 (93%) and IBM and have shown that patients with IBM have a very high frequency of MHC haplotypes bearing null alleles for C4. Each of these markers (DR3 and C4 null) are present on well-recognized ancestral haplotypes that have been associated with other autoimmune diseases. Because of the strong linkage disequilibrium exhibited by the alleles that mark these haplotypes, it is difficult to discern the primary association. We have also demonstrated a statistical association with the ApoE allele ε4. As is the case in AD, the presence of ApoE ε4 is neither sufficient nor necessary for the development of IBM. The genetic predisposition to IBM, as with most other idiopathic autoimmune diseases, is likely to be multifactorial. The presence of more than one predisposing genetic determinant may be necessary, and an additional effect of an environmental trigger may be required for disease development. The final manifestation of the disease seen as IBM may be reached via a number of separate paths, as seems to be the case in AD (42).

Discussion

Dalakas confirmed the absence of mutations in the βA4-encoding region of APP in his group of patients with IBM. Askanas emphasized the potential importance of the observation of an increased frequency of ApoE ε4 in sporadic IBM because of its crucial role in membrane repair and its potential role in deposition of βA4. Griggs commented that an analysis of 10 patients in his laboratory had not revealed such an association. The observation needs to be confirmed. Hohlfeld inquired as to the relative risk associated with DR3 in IBM. This is approximately 35–40 and is the highest yet reported for a DR3-associated disease. Dalakas suggested that the association with DR3 may be the best evidence that IBM is an autoimmune disease. The relative paucity of in vitro evidence for myocytotoxicity mediated by lymphocytes from these patients was pointed out by Garlepp and confirmed by Hohlfeld. Hohlfeld indicated that he and his colleagues had confirmed the very strong DR3 association with IBM. The fact that the B8/DR3 haplotype was associated with other autoimmune diseases was noted, and Garlepp pointed out the association with IgA deficiency and common variable immunodeficiency, the latter disease having been reported in association with IBM.

Acknowledgments

This work was supported by grants from the National Health and Medical Research Council of Australia, The Arthritis Foundation of Western Australia, and the Australian Neuromuscular Research Institute.

References

1. Dalakas MC. Polymyositis, dermatomyositis and inclusion-body myositis. *N Engl J Med* 1991, 325:1487–1498.
2. Askanas V, Engel WK, Mirabella M. Idiopathic inflammatory myopathies: inclusion body myositis, polymyositis and dermatomyositis. *Curr Opin Neurol* 1994, 7:448–456.
3. Chou SM. Inclusion body myositis. *Bailliere's Clinical Neurology* 1993, 2:557–577.
4. Arahata K, Engel AG. Monoclonal antibody analysis of mononuclear cells in myopathies. IV. Cell mediated cytotoxicity and muscle fibre necrosis. *Ann Neurol* 1988, 23:168–173.
5. Karpati G, Carpenter S. Pathology of the inflammatory myopathies. *Bailliere's Clinical Neurology* 1993, 2:527–556.
6. Hohlfeld R, Engel AG. Coculture with autologous myotubes of cytotoxic T cells isolated from muscle in inflammatory myopathies. *Ann Neurol* 1991, 29:498–507.
7. Sekul EA, Dalakas MC. Inclusion body myositis: new concepts. *Semin Neurol* 1993, 13:256–263.
8. Garlepp MJ. Immunogenetics of inflammatory myopathies. *Bailliere's Clinical Neurology* 1993, 2:579–597.
9. Plotz P. Current concepts in the idiopathic inflammatory myopathies: polymyositis, dermatomyositis and related disorders. *Ann Intern Med* 1989, 111:143–157.
10. Garlepp MJ, Laing B, Zilko PJ, Ollier W, Mastaglia FL. HLA associations with inclusion body myositis. *Clin Exp Immunol* 1994, 98:40–45.
11. Leclerc A, Tomé FMS, Fardeau M. Ubiquitin and β-amyloid protein in inclusion body myositis (IBM), familial IBM-like disorder and oculopharyngeal muscular dystrophy: an immunocytochemical study. *Neuromusc Disord* 1993, 3:283–291.
12. Campbell RD, Trowsdale J. Map of the human MHC. *Immunol Today* 1993, 14:349–352.
13. Germain RN, Margulies DH. The biochemistry and cell biology of antigen processing and presentation. *Ann Rev Immunol* 1993, 11:403–450.
14. Wu X, Zhang WJ, Witt CS, Abraham LJ, Christiansen FT, Dawkins RL. Haplospecific polymorphism between HLA-B and TNF: genomic conservation and ancestral haplotypes. *Hum Immunol* 1992, 33:88–97.

15. Garlepp MJ, Wilton AN, Dawkins RL, White PC. Rearrangement of 21-hydroxylase genes in disease-associated MHC supratypes. *Immunogenetics* 1986, 23:100–105.
16. Dawkins RL, Christiansen FT, Kay PH, Garlepp M, McCluskey J, Hollingsworth PN, Zilko PJ. Disease associations with complotypes, supratypes and haplotypes. *Immunol Rev* 1983, 70:5–22.
17. Bigazzi P, Rose NR. Autoimmune thyroid disease. In *The Autoimmune Diseases*; Rose NR, Mackay IR (eds). London, Academic Press, 1985, pp. 161–201.
18. Goldstein R, Duvic M, Targoff IN, Reichlin M, McMenemy AM, Reveille JD, Warner NB, Pollack MS, Arnett FC. HLA-D region genes associated with autoantibody responses to histidyl-transfer RNA synthetase (Jo-1) and other translation-related factors in myositis. *Arthritis Rheum* 1990, 33:1240–1248.
19. Kelly H, McCann V, Kay PH, Wilton A, McCluskey J, Christiansen FT, Dawkins RL. Susceptibility to IDDM is marked by MHC supratypes rather than individual alleles. *Immunogenetics* 1985, 22:643–651.
20. French MAH, Dawkins RL. Central MHC genes, IgA deficiency and autoimmune disease. *Immunol Today* 1990, 11:271–274.
21. Howe HS, So AK, Farrant J, Webster AD. Common variable immunodeficiency is associated with polymorphic markers in the human major histocompatibility complex. *Clin Exp Immunol* 1991, 83:387–390.
22. Volkanis JE, Zhu Z-B, Schaffer FM, Macon KJ, Palermos J, Barger BO, Go R, Campbell RD, Schroeder HW, Cooper MD. Major histocompatibility complex class III genes and susceptibility to immunoglobulin A deficiency and common variable immunodeficiency. *J Clin Invest* 1992, 89:1914–1922.
23. Olerup O, Edvard-Smith CI, Björkander J, Hammarstrom L. Shared class II-associated genetic susceptibility and resistance, related to the HLA-DQB1 gene, in IgA deficiency and common variable immunodeficiency. *Proc Natl Acad Sci USA* 1992, 89:10653–10657.
24. Lindberg C, Persson LI, Björkander J, Oldfors A. Inclusion body myositis: clinical, morphological, physiological and laboratory findings in 18 cases. *Acta Neurol Scand* 1994, 89:123–131.
25. Dalakas MC, Illa I. Common variable immunodeficiency and inclusion body myositis: a distinct myopathy mediated by natural killer cells. *Ann Neurol* 1995, 37:808–810.
26. Altmann DM, Sansom D, Marsh SGE. What is the basis for HLA-DQ associations with autoimmune disease? *Immunol Today* 1991, 12:267–270.
27. Christiansen FT, Zhang WJ, Griffiths M, Mallal S, Dawkins RL. Major histocompatibility complex (MHC) complement deficiency, ancestral haplotypes and systemic lupus erythematosus (SLE): C4 deficiency explains some but not all of the influence of the MHC. *J Rheumatol* 1991, 18:1350–1358.
28. Pociot F, Briant L, Jongeneel CV, Molvig J, Worsaae H, Abbal M, Thomsen M, Nerup J, Cambon-Thomsen A. Association of tumour necrosis factor (TNF) and class II major histocompatibility complex alleles with the secretion of TNF-α and TNF-β by human monocluear cells: a possible link to insulin-dependent diabetes mellitus. *Eur J Immunol* 1993, 23:224–231.
29. Leelayuwat C, Degli-Esposti M, Townend DC, Abraham LJ, Dawkins RL. A new polymorphic and multicopy MHC gene family related to non-mammalian class I. *Immunogenetics* 1994, 40:339–351.

30. Maury CPJ. Molecular pathogenesis of β-amyloidosis in Alzheimer's disease and other cerebral amyloidoses. *Lab Invest* 1995, 72:4–16.
31. DeArmond SJ, Prusiner SB. Etiology and pathogenesis of prion diseases. *Am J Pathol* 1995, 146:785–811.
32. Palmer MS, Dryden AJ, Hughes JT, Collinge J. Homozygous prion protein genotype predisposes to sporadic Creutzfeldt-Jakob disease. *Nature* 1991, 352:340–342.
33. Saunders AM, Strittmater WJ, Schmechel D, St George-Hyslop PH, Pericak-Vance MA, Joo SH, Rosi BL, Gusella JF, Crapper-Maclachlan DR, Alberts MJ, Hulette C, Crain B, Goldgaber D, Roses AD. Association of apolipoprotein E allele ε4 with late-onset familial and sporadic Alzheimer's disease. *Neurology* 1993, 43:1467–1472.
34. Poirier J, Davignon J, Bouthillier D, Kogan S, Bertrand P, Gauthier S. Apolipoprotein E polymorphism and Alzheimer's disease. *Lancet* 1993, 342:697–699.
35. Garlepp MJ, Tabarias H, van Bockxmeer FM, Zilko PJ, Laing B, Mastaglia FL. Apolipoprotein E ε4 in inclusion body myositis. *Ann Neurol* 1995, 38:957–959.
36. Harrington CR, Anderson JR, Chan KK. Apolipoprotein E type ε4 allele frequency is not increased in patients with sporadic inclusion-body myositis. *Neurosci Lett* 1995, 183:35–38.
37. Strittmatter WJ, Weisgraber KH, Huang D, Dong L-M, Salvesen GS, Pericak-Vance M, Schmechel D, Saunders AM, Goldgaber D, Roses AD. Binding of human apolipoprotein E to βA4 peptide: isoform-specific effects and implications for late-onset Alzheimer's disease. *Proc Natl Acad Sci USA* 1993, 90:1977–1981.
38. Roses AD. Apolipoprotein E affects the rate of Alzheimer disease expression: β-amyloid burden is a secondary consequence dependent on APOE genotype and duration of disease. *J Neurol Neuropathol Exp Neurol* 1994, 53:429–437.
39. Mahley RW. Apolipoprotein E: cholesterol transport protein with expanding role in cell biology. *Science* 1988, 240:622–630.
40. Kelly ME, Clay MA, Mistry MJ, Hsieh-Li HM, Harmony JA. Apolipoprotein E inhibition of proliferation of mitogen-activated T lymphocytes: production of interleukin 2 with reduced biological activity. *Cell Immunol* 1994, 159:124–139.
41. Mistry MJ, Clay MA, Kelly ME, Steiner MA, Harmony JA. Apolipoprotein E restricts interleukin-dependent T lymphocyte proliferation at the G1A/G1B boundary. *Cell Immunol* 1995, 160:14–23.
42. Harrison PJ. S182: from worm sperm to Alzheimer's disease. *Lancet* 1995, 346:388.

Part IV

Hereditary Inclusion-Body Myopathies:
Clinical and Diagnostic Considerations

10

Hereditary Inclusion-Body Myopathy in Jews of Persian Origin: Clinical and Laboratory Data

MENACHEM SADEH AND ZOHAR ARGOV

In 1984, Argov and Yarom (1) reported an unusual myopathy in 18 patients from six different families of Iranian Jews. Because of the combination of the typical histology with a unique clinical feature, this disorder was termed "rimmed-vacuole myopathy sparing the quadriceps." The clinical and laboratory features of this neuromuscular disorder were further elaborated by Sadeh et al. (2) in 1993. Those authors noted a very similar familial myopathy, not only in Jews of Persian origin but also in Jews from other ethnic communities (Egypt, Afghanistan, and Iraq). The notion that this "vacuolar myopathy sparing the quadriceps" is in fact a familial form of inclusion-body myopathy was first suggested by Massa et al. (3) in a study of a family of Iranian Kurdish (Iraq-based community) background. The disorder is now termed hereditary (or familial) inclusion-body myopathy (h-IBM) and has been diagnosed in Jews of Persian origin worldwide (4; Z. Argov, unpublished data).

We will review our combined experience with 49 patients from 31 different Jewish families of Persian origin.

Clinical Features

Age at Onset

The age at onset has varied widely in our patients, even within a given family. As with any slowly progressive adult neuromuscular disease, the reported age at weakness onset is a very subjective feature. However, we have examined patients in their early twenties, with the reported onset being as low as 17 years of age. We have also identified patients whose weakness started in their fifth decade (as late as 48 years of age). The majority of patients (80%) had their onset earlier than 35 years, with the mean being 30 ± 8.3 years. Intrafamilial variations were very marked in one family (see Figure 11.1, Chapter 11, this volume), where three members began noting weakness relatively early, at 27–28 years of age, whereas for four other members it was at 40–43 years. This late and variable age of onset created a problem in our attempt to verify unaffected members for linkage studies (Chapter 11, this volume).

Mode of Onset

Practically all of our patients noted the first symptoms of weakness in their legs. In 14 it was clearly recorded to be in the distal muscles of the legs; more precisely the isolated foot extensors (Figure 10.1). This distal onset, also anamnestically reported by other patients, resulted in steppage gait as the first sign. Such a mode of onset led to an erroneous initial diagnosis of peroneal muscular atrophy, or Charcot-Marie-Tooth (CMT) disease. This distal onset, continuing for several years in some patients, mimics other forms of distal myopathies. This may have relevance to other distal myopathies with IBM-like histologic features (5; Chapter 13, this volume). In most patients, however, the onset is in both the distal muscles and the hip flexors, leading to difficulties in climbing stairs, as well as frequent stumbling, and creating a general complaint of "gait problems."

Weakness Distribution

Because patients are examined at various stages of their disease, it is difficult to draw conclusions about the frequencies of involvement of various muscles. In some patients the disease remains limited to leg

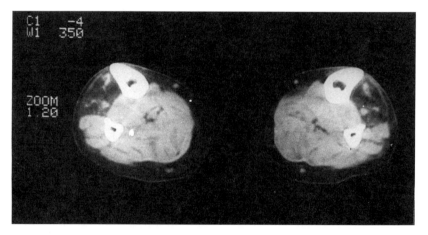

Figure 10.1.   CT of the lower leg muscles in a patient in the early stage of the disease. Note the isolated involvement of the foot dorsiflexors.

muscles for more than a decade, whereas in others upper-limb involvement is detected at earlier stages. As the disorder is termed "quadriceps-sparing myopathy," the lower-limb involvement is described first. Although the weakness at onset may be limited to the peroneal muscles and the hip flexors, the most common pattern is marked weaknesses of similar degrees (usually grade 3 or less on the 5-grade MRC scale) of the hip flexors (iliopsoas), extensors (the glutei group), and knee flexors (hamstrings). The foot extensors usually are very weak or paralyzed at this stage, with the foot flexors (gastrocnemius-soleus) being either similarly involved or at times unaffected. With such severe proximal weakness in the legs, it was so surprising to find that the hip extensors (quadriceps) were unaffected, even at very advanced stages of the disease, that the eponym "quadriceps-sparing myopathy" was given to this disease. Two of our patients have reached the ages of 70 and 75 years and are severely crippled (basically limited to their beds) by the combined weaknesses of upper- and lower-limb muscles, but their quadriceps muscles still have normal power on manual testing (subjects F2 II5 and F2 III3 in Figure 11.1, Chapter 11, this volume).

Three of our patients have also had quadriceps weakness. This phenotypic variant was recently reported by Neufeld et al. (6) in one Iranian Jewish family with two affected siblings. The other two known patients with quadriceps weakness (F2 III6 in Figure 11.1 and F1 III2 in Figure 11.2, Chapter 11, this volume) belong to large kindreds of familial IBM with typical weakness distributions in all other affected members. Such patients become wheelchair-bound at an early stage of their disease, unlike most of our patients, who can still walk after 15–20 years of disease. Not only do the vast majority of patients have quadriceps sparing, but this feature was recently described in two non-Jewish h-IBM families (7). The identification of patients without quadriceps sparing in the Persian Jewish community suggests that the h-IBM without quadriceps sparing that appears in other ethnic groups may still be the same genetic disorder. Furthermore, sporadic reports of patients with IBM and no inflammation, as was reported in nonfamilial IBM (8), may in fact represent single cases of h-IBM (9). The final status of these patients can be determined only after the h-IBM gene and its mutations have been defined.

In the upper limbs, involvement usually is limited initially to the scapular muscles (serratus, spinati, rhomboids). This pattern of scapular involvement with peroneal weakness led to the descriptive diagnosis of scapuloperoneal syndrome in some patients (1). Patients with sporadic IBM may also have such a weakness distribution (9). Distal hand muscles also become involved in the later stages of h-IBM in Jews of Persian origin. However, this is not an early distinctive feature as in the sporadic form of IBM.

Progression and Prognosis

h-IBM is a very slowly progressive neuromuscular disorder. We have followed several patients for 15 years and have seen little progression in their disability. Other patients have shown progression from only lower-limb involvement to more diffuse weakness over slightly more than a decade. Seven of our patients are in their sixth decade of life, and two are past 70 years of age. Many of the patients in their fifties can still walk on flat surfaces for short distances, and only the very old patients with about 40 years of disease history are bedridden. Death related to complications of diffuse muscle weakness has occurred in only two of our patients: a woman at 55 years of age and a man in his mid-sixties.

Other Features

None of our patients has had signs of disease of the central nervous system (CNS). Because of the reported association of brain white-matter disease with familial IBM in one family of non-Iranian Jews (10), we carried out magnetic-resonance imaging (MRI) of brain in two patients and found no such lesions. It must be noted, however, that they were young patients (30 and 35 years), and theoretically, MRI might later reveal changes. But even our two old patients (70 and 75 years) had no evidence of dementia or other abnormal CNS signs on clinical testing. In two families, siblings of patients were reported to manifest disturbed behavior. Although those persons refused any testing, weakness was not detectable in three of them. It is our impression that CNS involvement is not a part of the h-IBM syndrome, but a formal study of this has not been performed.

Laboratory Testing

Not all our patients would agree to laboratory testing, especially to biopsy, if several members of the family were affected and if their muscle-weakness distribution was typical. However, in all our families at least one member had complete evaluation to rule out any other causes of myopathies (hormonal disturbances, presence of autoimmune disorders, cancer, etc.).

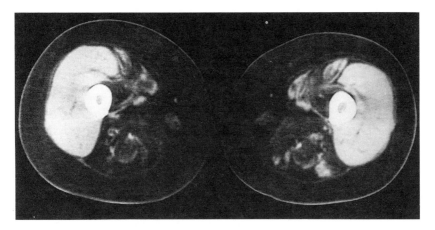

Figure 10.2. CT of the thigh muscles in an advanced-stage patient. Note the severe fatty degeneration of all muscles except the preserved vastus lateralis (which is completely white, i.e., normal).

Computed Tomography

Muscle CT was performed in nine patients (2). It confirmed the lack of involvement of the quadriceps muscle. In very advanced stages, however, only the vastus lateralis was truly spared, whereas other muscles of the quadriceps group were mildly involved (Figure 10.2). CT of the calf muscles revealed that the soleus was much more affected than the gastrocnemius (Figure 10.3), a situation that cannot be detected clinically

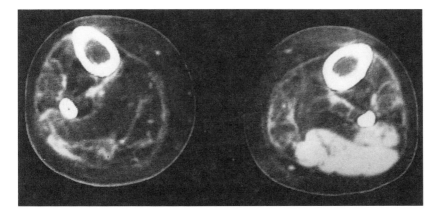

Figure 10.3. CT of the calf muscles in the advanced-stage patient in Figure 10.2, showing marked involvement of all muscles.

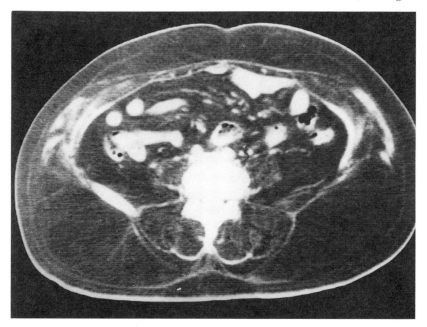

Figure 10.4. CT of the pelvis, showing the severe involvement of the paraspinal, glutei, and abdominal-wall muscles.

and is difficult to assess electrophysiologically or by histologic studies. Paraspinal and anterior abdominal muscles were clearly affected, as shown by CT (Figure 10.4), in addition to the previously mentioned limb muscles. We have no explanation for the particular pattern of muscle involvement in this familial IBM, and such a pattern has not been seen in other myopathies studied by us and others.

Creatine Kinase

In most patients, the serum concentrations of CK were only mildly elevated (about twice the upper limit of the control value). In a few (<15%) it was normal. Only one patient had a CK concentration greater than four times the upper limit of the control value.

Electromyography

Nerve-conduction studies (motor and sensory) yielded normal findings in all tested patients. Conventional concentric needle EMG showed spontaneous activity (abundant fibrillations and positive sharp waves, and, at times, bizarre high-frequency discharges) in the tibialis anterior in most tested patients. Spontaneous activity was rare in other muscles. In most of the tested muscles, many units were small and polyphasic. However, reduced recruitment, with prolonged large or even polyphasic units, was recorded in a few affected muscles. Thus, the EMG picture was reported as a mixture of "neurogenic" and "myopathic" patterns. This mixed EMG pattern and the small-to-moderate elevations in CK raised the possibility that h-IBM might be a neurogenic process rather than a primary myopathic process, or at least might have a neurogenic component to it (1). More recent quantitative EMG studies (2) have shown reductions in the sizes and durations of motor-unit action potentials, more pronounced in the severely affected muscles (Table 10.1). In the most severely affected tibialis anterior muscle, the turns/amplitude analysis also suggested an increase in polyphasia and an increase in the number of small amplitude waves (Table 10.1). Single-fiber EMG showed only a mild increase in fiber density. These electrophysiologic observations led to the conclusion that this disorder is primarily myopathic. The sometimes-observed large motor-unit potentials may reflect the presence of compensatory hypertrophied muscle fibers in the early myopathic stage. The pattern of "myopathic" potentials with spontaneous activity is often encountered in inflammatory myopathies. Inflammatory involvement of intramuscular nerves, which has been suggested as an explanation for the presence of fibrillations in polymyositis, cannot be the cause of the EMG pattern in h-IBM, where muscle inflammation is absent, as discussed later. Myogenous denervation by segmental ne-

Table 10.1 *Quantitative EMG findings in a group of 10 h-IBM patients*

Parameter	Tibialis anterior	Deltoid
Duration (msec)	6.9 ± 1.0[a]	8.4 ± 1.4[a]
	(15.7 ± 2.4)[b]	(11.7 ± 1.2)
Amplitude (mV)	362 ± 57[a]	459 ± 68[a]
	(916 ± 180)	(566 ± 104)
Turns/mean amplitude ($1/\mu V \cdot$ sec)	1.12 ± 0.2[c]	1.06 ± 0.23[d]
	(0.47 ± 0.07)	(0.84 ± 0.1)

[a]Different from control at $p < .05$
[b]Normal-control values.
[c]Different from control at $p < .005$
[d]Not significantly different from control.

crosis, disconnecting part of the muscle fiber from the endplate, may be a possible mechanism. However, in myopathies in which necrosis is widespread and active (e.g., Duchenne muscular dystrophy), the presence of fibrillations is much less prominent than in h-IBM. Furthermore, the amount of fiber necrosis in h-IBM, as judged by both histologic observations and serum CK determinations, is small. The determination of the gene product should settle the myopathic-versus-neurogenic origin of this disease.

Histology

Diagnostic muscle biopsy was carried out in 39 of our 49 patients, but at different stages of the disease. In a few patients, quadriceps biopsy was carried out before the concept of quadriceps-sparing myopathy had been described. Histologic examination of this muscle showed normal findings or minimal changes (few central nuclei, mainly). The most informative muscles were the tibialis anterior in the leg and the biceps in the upper limb. Biopsy of the tibialis can be technically difficult, and in some patients this muscle shows a very advanced nonspecific disease ("end-stage muscle"). On the other hand, when upper-limb involvement is mild or is confined to scapular muscles, biceps (or deltoid) biopsy may not show the diagnostic features. Thus the choice of site for muscle biopsy can be difficult. We suggest biopsy of the biceps if it is clearly weak, and tibialis biopsy if the disease is in its initial stages (first 5 years). In some patients the site for biopsy should be determined by imaging, showing the state of the tissue. In one 67-year-old patient undergoing abdominal surgery for ovarian carcinoma, the anterior abdominal muscles were sampled and showed the typical features of h-IBM.

In none of the biopsied patients was inflammation present, even in minimal amount. The number of fibers with vacuoles varied from very few in lower-magnification fields to 20% of the total. For diagnostic purposes, more than three fibers with rimmed vacuoles had to be visible in a medium-magnification field for the sample to be included in our series. In many fibers, few, usually small, rimmed vacuoles were seen, but in a few fibers a large single vacuole occupied the center of the fiber. Many vacuoles contained concentric structures reminiscent of "autophagic" vacuoles; however, the vacuoles were not membrane-bound, and the term "autophagic" may be incorrect in h-IBM. Only occasional fibers undergoing necrosis or regeneration were seen.

Muscle electron microscopy for all 12 of the recently biopsied patients (belonging to 11 different families) showed the typical inclusions, composed of filamentous structures, in the cytoplasm. Nuclear filaments were more difficult to detect in our patients, but were observed in a few.

Acknowledgments

All of the patients reported here were evaluated at one time or another by one of us (or both). However, many of the patients were referred to us by various colleagues, who continue to take care of them. We would like to thank especially Professor N. Gadoth (Beilinson Hospital, Petah Tikva, Israel), Professor E. Kahana (Ashkelon Hospital, Israel), and Dr. P. Matthews (Montreal Neurological Institute, Canada) for allowing us access to their patients.

References

1. Argov Z, Yarom R. "Rimmed vacuole myopathy" sparing the quadriceps: a unique disorder in Iranian Jews. *J Neurol Sci* 1984, 64:33–43.
2. Sadeh M, Gadoth M, Hadar H, Ben-David E. Vacuolar myopathy sparing the quadriceps. *Brain* 1993, 16:217–232.
3. Massa R, Weller B, Karpati G, Shoubridge E, Carpenter S. Familial inclusion body myositis among Kurdish-Iranian Jews. *Arch Neurol* 1991, 48:519–522.
4. Askanas V, Engel WK. New advances in inclusion body myositis. *Curr Opin Rheumatol* 1993, 5:732–741.
5. Nonaka I, Sunohara N, Ishiura S, Satoyoshi E. Familial distal myopathy with rimmed vacuole and lamellar (myeloid) body formation. *J Neurol Sci* 1981, 51:141–155.
6. Neufeld MY, Sadeh M, Assa B, Kushnir M, Korczyn AD. Phenotypic heterogeneity in familial inclusion body myopathy. *Muscle Nerve* 1995, 18:546–548.
7. Sivakumar K, Dalakas MC. Quadriceps-sparing (QS) myopathy: an autosomal recessive, early onset, familial inclusion body myopathy (F-IBM) in non-Iranian-Jewish families. *Neurology* (*suppl 4*), 45:A209.
8. Figarella-Branger D, Pellissier JF, Bianco N, DeVictor B, Toga M. Inflammatory and non-inflammatory inclusion body myositis. *Acta Pathol* 1990, 79:528–536.
9. Schlesinger I, Soffer D, Lossos A, Meiner Z, Argov Z. Inclusion body myositis – atypical clinical presentations. *Eur Neurol* 1996, 36:82–93.
10. Cole AJ, Kuzniecky RR, Karpati G, Carpenter S, Andermann E, Andermann F. Familial myopathy with changes resembling inclusion body myositis and periventricular leucoencephlopathy. *Brain* 1988, 111:1025–1037.

11

Hereditary Inclusion-Body Myopathy with Quadriceps Sparing: Epidemiology and Genetics

ZOHAR ARGOV AND
STELLA MITRANI-ROSENBAUM

Clinical Genetics

The most frequent form of hereditary inclusion-body myopathy (h-IBM) is the unique quadriceps-sparing myopathy most often encountered in Persian Jews (Chapter 10, this volume). When first described in 1984, three of the six original families each had an affected parent and two affected offspring (1). However, the condition was reported as an autosomal-recessive disorder because of the following facts: The parents in the aforementioned three families were first cousins. There were two other patients who constituted isolated cases in large families. One of the six aforementioned families had two affected siblings only.

The assumption that h-IBM in Iranian Jews was a recessive disorder was, however, never proved beyond doubt. In family 2 (Figure 11.1) three generations were affected. Two members of each of the currently living adult generations in that family (generations III and IV) have biopsy-proven h-IBM with quadriceps sparing. Thus a dominant disorder can clearly be considered for family 2. The lack of information about subject I2, who was born in Iran more than 120 years ago and died there decades ago, does not rule out this possibility. Dominant inheritance in familial IBM has been described (2). Although that was a caucasian kindred and the biopsy showed mild inflammation (which is not found in the Persian Jews' disease), other features were typical for h-IBM. In that family, parent-child transmission was found in two separate lines of the pedigree. It is important, however, to note that one of those parents was unaware of her muscle disease at the age of 61 years, and her disorder was detected only during careful family screening. If one looks at the pedigree of another family of ours (family 1, Figure 11.2), a very similar situation is seen. The 60-year-old woman II2 allowed only clinical examination, in which the findings were normal. She may, however, have had only a mild histologic disease. Thus, theoretically, a dominant disorder with partial penetrance

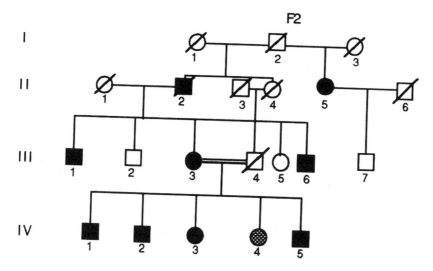

Figure 11.1. A Persian Jewish family with biopsy-proven IBM and a dominant-like pedigree. Individuals are designated with generation and pedigree numbers. Disease status: affected, filled symbols; unaffected, open symbols; unknown status, speckled symbols. Deceased individuals are denoted by slash marks through symbols.

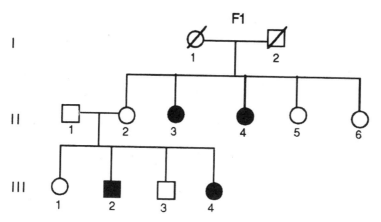

Figure 11.2. A pedigree of an h-IBM family that could be interpreted as dominant inheritance with partial penetrance, since subject II2 may be clinically asymptomatic. Symbols as in Figure 11.1.

can also be considered for h-IBM in Persian Jews. On the other hand, our family 5 (Figure 11.3) was much more suggestive of a recessive disease, because two parental couples who were clinically healthy had few affected offspring. Pedigree analysis alone has not settled the issue whether or not h-IBM with quadriceps sparing is indeed a recessive disorder.

History of Persian Jews

The history of the Persian Jewish community is relevant to the genetic analysis of h-IBM in this and related ethnic groups. Many details of Jewish history in Persia are missing, and only the major bits of information will be mentioned here, based on the work of Netzer (3).

It is probable that the first Jews arrived in old Persia after the destruction of the First Temple in the sixth century B.C. However, the first written documents about Jewish life in Persia are from the first Islamic period, around the seventh century A.D. There was massive destruction of almost all civilized life in Persia around 1220 A.D. during the Mongol invasion. There are fragmentary reports of a few hundred thousand Jews living in Persian cities some 50 years earlier, but those cities were completely destroyed by the Mongols. Many persons, not only Jews, took refuge in the mountainous areas of the neighboring regions (being, today, Afghanistan, Iraq, and the Islamic states around the Caspian Sea). More direct persecutions of the Jews occurred in the seventeenth century, with the rise to power of the Shiite Moslems. Many Jews were forced to convert to Islam or leave their places of residence. Although many did convert, they appear to have later returned to Judaism. During the Shiite persecutions from the seventeenth through the nineteenth centuries, written reports describe Jews taking shelter in the Afghanistan area, along the eastern border of Iran. In fact, the language spoken by Afghani Jews is very similar to the Persian language, and we have records of h-IBM families in which there was intermarriage between Iranian and Afghani Jews. In the western Iraq border area, Kurdish Jews also had cultural ties with Persia, and some of their poetry has similarities to the poetry of Persia. Farther away, in Egypt, there has been a continuing presence of Jews of Persian origin in Cairo since at least the tenth century. Some of the most important religious and secular texts from the Persian Jewish cultures survived only in Cairo. The Persian Jews living in Egypt maintained strong ties with their families in Persia as they carried on extensive trade around North Africa. Jewish migration from Iran to Israel occurred in two major waves: one in the 1950s and another after

F5

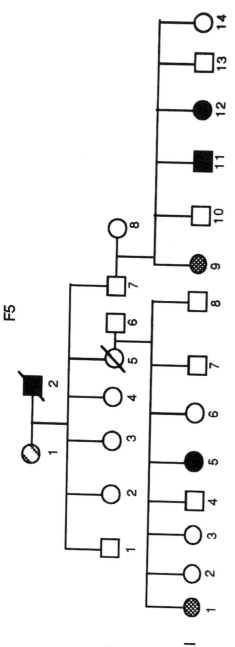

Figure 11.3. A family tree compatible only with h-IBM as a recessive disorder. Symbols as in Figure 11.1.

the fall of the Shah in 1978. In the latter period, many Iranian Jews settled in the United States, particularly in the Los Angeles area.

These historical facts about Persian Jews are important for the following reasons:

1. This is an ancient community, and the spread of the defective gene may have begun a long time ago. That could have resulted in many polymorphic changes around the gene site.
2. The Jewish communities in adjacent countries have stemmed from the Persian Jews or have had close ties to them. Thus, similar disorders are to be expected in Afghani and Kurdish-Iraqi Jews.
3. It is also possible that Egyptian Jews may show a similar disease.
4. Most of the former Iranian Jews reside in Israel and in the Los Angeles area, where most of the known h-IBM patients have been diagnosed.

All of these assumptions have in fact been supported by our clinical and genetic observations, as will be described later. We have no data on similar muscle diseases in the Moslem community of modern Iran.

Epidemiology of h-IBM in Persian Jews

In 1948 the Jewish community in Iran was estimated to number around 100,000. After the creation of the state of Israel in 1948, about 70,000 of them left Iran for Israel. In 1978, the population of Jews in Iran had rebounded to around 80,000. With the fall of the Shah, about 50,000 of them left (25,000 to the United States, 20,000 to Israel, and 5,000 elsewhere). The onset of h-IBM usually occurs around 30 years of age. Thus, for calculation of its prevalence, one needs to know the number of adult Jews of Persian ancestry. We estimate that there are around 150,000 Persian Jews older than 30 years outside of Iran.

It is difficult to estimate the number of Persian Jews afflicted with h-IBM, as many of them do not seek expert medical advice. Many of these patients have been given the diagnosis of "progressive muscular dystrophy," and no further evaluation has been carried out. Also, because of the hereditary nature of this muscle disease, its diagnosis has sometimes caused familial hostility and estrangement, and not all patients have come forward with full family histories about other relatives with similar diseases. We therefore believe that there are numerous patients with h-IBM who remain undiagnosed. The number of patients that we report here is 49 (Chapter 10, this volume). But we know of about 15 more patients who probably have h-IBM – either we have examined them at some time in the past (Z. Argov, unpublished data), or we are aware of them through descriptions by their relatives (some live outside of Israel). In the United States, 20 additional patients have been diagnosed (V. Askanas, personal communication). Taking into account those estimates concerning undiagnosed patients, we believe that the number of adult Persian Jews afflicted with h-IBM may be around 100 outside of Iran. Thus, the prevalence of this disease appears to be about 1 : 1,500 in this ethnic group.

The estimated prevalence of 1 : 1,500 is relatively high for such a "rare" muscle disease. One factor contributing to the high frequency of h-IBM in the Iranian Jewish community is the very high number of intrafamilial marriages. It is a well-established tradition among Jews of Persian origin. Its origins are not clear, but one possible factor has been suggested: the desire to preserve family wealth. Also, because this community was so long relatively isolated and small, with religious rules that did not permit marriage to persons of other religions, consanguineous marriage was very common. Interestingly, it is still practiced today in this community, even in the young generations living in modern countries. In one recently identified family with h-IBM, 5 of 10 genetically "informative" marriages were with relatives (usually first cousins). Some other rare genetic diseases are also frequent among Jews of Persian origin, and other explanations may be possible (4). The need for molecular markers that could be used for genetic counseling in this community is very clear.

h-IBM in Other Jewish Communities

When faced with an isolated patient who has biopsy-proven IBM without inflammation, it is difficult to decide whether the condition is h-IBM or a sporadic form of inclusion-body myositis (5). Defining other Jewish communities with familial IBM must be carried out according to strict guidelines, and only families with more than one affected member are considered here. However, we suspect that some of the reported patients with "sporadic" inclusion-body myositis without inflammation in fact have an h-IBM variant.

Afghani Jews. There are two clearly diagnosed families with h-IBM in this community. One was reported by Sadeh et al. (6), with 7 affected members of two generations. The other was recently identified (Z. Argov, unpublished data), with 6 affected members of two generations. At least two more isolated cases are known to us (M. Sadeh and Z. Argov, unpublished data). All these patients have the typical syndrome of adult-onset, quadriceps-sparing, biopsy-proven IBM. Because of this and the common history of Jews in Afghanistan and Iran, we suspect it to be the same genetic disorder.

Egyptian Jews. One family with two affected siblings was reported by Sadeh et al. (6). There is at least one other isolated case of noninflammatory IBM with quadriceps sparing in an Egyptian Jewish patient (Z. Argov, unpublished data).

Kurdish-Iraqi Jews. One family of mixed Kurdish-Iranian origin was reported by Massa et al. (7). This family was again examined by us, and the clinical features are identical with those of other patients with h-IBM. The biopsy specimen was thoroughly evaluated by Massa et al. (7), who were the first to call this disorder familial IBM instead of "vacuolar myopathy sparing the quadriceps." Few members of this family were included in our linkage analysis. An isolated patient of Iraqi Jewish origin was also reported by Sadeh et al. (6).

When molecular-genetic probes become more accurate for diagnosis of h-IBM, such small families and other isolated patients from different communities (8) will be better defined.

Quadriceps-sparing Myopathy in Non-Jews

Recently, Sivakumar and Dalakas (9) reported two families with biopsy-proven h-IBM that was quadriceps-sparing. One family was from India, with few affected members, and the other was caucasian, residing in the United States. The clinical and histologic features were identical with those of h-IBM in Iranian Jews. These cases may represent a single disease with the same mutation or with allelic disorders affecting different parts of the same gene. Future genetic studies will have to determine the nature of these other forms of h-IBM and distal myopathies with similar histologic findings, but without the clinical features reported in other ethnic groups.

Genetic-Linkage Analysis of h-IBM in Persian Jews

In an effort to identify the genetic nature of h-IBM, nine families of Persian Jewish descent were selected for our study. At least one member of each of these families was diagnosed with h-IBM, based on the accepted criteria, as recently redefined by the IBM Workshop (10). History and clinical evaluation performed by one of us (Z. Argov) identified 29 affected family members. Nineteen of 24 affected individuals available for this study exhibited their disease before age 35. Based on this finding, a disease-gene penetrance of 80% at ages above 35 years was assumed for linkage-analysis purposes. Unaffected individuals below age 35 were not included in these linkage studies. Thus, only 54 healthy family members were used in our calculations.

Two modes of inheritance for IBM could be postulated based on pedigree analyses of these families: recessive and dominant with partial penetrance. Data were analyzed for both models initially, until it became clear that only the recessive model gave positive linkage.

Candidate Genes

We started our linkage analysis with studies of the few genes that theoretically could be involved in h-IBM.

Alzheimer genes. Because h-IBM muscle biopsies show accumulations of β-amyloid precursor protein, and the IBM filamentous inclusions are similar to those observed in neurons of the CNS degenerative disorder Alzheimer disease (neurofibrillary tangles), the known Alzheimer-related sites on chromosomes 14 and 21 were tested and excluded.

Prion gene. Because of the increase in normal prion protein in the muscle fibers of patients with inclusion-body myositis, we tested for markers in the region of the prion disease (Creutzfeldt-Jakob disease). Again, this gene was clearly excluded.

Scapuloperoneal syndrome. Some patients with h-IBM show the clinical features of muscle involvement seen in the scapuloperoneal syndrome. Dr. Wilhelmsen (Columbia University, New York) provided us with markers that showed linkage with the disease in one Italian-American family (11). This site was also excluded for h-IBM.

At that stage, there were no further obvious candidate genes to analyze, and therefore a genome-wide linkage-analysis approach was taken.

Genetic-Linkage Analysis

Genetic-linkage analyses were carried out using standard methods for mapping autosomal-recessive disease loci. Highly polymorphic loci containing short tandem-repeat sequences were selected for study, based on their locations throughout the genome and their polymorphism information content. LOD scores were calculated to be less than -2 in analyses of each of 74 loci, thereby excluding approximately 40% of the human genome. In contrast, analysis with *D9S165* yielded a LOD score of 4.93 ($\Theta = 0.01$), providing odds of more than 85,000 : 1 that the disease gene maps to chromosome 9p1. Using other markers, we could narrow the gene location to about 10 cM in the centromere region of chromosome 9 (9p1-q1) (12).

Our data show that the h-IBM found in Persian Jews is an autosomal-recessive disorder, with an age-related penetrance, that maps to chromosome 9p1-q1. We have not yet demonstrated linkage disequilibrium with any DNA loci, but we anticipate that this powerful technique will lead to further localization of the disease gene. We are not aware of any candidate genes encoding known muscle proteins in this region. However, localization of h-IBM to chromosome 9p1-q1 will enable us to determine the genetic relationship between h-IBM and other clinically related heritable myopathies. We are currently testing h-IBM in Afghani Jews and non-Jews originating from India.

Certainly the isolation and characterization of the disease gene may also provide insight into the pathogenesis of h-IBM. Such insight may have relevance to cell degenerative processes in other diseases, especially the neurodegenerative diseases with amyloid and fibrillary-material accumulations. This may be one of the final common pathways of cell degeneration (whether muscle or neuron). The more frequent sporadic inclusion-body myositis may also share such a degenerative process. Only when the gene product of the h-IBM gene has been clearly defined and its mutations have become known, will we be able to define the final status of the various muscle diseases described in this volume.

Acknowledgments

Genetic-linkage studies were conducted during Dr. Mitrani-Rosenbaum's sabbatical leave to work with Drs. J. Seidman and C. Seidman at Harvard Medical School in Boston. Part of this work was supported by grants to the Seidman laboratory from the National Institutes of Health and the Howard Hughes Medical Institute.

We appreciate the efforts of all the family members without whose willing participation these studies would have been impossible. During the years of our research into this disease, many colleagues from our hospital and medical school have helped us. In particular, we thank Dr. J. Zlotogora (Department of Genetics), Dr. R. Gabizon (Department of Neurology), and Dr. A. Blumenfeld (Unit for Development of Molecular Biology & Genetic Engineering). We are grateful to Barbara McDonough, Mohammed Miri, and Hana Rosenmann for technical assistance.

Addendum

Since the time this chapter was first submitted for publication, some major advances in the molecular genetics of h-IBM have occurred:

1. We have been able to narrow the region of the h-IBM gene down to 2 cM. Using new markers from this region, we have achieved a LOD score of more than 10 and obtained a clear linkage disequilibrium with one of these markers. In 47 of 49 patients tested, a similar haplotype was obtained. Pedigree analysis with these haplotypes now proves beyond doubt that h-IBM is transmitted as a recessive trait in Jews of Persian, Afghani, Iraqi and Egyptian origin, as well as in non-Jews from India.

2. Using these markers, we have been able to confirm that the h-IBM in Afghani Jews (we now have five families from this community) maps to the same site as the disease in Iranian Jews (13). Furthermore, in a large kindred group from India (non-Jews), we also showed that quadriceps sparing h-IBM is linked to the same site (13). A recent report suggests that a Japanese form of distal myopathy also maps to a region on chromosome 9p1-q1 (14). These findings suggest that in addition to the disease in Jewish communities related to Persia, a similar (allelic?) disease exists in non-Jews, most probably resulting from defects in the same gene.

3. In addition, we now have data from smaller families of Iraqi Jews (13) and Egyptian Jews (15), where a positive LOD score suggests that h-IBM in these communities maps to the same region. By contrast, the recessive gene of h-IBM with CNS white matter changes in one family of French Canadians is excluded from the site of chromosome 9p1-q1 (13).

References

1. Argov Z, Yarom R. "Rimmed vacuole myopathy" sparing the quadriceps: a unique disorder in Iranian Jews. *J Neurol Sci* 1984, 64:33–43.
2. Neville HE, Baumbach LL, Ringel SP, Russo LS, Sujansky E, Garcia CA. Familial inclusion body myositis: evidence for autosomal dominant inheritance. *Neurology* 1992, 42:897–902.

3. Netzer A. The Jewish communities in Iran. In *Iranian Jews*. Tel Aviv, Koresh House–World Center of Iranian Jews in Israel, pp. 3–20.

4. Zlotogora J. Hereditary disorders among Iranian Jews. *Am J Med Genet* 1995, 58:32–37.

5. Figarella-Branger D, Pellissier JF, Bianco N, DeVictor B, Toga M. Inflammatory and non-inflammatory inclusion body myositis. *Acta Pathol* 1990, 79:528–536.

6. Sadeh M, Gadoth M, Hadar H, Ben-David E. Vacuolar myopathy sparing the quadriceps. *Brain* 1993, 16:217–232.

7. Massa R, Weller B, Karpati G, Shoubridge E, Carpenter S. Familial inclusion body myositis among Kurdish-Iranian Jews. *Arch Neurol* 1991, 48:519–522.

8. Schlesinger I, Soffer D, Lossos A, Meiner Z, Argov Z. Inclusion body myositis - atypical clinical presentations. *Eur Neurol* 1996, 36:89–93.

9. Sivakumar K, Dalakas MC. The spectrum of familial inclusion body myopathies in 13 families and a description of a quadriceps-sparing phenotype in non-Iranian Jews. *Neurology* 1996, 47:977–984.

10. Griggs RC, Askanas V, DiMauro S, Engel A, Karpati G, Mendell JR, Rowland LP. Inclusion body myositis and myopathies. *Ann Neurol* 1995, 38:705–715.

11. Wilhelmsen KC, Blake DM, Linch T, Mabutas J, De Vera M, Neystat M, Bernstein M, Hirano M, Gilliam TC, Murphy PL, Sola MD, Bonilla E, Schotland DL, Hays AP, Rowland LP. Chromosome 12-linked autosomal dominant scapuloperoneal muscular dystrophy. *Ann Neurol* 1996, 39:507–520.

12. Mitrani-Rosenbaum S, Argov Z, Blumenfeld A, Seidman CE, Seidman JG. Recessively-inherited inclusion body myopathy in Iranian Jews maps to chromosome 9p11–p21. *Hum Mol Genet* 1996, 5:159–163.

13. Argov Z, Tiram T, Eisenberg I, Sadeh M, Seidman CE, Seidman JG, Karpati G, Mitrani-Rosenbaum S. Various forms of hereditary inclusion body myopathies map to chromosome 9p1–q1. *Ann Neurol* 1997, 41:548–551.

14. Ikeuchi T, Asaga T, Saito M, Tanaka H, Higuchi S, Tanaka K, Saida K, Uyama E, Mizusawa H, Fukahara Y, Nonaka I, Takamori M, Tsuji S. Autosomal recessive distal myopathy with rimmed vacuoles (Nonaka myopathy) maps to chromosome 9 (abstract). *Am J Hum Genet* 1996, 59 (suppl. 4):1274.

15. Argov Z, Sadeh M, Karpati G, Eisenberg I, Mitrani-Rosenbaum S. New forms of hereditary inclusion body myopathy (HIBM) and their genetic spectrum (abstract). *Neurology* 1997, 48 (sup 3): A331.

12

Familial Autosomal-Recessive Inclusion-Body Myositis with Asymptomatic Leukoencephalopathy

FAYCAL HENTATI, CHRISTIANE BEN HAMIDA, SAMIR BELAL, FERNANDO TOMÉ, MICHEL FARDEAU, AND MONGI BEN HAMIDA

Inclusion-body myositis (IBM) is a progressive and usually sporadic muscle disorder that usually occurs after the age of 50 years, with a slight predominance in males (1–3). It is characterized by the presence of rimmed vacuoles and typical fibrillary inclusions in muscle fibers, in addition to variable involvements of inflammatory lesions, as in common myositis (1–3). Several reports have described the pathologic findings in IBM in young patients (4–7) and in apparent familial cases (8–10). The patients reported as having distal myopathy with rimmed vacuoles in Japan showed histologic findings similar to those seen in IBM (11–16). Cole et al. (10) described five male siblings with familial IBM of childhood onset associated with asymptomatic leukoencephalopathy, as revealed by computed tomography (CT) and magnetic-resonance imaging (MRI) of the brain.

The cause of IBM and the significance of its filamentous inclusion remain enigmatic. Demonstration of the amyloidogenic properties of the filaments (17,18) suggested the possibility of a relationship between IBM and prion diseases. The aim of this chapter is to analyze the prion-protein (PrP) gene in some members of a large kindred with five affected patients suffering from progressive myopathy that shows the typical features of IBM, with variable degrees of asymptomatic periventricular leukoencephalopathy seen at brain CT, in order to assess the possible relationship between IBM and a PrP gene mutation.

Patients and Methods

The five patients were born to two highly consanguineous parents who had no neurologic impairments. The inheritance clearly was of the autosomal-recessive type (Figure 12.1). All the patients developed progressive difficulty in walking with similar clinical neurologic features, but variable courses and severities: waddling and steppage gait and moderate muscle weakness in the proximal upper-limb muscles, in the proximal lower-limb muscles, and in the peroneal muscles. For three of the patients, ankle reflexes were absent. All of the other tendon reflexes were normal. There was no involvement of facial or neck muscles.

Case Studies

The clinical and laboratory data are summarized in Table 12.1.

- Salah, the propositus (patient IV-9) (Figure 12.2), a 33-year-old man, developed weakness in the proximal muscles in his lower limbs, with relative sparing of the quadriceps. The peroneal muscles were severely affected. He became bedridden at the age of 27 years.
- Hadba (patient IV-4), 55 years old, a housewife, on examination showed waddling and steppage gait, with lordosis and winging of the scapulae.
- Zohra (patient IV-5), 47 years old, a housewife, had severe weakness in her distal peroneal muscles.

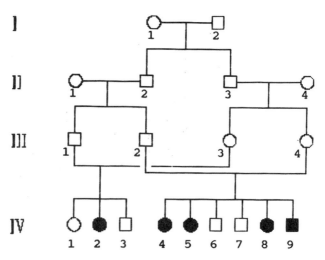

Figure 12.1. Pedigree of the family, showing the high degree of consanguinity and the autosomal-recessive inheritance.

Table 12.1. *Clinical and laboratory data*

Parameter	Patient IV-9	Patient IV-4	Patient IV-5	Patient IV-8	Patient IV-2
Age (years)	33	55	47	35	42
Age at onset (years)	19	25	35	30	31
Muscle strength[a]					
Sternocleidomastoid	3	5	5	5	5
Humeral muscles	2	3	4	5	4
Hand muscles	4	4	5	5	5
Iliopsoas muscles	2	2	2	4	3
Gluteus muscles	2	2	3	4	3
Quadriceps	4	4	4	5	4
Peroneal muscles	2	2	1	1	2
Gastrocnemius	4	4	4	4	4
Ankle reflexes	Absent	Absent	Absent	Present	Present
CK (UI/L)	482	80	83	86	99
Proteinorrachia	0.20	0.22	0.21	0.21	0.20
EMG pattern	Mixed	Mixed	Myopathic	Myopathic	Myopathic
Peroneal motor-nerve conduction	NP[b]	1.3	0.15	0.10	NP
Amplitude Conduction velocity (m/s)	40	46	50	40	48
Saphenous sensory-nerve conduction	NP	17	22	22	NP
Amplitude Conduction velocity (m/s)	NP	50	32	33	NP

[a] Muscle strength expressed on a scale from 0 to 5.
[b] NP, not performed.

- Fatma (patient IV-8), a 35-year-old woman, showed steppage gait and moderate weakness in her peroneal muscles. Her upper-limb strength was normal.
- Khedija (patient IV-2), a 42-year-old woman, showed waddling and steppage gait, mild proximal muscle weakness in the upper limbs, moderate weakness in the pelvic-girdle muscles, and marked asymmetrical weakness of the peroneal muscles.

Muscle Biopsy Studies

Peroneus brevis muscle biopsy was performed in the five patients, and the specimens were studied by routine histochemical and electron-microscopic (EM) techniques (19). Frozen sections stained with hematoxylin

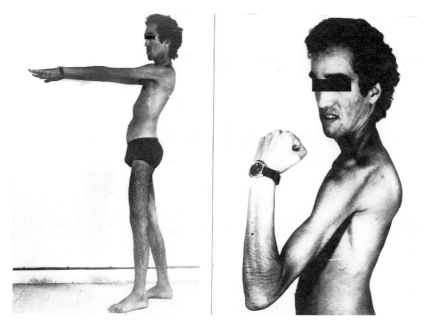

Figure 12.2. The propositus when he was 25 years old: proximal muscle atrophy in the upper limbs and distal and proximal muscle atrophy in the lower limbs.

and eosin (H&E) and Gomori trichrome were analyzed for quantification of fibers with rimmed vacuoles, necrosis, and perivascular inflammatory and atrophic fibers. Those lesions were quantified at examination on four low-power fields at magnification 75 as follows: (0), absence of lesions; (+), presence of rare lesions; (++), presence, on average, of 1–2 lesions per low-power field; (+++), presence, on average, of 3 or more lesions per low-power field.

Results

Muscle Biopsy Studies

The findings at muscle biopsy are summarized in Table 12.2. Each of the affected patients demonstrated the characteristic findings of IBM on histochemical and EM examination of muscle biopsy specimens. Histochemical study revealed, in all the biopsies, the presence of rimmed vacuoles and atrophic and necrotic fibers (Figure 12.3, Table 12.2), variations in fiber size, increased numbers of central nuclei, and predomi-

Table 12.2. *Muscle biopsy findings*

Finding	Patient IV-9	Patient IV-4	Patient IV-5	Patient IV-8	Patient IV-2
Fibers with rimmed vacuoles	+ +	+	+ + +	+	+ +
Necrotic fibers	+ +	+	+	+	+
Atrophic fibers	+	+	+	+	+
Perivascular inflammation	+	0	+	0	0
Abnormal 15–18-nm cytoplasmic filaments	+	+	+	+	+

nance of type I fibers (Figure 12.4). Inflammatory perivascular infiltrates were noted in two patients (IV-9 and IV-5) (Figure 12.3). Oxidative reactions showed lobulated fibers in two muscle specimens (patients IV-4 and IV-5) (Figure 12.4). At EM, all five muscle biopsy specimens showed autophagic vacuoles filled with membranous whorls and accumulations

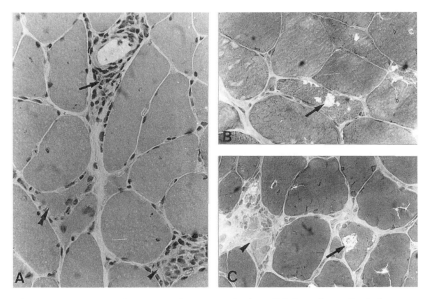

Figure 12.3. Muscle biopsy specimens. A: Patient IV-5: perivascular inflammatory cells (arrow), necrotic fiber invaded by mononuclear inflammatory cells (arrowhead), and regenerating fibers (double arrowheads) (H&E, ×360). B: Patient IV-4. C: Patient IV-5: rimmed vacuoles (arrow) and foci of necrotic fibers (arrowhead) (modified trichrome stain, ×3,500).

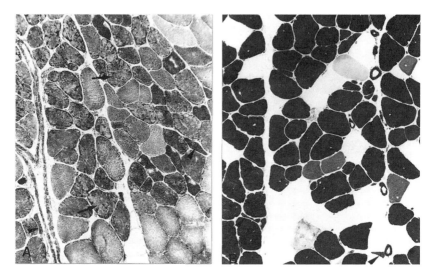

Figure 12.4.   Muscle biopsy specimens. A: Patient IV-4: lobulated aspect of some fibers (arrow) and atrophic fibers (arrowhead) (NADH–tetrazolium reductase, ×200). B: Patient IV-4: fiber-size variation, internal nuclei, type I fiber predomi-nance, and atrophic fibers (arrowhead) (ATPase stain, 4, 35pH preincubation, ×200).

of characteristic 15–18-nm filaments in the cytoplasm (Figure 12.5). No filamentous inclusions were noted in the nuclei of muscle fibers.

Cranial CT

Cranial CT was carried out in four patients (IV-2, IV-4, IV-5, IV-8) and revealed white-matter hypodensities in three patients. The hypodensity was marked in patients IV-4 and IV-5 (Figure 12.6) and was mild in patient IV-2. The CT findings were normal in patient IV-8.

PrP Gene Study

The sequencing of the PrP gene for patient IV-5 did not reveal any mutation. The gene is homozygous for the more common methionine at position 129. Members III3, IV7, and IV4 are heterozygous for a deletion of one octarepeat in the PrP gene. This mutation was not associated with the disease state.

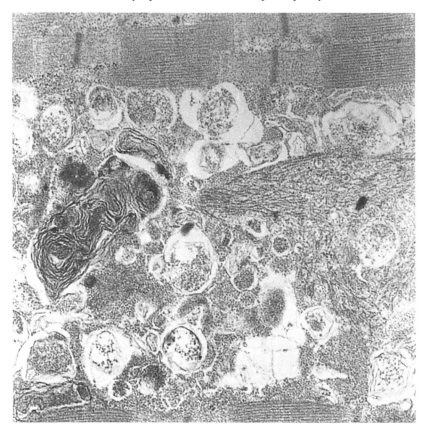

Figure 12.5. Muscle biopsy of patient IV-4: electron micrograph showing a collection of abnormal filaments (arrow) in muscle fiber and some membranous whorls.

Comments

The five patients presented with an autosomal-recessive, progressive, juvenile-onset (or adult-onset) myopathy with symmetrical proximal and distal weaknesses (with relative sparing of the quadriceps) in the lower limbs; there were an important variabilities in their clinical courses, and there was CT evidence of abnormal cerebral white matter in three of four patients. The pathologic changes seen at muscle biopsy were consistent with a diagnosis of IBM: variations in fiber diameter, perivascular inflammation, necrotic fibers, rimmed vacuoles, membranous whorls, and inclusions composed of 15–18-nm-diameter filaments. The clinical features observed in our patients differed in significant respects from the usual

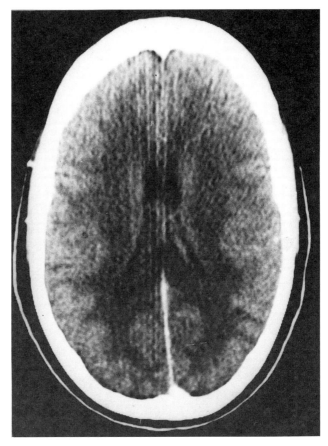

Figure 12.6. Contrast-enhanced cranial CT image from patient IV-5 showing white-matter hypodensity.

presentation of IBM, which ordinarily begins in the sixth or seventh decade and is never familial (2,3).

Our cases can be discussed in the frame of reference of the reported familial myopathies that meet the pathologic criteria for diagnosis of IBM. The "distal myopathy with rimmed-vacuole formation," described especially in Japan (11–15) and showing an autosomal-recessive inheritance, is distinguishable by its onset exclusively in the distal muscles of the legs, by its involvement of the neck and the small muscles of the hands, and by its lack of perivascular inflammatory cells at muscle biopsy (16).

The patients reported by Argov and Yarom (9), encountered among Iranian Jews, showed clinical features similar to those of our patients, but

15–18-nm filamentous inclusions and cerebral white-matter changes were not mentioned in their original paper. The Iranian Jewish woman examined by Cole et al. (10) had typical 15–18-nm filamentous inclusions seen at muscle biopsy, but normal brain MRI findings. The six siblings with "familial inclusion-body myositis and periventricular leukoencephalopathy" reported by Cole et al. (10) differed from our patients in having an earlier age of onset and in being all males. In fact, the clinical variability observed in our patients – variability in age at onset and variability in clinical courses (patient IV-9 bedridden since age 27, patient IV-4 still walking at age 55), as well as the inconsistent leukoencephalopathy (in 3 of our 4 studied patients) – suggested that all cases of familial autosomal-recessive IBM may belong to a single unique genetic disorder with phenotypical variability. The amyloidogenic properties of the filamentous inclusions observed in sporadic IBM, the association of amyloid deposits with autophagic vacuoles, and the presence of sporadic and familial forms of IBM suggest the possibility (17) that IBM may be related to some prion disease (20–22). But the absence of any pathologic mutation in the PrP gene in our patients excludes that possibility. An international effort to find and study families with familial IBM would seem to be the only way to localize and identify the gene or genes responsible for these disorders. Such an effort would allow us to clarify the pathogenesis of the sporadic and more frequent form of IBM.

Acknowledgments

We are grateful to Professor Stanley B. Prusiner (University of California, San Francisco) for the prion gene analysis. This work was supported by grant from Tunisian Secretary of Research, MDA and IAEN.

References

1. Carpenter S, Karpati G, Heller I, Eisen A. Inclusion body myositis. A distinct variety of idiopathic inflammatory myopathy. *Neurology (Minneap.)* 1978, 28:8–17.
2. Lotz BP, Engel AG, Nishino H, Stevens JC, Litchy WJ. Inclusion body myositis: observations in 40 patients. *Brain* 1989, 112:727–747.
3. Ringel SP, Kenny CE, Neville HE, Giorno R, Carry MR. Spectrum of inclusion body myositis. *Arch Neurol* 1987, 44:1154–1157.
4. Sato O, Walker DL, Peters HA, Chou SM. Myxovirus-like inclusion bodies in chronic polymyositis: electronmicroscopic and vival studies. *Trans Am Neurol Assoc* 1969, 94:339–341.

5. Yunis EJ, Samaha FJ. Inclusion body myositis. *Lab Invest* 1971, 25:240–248.

6. Tomé FMS, Fardeau M, Lebon P, Chevallay M. Inclusion body myositis. *Acta Neuropathol (Berlin), (suppl)* 1981, 7:287–291.

7. Riggs JE, Schochet SS, Gutmann L, Lerfald SC. Childhood onset inclusion body myositis mimicking limb-girdle muscular dystrophy. *J Child Neurol* 1989, 4:283–285.

8. Eisen A, Berry K, Gibson G. Inclusion body myositis (IBM): Myopathy or neuropathy? *Neurology (Cleveland)* 1983, 33:1109–1114.

9. Argov Z, Yarom R. Rimmed vacuole myopathy sparing the quadriceps: a unique disorder in Iranian Jews. *J Neurol Sci* 1984, 64:33–43.

10. Cole AJ, Kuzniecky R, Karpati G, Carpenter S, Andermann E, Andermann F. Familial myopathy with changes resembling inclusion body myositis and periventricular leucoencephalopathy. *Brain* 1988, 111:1025–1037.

11. Markesbery WR, Griggs RC, Herr B. Distal myopathy. Electron microscopic and histochemical studies. *Neurology (Minneap.)* 1977, 27:727–735.

12. Fukuhara N, Kumamoto T, Tsubaki T, Mayuzumi T, Nitta H. Oculopharyngeal muscular dystrophy and distal myopathy. *Acta Neurol Scand* 1982, 65:458–467.

13. Matsubara S, Tanabe H. Hereditary distal myopathy with filamentous inclusions. *Acta Neurol Scand* 1982, 65:363–368.

14. Nonaka I, Sunohara N, Ishura S, Satoyoshi E. Familial distal myopathy with rimmed vacuole and lamellar (myeloid) body formation. *J Neurol Sci* 1981, 51:141–155.

15. Nonaka I, Sunohara N, Satoyoshi E, Terasawa K, Yonemoto K. Autosomal recessive distal muscular dystrophy: a comparative study with distal myopathy with rimmed vacuole formation. *Ann Neurol* 1985, 17:51–59.

16. Sunohara N, Nonaka I, Kamaei N, Satoyoshi F. Distal myopathy with rimmed vacuoles formation. *Brain* 1989, 112:65–89.

17. Mendell JR, Sahenk Z, Gales T, Paul L. Amyloid filaments in inclusion body myositis: novel findings provide insight into the nature of filaments. *Arch Neurol* 1991, 48:1929–1934.

18. Askanas V, Engel WK, Alvarez RB, Glenner GG. β-amyloid protein immunoreactivity in muscle of patients with inclusion-body myositis. *Lancet* 1992, 339:560–561.

19. Dubowitz V, Brooke MH. *Muscle Biopsy. A Modern Approach.* London, Saunders, 1973.

20. Prusiner SB, McKinley MP, Bowman KA, et al. Scrapie prions aggregate to form amyloid-like birefringent rods. *Cell* 1983, 35:349–358.

21. Prusiner SB. Prions and neurodegenerative diseases. *N Engl J Med* 1987, 317:1571–1581.

22. Prusiner SB. Scrapie prions. *Ann Rev Microbiol* 1989, 43:345–374.

13

Welander Distal Myopathy: Clinical, Pathophysiologic, and Molecular Aspects

KRISTIAN BORG, GABRIELLE ÅHLBERG,
MARIA ANVRET, AND LARS EDSTRÖM

In 1951, Welander (1) described a distal myopathy (249 cases from 72 pedigrees) with an autosomal-dominant mode of inheritance. The disorder is considered to be the world's most common distal myopathy, but it is found almost exclusively in Sweden (2). On clinical, morphologic, and genetic grounds the disorder can be clearly distinguished from other distal myopathies, such as the distal myopathies described by Markesbery et al. (3) and Nonaka et al. (4), the Finnish tibial muscle dystrophy (5), and Miyoshi myopathy (6). The finding of "rimmed vacuoles" in muscle biopsy specimens from patients with Welander distal myopathy (WDM) constitutes one similarity to inclusion-body myositis (IBM).

Symptoms and Clinical Findings

Welander (1) considered the onset of WDM before the age of 30 years to be exceedingly rare, and onset before the age of 40 years to be uncommon. The onset is slow, and when young and middle-aged relatives of patients with WDM have been examined, clinical signs have been found (7). Often the diagnosis is significantly delayed because of the mild symptoms and their slow rates of progression.

The first symptom most often is weakness of the thumb and/or index finger, noticed as clumsiness in small precision movements. This clumsiness slowly spreads to the other fingers and results in inability to extend the fingers. Gradually, weakness of the distal parts of the lower extremities develops. The anterior tibial muscle is the most severely affected muscle, leading to inability to raise the toes (and making it difficult for the patient to stand with all weight on the heels), which leads to walking difficulties and steppage gait.

On clinical examination, weakness and muscle atrophy are evident in the small muscles of the hands and feet and the long extensor muscles of the arms and lower legs (i.e., the anterior tibial muscles). Tendon reflexes are weak or absent.

The posterior distal muscles of the lower extremities have been shown to be affected when studied by magnetic-resonance imaging (MRI) and at muscle biopsy (8), but weakness is seldom found in this muscle group. Welander reported the proximal limb muscles to be affected in some cases (1), but in other studies involvement of proximal muscles could not be detected by MRI or at muscle biopsy (8). Cardiac involvement has never been seen in patients with WDM.

Sensory abnormalities were reported in the original description by Welander, but were ascribed to aging and coincidental conditions (1). However, sensory impairments most pronounced for thermal stimuli in the distal parts of the upper and lower extremities were described by Borg et al. (9), and they have been found to precede other symptoms and signs of muscle abnormalities in the early stages of WDM (7). Creatine kinase (CK) values usually are normal or slightly elevated in WDM patients.

Neurophysiologic Findings

Nerve conduction velocities are normal in most WDM patients. Slight abnormalities can be found in severe cases. The electromyographic (EMG) changes are complex and include typical myogenic features as well as neurogenic features: small polyphasic motor-unit potentials, reduced interference patterns, giant motor-unit potentials, and spontaneous activity, including pseudomyotonia, fibrillations, and complex potentials (10). In the early stages of WDM, pure myopathic EMG changes have been found (7).

Quantitative determinations of somatosensory thresholds have revealed increased thermal and vibration thresholds in WDM patients (9).

In a study of autonomic cardiovascular responses there were no signs of dysfunction of the peripheral autonomic nerves (11). However, WDM patients have shown altered peripheral vasomotor responses following peripheral vasoconstriction, probably because of stronger activation of α- than of β-adrenergic receptors.

Morphologic and Ultrastructural Findings

The histopathologic changes in the affected muscles were described by Welander (1) as being typical of a primary myopathy and similar to those seen in other muscular dystrophies. However, neurogenic abnormalities have frequently been found (2,7,8,10,12–16).

The abnormalities seen at microscopy are increased variations in muscle-fiber diameters and the presence of centrally located nuclei, split fibers, group atrophy, and scattered atrophic fibers of both type I and type II. The atrophic muscle fibers are mainly angulated, but rounded atrophic fibers can also be found (Figure 13.1). The most prominent histopathologic finding is the presence of rimmed vacuoles, found in atrophic as well as in normal-size muscle fibers (Figure 13.2). Rimmed vacuoles are abundant in muscle biopsy specimens from patients with moderate and severe symptoms, but they were not found in one study of muscle biopsy specimens from the early stages of WDM (7). Inflammatory infiltrates have never been seen in muscle biopsy specimens from patients with WDM.

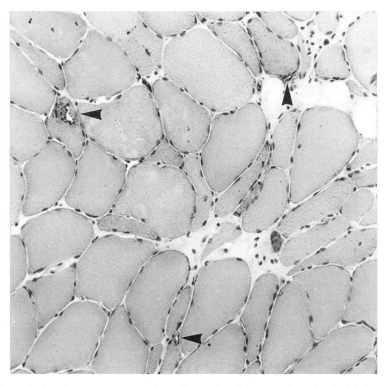

Figure 13.1. Cryostat cross section of anterior tibial muscle stained with H&E. Arrowheads mark rimmed vacuoles. Note also the scattered angulated atrophic muscle fibers (×150).

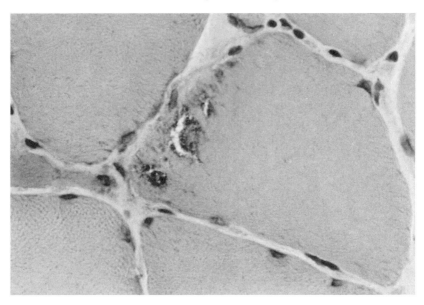

Figure 13.2. Cryostat cross section of anterior tibial muscle stained with H&E. A rimmed vacuole is seen in a normal-size muscle fiber (×1,000).

In an immunohistochemical study, various antibodies were applied, and normal staining for dystrophin, spectrin, and desmin in normal-size muscle fibers indicated normal cytoskeletal structure (16). However, increased immunoreactivities were found for desmin, spectrin, and Leu-19 (myoblast- and satellite-cell-related antigen) antibodies in atrophic muscle fibers. That staining pattern had earlier been seen under different neurogenic conditions (17), including patients who had had poliomyelitis (18), which suggests that these atrophic fibers are denervated.

On electron-microscopic examination, the rimmed vacuoles correspond to autophagic vacuoles containing membranous bodies, with the appearance of dense bodies and myelin figures intermingled with collections of glycogen and amorphous material (10,13,15,16,19) (Figure 13.3). The autophagic vacuoles are found in fibers of normal size and normal myofibrillar ultrastructure, as well as in atrophic fibers with disorganization of myofibrils.

Cytoplasmic filamentous inclusions are found in association with autophagic vacuoles (Figure 13.4). The filaments can be straight or gently curved and generally are randomly dispersed, but sometimes are arranged in parallel, forming an interlacing meshwork (10,19). The diame-

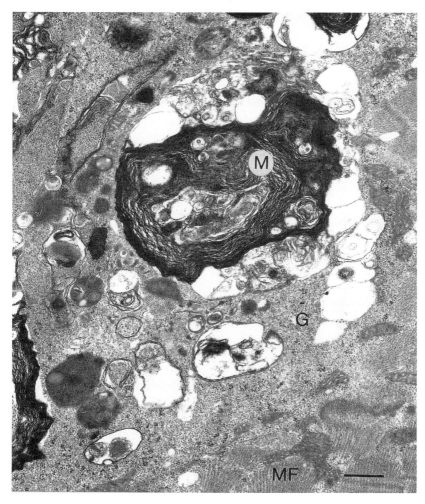

Figure 13.3. Electron micrograph of anterior tibial muscle showing an autophagic vacuole containing myelin bodies (M) and collections of glycogen (G) surrounded by myofilaments (MF) (bar = 400 nm).

ters of these filaments are 16–21 nm, and they correspond to the filaments described in IBM (10,20,21).

Less frequently, filamentous inclusions can be found within myofiber nuclei. Borg et al. (19) described intranuclear filamentous inclusions with diameters of 13–17 nm in multiple sites within a nucleus in an atrophic muscle fiber containing autophagic vacuoles. A similar finding was later reported in another case of WDM (16).

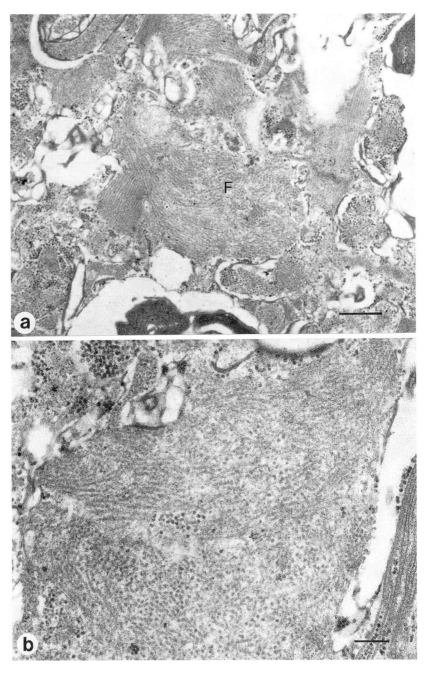

Figure 13.4. Electron micrographs of anterior tibial muscle showing (a) tubulofilamentous inclusions (F) (bar = 500 nm) and (b) tubulofilamentous inclusions at higher magnification (bar = 200 nm).

Fingerprint bodies identical with those reported by Engel et al. (22) and Tomé and Fardeau (23) were reported near nuclei in two atrophic muscle fibers in one WDM patient (19).

Other ultrastructural abnormalities reported have included dense collections of Z-disc material or streaming, double Z-discs, honeycomb structures, and abnormal mitochondria (13,15,16,19).

Sural-nerve biopsies performed in WDM patients (15) showed moderate losses of myelinated nerve fibers in two of five cases. The mean density of nerve fibers was decreased, as compared with normal controls. The mean nerve-fiber area and diameter were increased because of selective loss of small-diameter $(A\text{-}\delta)$ nerve fibers (15).

Molecular Genetics

In a large-scale mapping project, 62 WDM patients from six families were studied initially. For genotyping with micro-satellites, DNA was isolated from peripheral-blood lymphocytes, amplified with a polymerase chain reaction, separated by polyacrylamide-gel electrophoresis, and autoradiographed, as originally described by Weber and May (24). Initially, 105 CA-repeat markers were analyzed, the majority being of dinucleotide type, and a few of trinucleotide or tetranucleotide type.

WDM was analyzed as an autosomal-dominant trait with complete penetrance, a gene frequency of 0.0001, and no rate of new mutations. Two-point analysis was performed with the MLINK program. For exclusion mapping and for potential location of the WDM gene, the program EXCLUDE (25) was used, and about 60% of the autosomal genome has thus far been excluded.

Regarding specific regions of interest for distal myopathy, linkage to chromosome 2 has been excluded at 2p12 with D2S101, with a LOD score of -11.6, and at 2p13–16 with the marker D2S134. Chromosome-14 linkage was excluded with several markers on 14q; D14S50 at 14q11 gave a LOD score of -31.2, and D14S54 and D14S49 gave LOD scores of -19.2 and -18.8, respectively.

Discussion

On the basis of clinical, neurophysiologic, and morphologic findings, WDM can be clearly distinguished from the other distal myopathies (3–6). That can be further supported by genetic studies. The mapping studies thus far have excluded linkage to chromosome 2 (2p12–14), which is linked to the Miyoshi myopathy (26), and to chromosome 14, where the region on 14q between D14S49 and D14S72 has been assumed to house the gene of the distal myopathy described by Laing et al. (27). Around 60% of the autosomal genome has now been excluded, but another set of 160 CA-repeat markers has been genotyped to cover the previously unexamined gaps, and further work is thus in progress. However, although there are no clear indications, WDM might be a heterogeneous disorder.

There are some similarities between WDM, a hereditary disorder, and IBM, an acquired inflammatory myopathy. Both disorders feature a late and insidious onset, neurophysiologic changes, and morphologic abnormalities seen at muscle biopsy that are of mixed myopathic and neuropathic character. The most prominent similarity is the frequent finding of rimmed vacuoles in muscle biopsy specimens. However, there are also clear differences: WDM strictly affects distal muscles, whereas IBM affects proximal muscles. The course of IBM is rapid, but the progression in WDM is slow. In WDM, inflammatory changes are never seen in muscle.

The neurophysiologic changes are of mixed myopathic and neuropathic nature in both WDM and IBM. Furthermore, morphologic abnormalities of neurogenic character have been described at muscle biopsy in both WDM and IBM (2,7,8,10,12–16,20,21,28–30). In WDM, sensory dysfunctions and loss of small-diameter myelinated sural-nerve fibers have been reported, and a neurogenic cause or component has been suggested (9,15,16). Recently, sensory dysfunctions mainly affecting large-diameter myelinated nerve fibers were reported in IBM patients (31). On the basis of abnormalities seen at nerve biopsy, Schröder and Neudecker (32) described a peripheral neuropathy that was assumed to be associated with IBM.

The most obvious morphologic similarity between WDM and IBM is the finding of rimmed vacuoles that correspond to autophagic vacuoles at the ultrastructural level. In association with the autophagic vacuoles, filamentous inclusions are found. They have the same organization, appearance, and diameter as the filamentous inclusions found in IBM (10,20,21,28–30) and in other conditions, including myotonic dystrophy (33) and recessive distal myopathy (4). However, they contrast markedly with the intranuclear 8.5-nm-diameter filaments seen in oculopharyngeal muscular dystrophy (OPMD) (34). The nature of the filamentous inclusions is thus far unknown.

As the rimmed vacuoles and filamentous inclusions appear in disorders with possibly different causes, affecting muscle as well as nerve, they probably are nonspecific phenomena seen in degenerating muscle fibers, as suggested by Diehler and Schröder (33). It is only when they are frequently found and constitute a predominant change that they may be of significance for a given disease. This means that the filaments probably do not play a central role in the pathophysiologic process of WDM. The finding of the filamentous inclusions in WDM further supports the view expressed by several authors that the filamentous inclusions are not specific for IBM.

Thus, there are neurophysiologic and morphologic similarities between these two conditions, even though they obviously have different causes. One can speculate that the degenerative changes seen in the muscles of patients with WDM and IBM may, regardless of their causes, represent a common pathway of neuromuscular degeneration. The common denominator for WDM and IBM may, in this respect, be involvement of both nerve and muscle.

Acknowledgments

This study was supported by grants from the Swedish Medical Research Council (Project 3875) and the Karolinska Institute. We are indebted to Ms Birgitta Hedberg, Ms Lillebil Stuart, and Ms Birgitta Lindegren for excellent technical assistance.

References

1. Welander L. Myopathia distalis tarda hereditaria. *Acta Med Scand* 1951, 141:1–124.
2. Somer H. Distal myopathies. *Neuromusc Disord* 1995, 5:249–252.
3. Markesbery WR, Griggs RC, Leach RP, et al. Late onset hereditary distal myopathy. *Neurology* 1974, 23:127–134.
4. Nonaka I, Sunohara N, Ishiura S, Satoyosi E. Familial distal myopathy with rimmed vacuole and lamellar (myeloid) body formation. *J Neurol Sci* 1981, 51:141–155.
5. Udd B, Partanen J, Halonen P, et al. Tibial muscular dystrophy. Late adult onset distal myopathy in 66 Finnish patients. *Arch Neurol* 1993, 50:604–608.
6. Miyoshi K, Kawai H, Iwasa M, et al. Autosomal recessive distal muscular dystrophy as a new type of progressive muscular dystrophy: seven cases in eight families, including an autopsied case. *Brain* 1986, 109:31–54.
7. Borg K, Åhlberg G, Borg J, Edström L. Welander's, distal myopathy: clinical, neurophysiological and muscle biopsy observations in young and middle-aged adults with early symptoms. *J Neurol Neurosurg Psychiatry* 1991, 54:494–498.

8. Åhlberg G, Jakobsson F, Fransson A, Moritz Å, Borg K, Edström L. Distribution of muscle degeneration in Welander distal myopathy – a magnetic resonance imaging and muscle biopsy study. *Neuromusc Disord* 1994, 4:55–62.

9. Borg K, Borg J, Lindblom U. Sensory involvement in distal myopathy (Welander). *J Neurol Sci* 1987, 80:323–332.

10. Lindberg C, Borg K, Edström L, Hedström A, Oldfors A. Inclusion body myositis and Welander distal myopathy – a clinical, neurophysiological, structural and immunohistological comparison. *J Neurol Sci* 1991, 103:76–81.

11. Borg K, Sachs C, Kaijser L. Autonomic cardiovascular responses in distal myopathy (Welander). *Acta Neurol Scand* 1987, 76:261–266.

12. Edström L. Histochemical and histopathological changes in skeletal muscle in late-onset hereditary distal myoapthy (Welander). *J Neurol Sci* 1975, 26:147–157.

13. Thornell L-E, Edström L, Billeter R, Butler-Browne GS, Kjörell U, Whalen RG. Muscle fibre type composition in distal myopathy (Welander). An analysis with enzyme- and immuno-histochemical, gelelectrophoretic and ultrastructural techniques. *J Neurol Sci* 1984, 65:269–292.

14. Borg J, Grimby L, Hannerz J. Motor neuron firing range, axonal conduction velocity, and muscle fiber histochemistry in neuromuscular diseases. *Muscle Nerve* 1979, 2:423–430.

15. Borg K, Solders G, Borg J, Edström L, Kristensson K. Neurogenic involvement in distal myopathy (Welander). *J Neurol Sci* 1989, 91:53–70.

16. Borg K, Åhlberg G, Hedberg B, Edström L. Muscle fibre degeneration in distal myopathy (Welander) – ultrastructure related to immunohistochemical observations on cytoskeletal proteins at Leu-19. *Neuromusc Disord* 1993, 3:149–155.

17. Edström L, Thornell L-E, Borg K, Butler-Brown G. Expression of neonatal/fetal myosin related to a satellite cell marker (Leu-19) in neurogenic muscle atrophy of man. 1997, subm. for publ.

18. Borg K, Edström L. Prior poliomyelitis – an immunohistochemical study of cytoskeletal proteins and a marker for muscle fibre regeneration in relation to usage of remaining motor units. *Acta Neurol Scand* 1993, 87:128–132.

19. Borg K, Tomé FMS, Edström L. Intranuclear and cytoplasmic filamentous inclusions in distal myopathy (Welander). *Acta Neuropathol* 1991, 82:102–106.

20. Carpenter S, Karpati G, Heller I, Eisen A. Inclusion body myositis: a distinct variety of idiopathic inflammatory myopathy. *Neurology* 1978, 28:8–17.

21. Tomé FMS, Fardeau M, Lebon P, Chevallay M. Inclusion body myositis. *Acta Neuropathol (suppl 8)* 1981, pp. 287–291.

22. Engel AG, Angelini C, Gomez MR. Fingerprint body myopathy: a newly recognized congenital muscle disease. *Proc Mayo Clin* 1972, 47:377–382.

23. Tomé FMS, Fardeau M. "Fingerprint inclusions" in muscle fibres in dystrophia myotonica. *Acta Neuropathol* 1973, 24:62–67.

24. Weber WL, May PE. Abundant class of human DNA polymorphisms which can be typed using the polymerase chain reaction. *Am J Hum Genet* 1989, 44:388–396.

25. Edwards JH. Exclusion mapping. *J Med Genet* 1987, 24:539–543.

26. Bejaoui K, Hirabayashi K, Hentati F, et al. Linkage of Miyoshi myopathy (distal autosomal recessive muscular dystrophy) locus to chromosome 2p12–14. *Neurology* 1995, 45:768–772.
27. Laing NG, Laing BA, Meredith C, et al. Autosomal dominant distal myopathy: linkage to chromosome 14. *Am J Hum Genet* 1995, 56:422–427.
28. Lindberg C, Oldfors A, Hedström A. Inclusion body myositis: peripheral nerve involvement. Combined morphological and electrophysiological studies on peripheral nerve. *J Neurol Sci* 1990, 99:327–338.
29. Lotz BP, Engel AG, Nishino H, Stevens JC, Litchy WJ. Inclusion body myositis. Observations in 40 patients. *Brain* 1989, 112:727–747.
30. Yunis EJ, Samaha F. Inclusion body myositis. *Lab Invest* 1971, 25:240–248.
31. Borg K. Neurogenic involvement in inclusion body myositis – a study with muscle biopsies and determination of somatosensory thresholds. 1997, subm. for publ.
32. Schröder JM, Neudecker S. Peripheral neuropathy associated with inclusion body myositis: proof by sural nerve biopsies. Presented at XXth Oxford Symposium on Muscle Disease, Oxford, 1995.
33. Diehler R, Schröder JM. Lacunar dilatations of intrafusal and extrafusal terminal cisternae, annulate lamellae, confronting cisternae and tubulofilamentous inclusions within the spectrum of muscle and nerve fiber changes in myotonic dystrophy. *Path Res Pract* 1990, 186:371–382.
34. Tomé FMS, Fardeau M. Nuclear inclusions in oculopharyngeal dystrophy. *Acta Neuropathol* 1980, 49:85–87.

14

Tibial Muscular Dystrophy: Clinical, Genetic, and Morphologic Characteristics

BJARNE UDD, HANNU KALIMO,
PEKKA NOKELAINEN, AND HANNU SOMER

Tibial muscular dystrophy (TMD) is one of the most recently defined entities in the category of hereditary distal myopathies (1). The disease appears to be relatively common in Finland. A growing number of patients with TMD have been diagnosed since its discovery in the late 1980s.

Rimmed vacuoles (RVs) seen at muscle biopsy have been reported as major findings in many distal myopathies (2–6), but there are exceptions (7). RVs are inconsistently found in biopsy specimens from TMD patients. None of the 12 biopsied patients in the initially investigated large Larsmo kindred with 26 TMD patients showed RVs (8). In other families, RVs were detected in the muscle biopsy specimens of many patients, and some of those families were genealogically linked to the Larsmo kindred (9). In addition, one recently diagnosed TMD patient belonging to the Larsmo kindred showed a few RVs at muscle biopsy. These findings suggest that the presence or absence RVs does not indicate genetic heterogeneity of the disease. Further morphologic studies have been addressing the inconsistency in the presence of RVs and their role in the degradation of muscle fibers in TMD. Findings and progress from ongoing molecular-genetic investigations are also reported here.

Clinical and Laboratory Findings

TMD patients have no muscle symptoms until 35–40 years of age, when weakness occurs in regard to dorsal extension of the ankles. However, some males have complained of extraordinary muscle pain in their lower leg muscles after strenuous physical exercise while still in their twenties. The ability to walk on one's heels is lost some years after the onset, and the initial symptoms may be asymmetric. In some patients, the onset of weakness in the anterior-compartment muscles of the lower legs is delayed until the seventh decade. After 10–15 years of symptoms, the long toe extensors also become affected, causing bilateral mild to moderate foot-drop. The gait is clumsy, with flapping of the feet, and the knees are lifted slightly higher than normal. In many patients, no other signs occur, and in some patients the weakness is very mild, even at older ages, causing only inability to walk on one's heels, but no further disability. About 10% of the patients will develop mild to moderate weakness of the proximal leg muscles, but all patients have remained ambulant throughout their lifetimes.

The dominating feature on clinical examination is the reduced ability to execute dorsal extension of the ankles, with atrophy of the anterior tibial (TA) muscles, shown by the prominence of the ventral edge of the tibial bone (Figure 14.1). Usually all other muscles are clinically normal, such as shoulder muscles, upper-limb muscles, short toe extensors (EDB), and intrinsic muscles. All tendon reflexes are preserved, and there is no sensory loss.

Serum creatine kinase (CK) concentrations are normal or mildly elevated, up to three to four times the upper limit of normal. Nerve conduction velocities are normal, and there is no reduction of sensory action

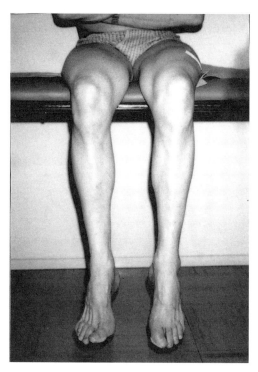

Figure 14.1. Lower legs of a 47-year-old male TMD patient showing atrophy of anterior tibial (TA) muscles.

potentials. Electromyography (EMG) shows profound changes in the TA muscles, consisting in decreased numbers of very low and short polyphasic potentials and some fibrillation activity. Other muscles usually show normal findings at EMG, although at later stages minor myopathic changes can be observed in posterior leg muscles and gluteal and shoulder muscles. There is no myotonia, and, notably, the EDB muscles are normal for the patient's age.

Computed tomography (CT) and magnetic-resonance imaging (MRI) provide very useful and conclusive information regarding the selective muscle involvement in TMD (10). Changes in the TA muscles can be detected by CT and MRI in the initial stages of ankle weakness, and after some additional years the TA muscles will show complete fatty degeneration, whereas other muscles will still be imaged as normal (Figure 14.2). In some patients the long toe extensors will try to compensate for the loss of function in the TA muscles and will bulge into the TA compartment, which can cause EMG and biopsy bias. At later stages of the disease, the long toe extensors will become degenerated, and many patients will also show patches or areas of fatty degeneration in other muscles: hamstrings, medial part of gastrocnemius, soleus, and tensor fasciae latae.

Morphologic Changes Seen at Muscle Biopsy

Histopathology

Because of the high degree of selectivity of the disease process in TMD, findings at muscle biopsy can vary greatly, depending on the muscle

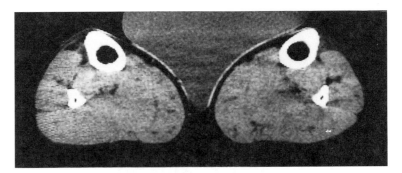

Figure 14.2. CT image of lower-leg muscles of a 54-year-old male TMD patient with almost normal gait, but inability to walk on his heels. Highly selective fatty degeneration of the TA muscles is shown on both sides, and extensor hallucis longus muscles bulge into the space of the TA muscles.

biopsied. Biopsy of the TA muscle usually shows severe nonspecific end-stage dystrophy. In addition to the presence of increased endomysial fatty and fibrous connective tissue, the remaining muscle fibers display markedly increased variations in fiber size, fiber splitting, internalized nuclei, and changes of the inner structure. However, fiber necrosis and phagocytosis are rare, and there are no inflammatory cells (Figure 14.3).

In biopsies of clinically unaffected muscles, such as the vastus lateralis or gastrocnemius, the morphologic findings at routine histochemistry will be normal or will show only slight increases in central nuclei or variations in fiber size. Immunohistochemical methods have been used to determine the expressions of dystrophin, spectrin, desmin, and laminin in affected muscles, all of which have proved normal. Another study with antibodies against adhalin, 43-kDa DAG (β-dystroglycan), the laminin M, A, B1, and B2 chains, and the *C*-terminal and *N*-terminal domains of dystrophin revealed no abnormalities.

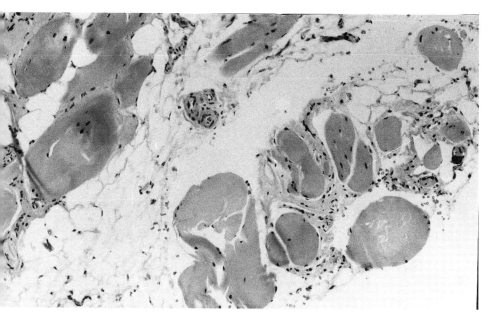

Figure 14.3. Muscle biopsy specimen from TA muscle of the TMD patient in Figure 14.2 showing nonspecific end-stage dystrophy, with increased adipose and connective tissues, variations in fiber size, fiber splitting, structural changes, and increased number of internal nuclei (H&E, ×250).

If a muscle specimen can be obtained from TA muscle before the transformation into end-stage degeneration, variable numbers of RVs will be seen in many, but not all, patients. The proportion of vacuolated fibers can vary from very few (0.1–0.5%) to considerable numbers (5–10%) (Figure 14.4).

Ultrastructural Findings

A recent study has confirmed that the RVs in TMD are ultrastructurally similar to those described in sporadic inclusion-body myositis (IBM). The space of the RV is filled with cellular debris, myeloid bodies, lamellar figures, droplets, amorphous material, smaller (probably secondary) lysosomal vesicles, and degenerating mitochondria. The space is definitely not membrane-bound, nor is the debris always gathered in a limited area, but very often is scattered between myofilaments and is distant from myonuclei (Figure 14.5). Cytoplasmic 15–20-nm filaments are occasionally present in RVs (Figure 14.6), but neither intranuclear 15–20-nm filaments nor cytoplasmic 6–9-nm filaments have been detected. Material consisting of cellular debris is not seen at the ultrastructural level if the biopsy specimen does not show RVs by light microscopy. The number of mitochondria between myofilaments is slightly increased in many biopsy specimens, and occasionally there will be groups of degenerating mitochondria with paracrystalline inclusions.

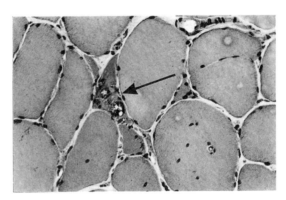

Figure 14.4. Muscle biopsy specimen from TA muscle of a 45-year-old female TMD patient with less advanced dystrophic abnormalities than those shown in Figure 14.3, with RVs in some muscle fibers (arrow) (H&E, ×250).

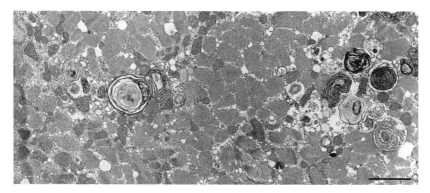

Figure 14.5. Electron micrograph of a TA muscle biopsy specimen from a TMD patient (which showed RVs at light microscopy) showing cellular debris: myeloid figures, small vesicular structures, and amorphous material scattered over a larger area between myofilaments and without any membrane boundary (bar 1 = 1 μm).

Enzyme Histochemical and Immunohistochemical Findings in the Rimmed Vacuoles in TMD

Acid phosphatase activity, studied with the naphthol method, is present in some, but not all, RVs. Specific antibodies to the lysosomal constituents lysozyme, a_1-antitrypsin, and a_1-antichymotrypsin have shown no immunoreactivity to these enzymes in RVs. These findings suggest that the lysosomal degradative system is only partly activated, possibly within the smaller membrane-bound vesicles in the RVs visible by electron microscopy.

On the other hand, many RVs in TMD are immunoreactive for ubiquitin, indicating that non-lysosomal degradative processing takes place in RVs. Positive Congo-red staining has not been detected in the RVs of more than 150 vacuolated muscle fibers examined, however, extremely faint positivity is rarely seen with the specific fluorescence enhancing technique (11). Beta-amyloid protein immunoreactivity has not been detected in RVs. Studies of τ-protein expression have also yielded negative findings (12).

Genetics and Epidemiology

The mode of inheritance of TMD is autosomal-dominant. In the whole patient cohort studied in Finland there have been some apparently spo-

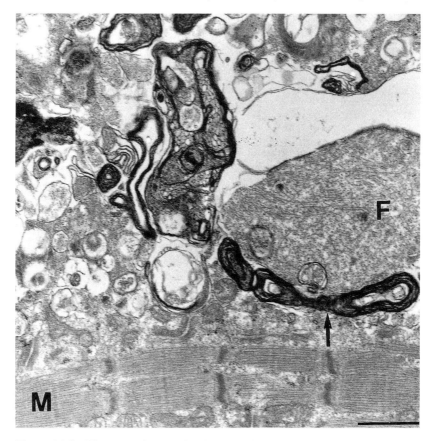

Figure 14.6. Electron micrograph of an RV in a TA muscle biopsy specimen from a TMD patient, showing a bundle of 15–20-nm filaments (F) among the cellular debris, with myeloid figures (arrow) adjacent to myofilaments (M) (bar = 1 μ m).

radic cases of patients without known affected relatives. However, comprehensive family studies have not been conducted in those families, and because TMD can be very mild in some patients, symptoms can easily be overlooked. No clear anticipation has been observed, although in one family with typical TMD in the mother and a son, a grandson has shown general muscle weakness in childhood. His muscle symptoms have not been progressive, thus resembling congenital myopathy, and his muscle biopsy showed RVs, but no other specific abnormalities.

Molecular-genetic-linkage studies have been carried out using mainly the initial large and very complex Larsmo kindred (13). All known loci for muscular dystrophies have been excluded as possible gene loci for TMD (14–19). A random search with 147 highly polymorphic micro-satellite markers has, thus far, not shown any definite linkage (20). Mitochondrial DNA from these patients has been screened for deletions, which have not been found.

The number of diagnosed TMD patients in Finland is still growing because of the increased awareness of TMD as a diagnostic possibility. At the end of 1996 there were more than 140 patients whose disease had been verified by neurologic examination, and they had about 70 known symptomatic relatives, not yet clinically examined. On the basis of those numbers, the prevalence appears to be at least 4/100,000. Patients outside the Finnish population have not been reported.

TMD patients are scattered all over Finland, but a study of the birthplaces of the oldest patients in all of the families affected has revealed an uncommon pattern of geographic origin. There is one cluster of families that originated in the eastern Savo-Karelia area, next to Russia, and another cluster with links to the west-coast region at the Gulf of Bothnia, opposite Sweden (Figure 14.7). The reason for the dual clustering is not known, and the clinical, laboratory, and muscle-biopsy findings are indistinguishable for patients from the two cluster regions (1).

Conclusion

TMD is a relatively mild muscle disease that usually causes clumsiness in walking and moderate foot-drop. Some patients with minor symptoms, occurring very late in life, may not even be aware of any disease, whereas patients with the most pronounced symptoms also develop mild to moderate weakness of the proximal leg muscles. Patients examined before TMD had been defined usually were given a diagnosis of atypical Charcot-Marie-Tooth (CMT) disease. Preserved reflexes, normal EDB muscles, normal nerve conduction velocities and sensory amplitudes, and an absence of chronic neurogenic potentials at EMG testing should help to differentiate TMD from CMT and other neurogenic disorders. The absence of clinically detectable muscle atrophy of upper-limb muscles or shoulder muscles will exclude Welander distal myopathy (21) and scapuloperoneal dystrophy (22). There has been only one family reported with similarities to TMD (23). The patients in that family of French-English ancestry showed more severe progressions of disease, with marked disability, and they also had involvement of upper-limb muscles and intrinsic muscles.

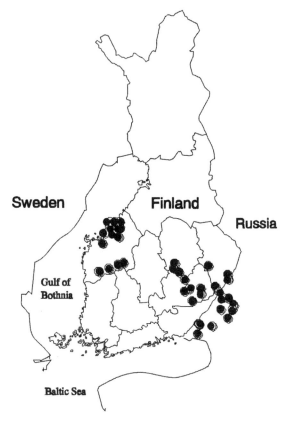

Figure 14.7.   Map of Finland, with dots representing the birthplaces of the oldest patients in the 35 different TMD families. There is one cluster of origins in the eastern Savo-Karelia region, and another one in the west-coast area.

The finding of RVs in TMD is rather peculiar. They are found at a very early stage, mainly in the TA muscle, and they disappear from that muscle later, as the muscle becomes increasingly replaced by fat and connective fibrous tissue. Such RVs share many properties with the RVs described in IBM and other vacuolar myopathies (24). Whether this indicates that they all have a common origin, or whether some RVs appear because of failure in the disposal system for cellular debris, and others because of increased formation of certain cellular debris, is not known. The degradation of muscle fibers in autosomal-recessive distal myopathy with RVs has been reported to be processed through both non-lysosomal and lysosomal pathways (25). A similar mechanism could explain the findings in TMD.

Some hereditary myopathies with RVs have been considered to fit into the concept of hereditary inclusion-body myopathy (26,27). Including TMD in such a category might not necessarily be helpful for further research, but is not harmful either. TMD is clinically well characterized and has some specific features, such as its extreme selectivity of muscle involvement, the clear change to nonspecific dystrophy at later stages, and the possible connection to a limb-girdle-phenotype muscular dystrophy in possible homozygotes. Moreover, we have not been able to clearly demonstrate β-amyloid protein in the RVs of TMD, whereas that protein is considered a hallmark of IBM (28,29). These controversies involving the concept of hereditary inclusion-body myopathy can by no means diminish the importance of the fact that advances to come in molecular-genetic research on the hereditary entities probably will provide useful insights to elucidate the mysteries of IBM.

Acknowledgments

Dr. Fernando Tomé, from the Institut National de la Santé et de la Recherche Médicale in Paris, France, has kindly performed the immuno-cytochemical studies with antibodies against adhalin, 43-kDa DAG, the laminin M, A, B1, and B2 chains, and the *C*-terminal and *N*-terminal domains of dystrophin.

References

1. Udd B, Partanen J, Halonen P, et al. Tibial muscular dystrophy – late adult onset distal myopathy in 66 Finnish patients. *Arch Neurol* 1993, 50:604–608.
2. Griggs R, Markesbery W. Distal myopathies. In: Engel AG, Franzini-Armstrong C (eds), *Myology*, 2nd ed. New York; McGraw-Hill, 1994; pp. 1246–1257.
3. Borg K, Ahlberg G, Hedberg B, Edström L. Muscle fiber degeneration in distal myopathy (Welander) – ultrastructure related to immunohistochemical observations on cytoskeletal proteins and Leu-19 antigen. *Neuromusc Disord* 1993, 3:149–155.
4. Borg K, Tomé F, Edström L. Intranuclear and cytoplasmatic filamentous inclusions in distal myopathy (Welander). *Acta Neuropathol* 1991, 82:102–106.
5. Nonaka I, Sunohara N, Ishiura S, Satoyoshi E. Familial distal myopathy with rimmed vacuoles and lamellar (myeloid) body formation. *J Neurol Sci* 1981, 151:141–155.
6. Villanova M, Kawai M, Lübke U, et al. Rimmed vacuoles of inclusion body myositis and oculopharyngeal muscular dystrophy contain amyloid precursor protein and lysosomal markers. *Brain Res* 1993, 603:343–347.

7. Miyoshi K, Kawai H, Iwasa M, Kusaka K, Nishino H. Autosomal distal dystrophy as a new type of progressive muscular dystrophy. *Brain* 1986, 109:31–54.

8. Udd B, Rapola J, Nokelainen P, Arikawa E, Somer H. Nonvacuolar myopathy in a large family with both late adult onset distal myopathy and limb-girdle type muscular dystrophy. *J Neurol Sci* 1992, 113:214–221.

9. Udd B, Somer H. Tibial muscular dystrophy. *Neurology* 1993, 43:A202 (abstract).

10. Udd B, Lamminen A, Somer H. Imaging methods reveal unexpected patchy lesions in late onset distal myopathy. *Neuromusc Disord* 1991, 1:271–280.

11. Askanaz V, Engel WK, Alvarez M. Enhanced detection of Congo-red-positive amyloid deposits in muscle fibers in inclusion body myositis and brain of Alzheimer's disease using fluoroscence technique. *Neurology* 1993, 43:1265.

12. Udd B, Somer H, Kalimo H. Tibial muscular dystrophy – rimmed vacuoles with irregular lysosomal activity. *Eur J Neurol* 1995, 2:118.

13. Udd B. Limb-girdle type muscular dystrophy in a large family with distal myopathy: homozygous manifestation of a dominant gene? *J Med Genet* 1992, 29:383–389.

14. Bejaoui K, Hirabayashi K, Hentati F, et al. Linkage of Miyoshi myopathy (distal autosomal recessive muscular dystrophy) to chromosome 2p12–14. *Neurology* 1995, 45:768–72.

15. Laing NG, Laing BA, Meredith C, et al. Autosomal dominant myopathy: linkage to chromosome 14. *Am J Hum Genet* 1995a, 56:422–27.

16. Abizi K, Bachner L, Beckman J, Matsumura K, Hamouda E, Chanouch M, Chanouch A, Ait-Ouarab R, Vignal A, Weissenbach J, Vinet M-C, Leturq F, Collin H, Tomé FMS, Reghis A, Fardeau M, Campbell KP, Kaplan J-C. Severe childhood autosomal recessive muscular dystrophy with deficiency of the 50kDa dystrophin-associated glycoprotein maps to chromosome 13q12. *Hum Molec Gen* 1993, 2: 1423–1428.

17. Speer M, Yamaoka L, Gilchrist J, Gaskell C, Stajich J, Vance J, Kazantsev A, Lastra A, Haynes C, Beckman J, et al. Confirmation of genetic heterogeneity in limb-girdle muscular dystrophy: linkage of an autosomal dominant form to chromosome 5q. *Am J Hum Genet* 1992, 6:1211–1217.

18. Fougerousse F, Broux O, Richard I, Allamand V, Pereira de Souza A, Bourg N, Brenguier L, Devaud C, Pasturaud P, Roudaut C, Chiannikulchai N, Hillaire D, Bui H, Chumakov I, Weissenbach J, Cherif D, Cohen D, Beckman J. Mapping of a chromosome 15 region involved in limb girdle muscular dystrophy. *Hum Molec Genet* 1994, 3:285–293.

19. Love D, Hill D, Dickson G, Spurr N, Byth C, Marsden R, Walsh F, Edwards Y, Davis K. An autosomal transcript in skeletal muscle with homology to dystrophin. *Nature* 1989, 339:55–58.

20. Nokelainen P, Udd B, Somer H, Peltonen L. Linkage analyses in a novel muscular dystrophy. *Human Heredity* 1996, 46:98–107.

21. Welander L. Myopathia distalis tarda hereditaria. *Acta Med Scand* 1951, 141:1–124.

22. Thomas P, Schott G, Morgan-Hughes J. Adult onset scapuloperoneal myopathy. *J Neurol Neurosurg Psychiatry* 1975, 38:1008–1015.

23. Markesbery W, Griggs R, Leach L, Lapham L. Late onset hereditary distal myopathy. *Neurology* 1974, 23:127–134.

24. Engel AG, Banker B. Focal cytoplasmic degradation and autophagic mechanisms. In: Engel AG, Franzini-Armstrong C (eds), *Myology*, 2nd ed. New York; McGraw-Hill, 1994, pp. 966–975.
25. Kumamoto T, Ueyama H, Watanabe S, Kominami E, Ando M. Muscle fiber degradation in distal myopathy with rimmed vacuoles. *Acta Neuropathol* 1994, 87:143–148.
26. Neville H, Baumbach L, Ringel S, Russo L, Sujansky E, Garcia L. Familial inclusion body myositis: evidence for autosomal dominant inheritance. *Neurology* 1992, 42:897–902.
27. Sadeh M, Gadoth N, Hadar H, Ben-David E. Vacuolar myopathy sparing the quadriceps. *Brain* 1993, 116:217–232.
28. Mendell J-R, Sahenk Z, Gales T, Paul L. Amyloid filaments in inclusion body myositis. Novel findings provide insight into nature of filaments. *Arch Neurol* 1991, 48:1229–1234.
29. Askanas V, Engel WK, Alvarez RB, Glenner GG. Beta-amyloid protein immunoreactivity in muscle of patients with inclusion-body myositis. *Lancet* 1992, 339:560–561.

15

Distal Myopathy with Rimmed Vacuoles, Inclusion-Body Myositis, and Related Disorders in Japan

EIJIRO SATOYOSHI, NOBUHIKO SUNOHARA, AND IKUYA NONAKA

Rimmed-vacuole formation is a nonspecific pathologic feature seen in a variety of neuromuscular disorders, but it may be pathognomonic for several diseases, including inclusion-body myositis (IBM) and distal myopathy with rimmed-vacuole formation (DMRV), because in these two diseases there is no other change that could explain the muscle atrophy. At the 11th International Meeting on Neuromuscular Diseases, held in Marseille in 1992, we discussed the possible significance of "rimmed" vacuoles in a variety of neuromuscular disorders (1–3). Of 3,260 muscle biopsies studied in our National Center of Neurology and Psychiatry over the past 14 years there were 82 that showed more than three muscle fibers with rimmed vacuoles in a single low-power microscopic field (magnification, ×20). Among those biopsy specimens, rimmed vacuoles were most frequently found in specimens from IBM, DMRV, oculopharyngodistal myopathy, Marinesco-Sjögren syndrome, and the glycogen-storage diseases. However, there were only five cases of IBM (Table 15.1).

IBM is much less frequent in Japan than in Western countries, whereas DMRV is much more common. The reason for this difference is not known. Racial, nutritional, or environmental factors may play some role, but the differing diagnostic criteria for IBM may be an important factor. We have attempted to get a more accurate estimate of the incidences of IBM, DMRV, and other myopathies with rimmed vacuoles in Japan by surveying the experience with such diseases in our major hospitals and institutions over the past 10 years.

Materials and Methods

We obtained clinical and pathologic information on 248 patients with myopathies involving rimmed vacuoles at 53 hospitals and institutions;

Table 15.1. *Incidence of inflammatory myopathies in NCNP*[a]

Diseases	Numbers of patients	Percentage
IBM	5	3.5
Polymyositis	75	52.4
Dematomyositis	53	37.1
Others	10	7.0
Total	143	

[a]Incidence of inflammatory myopathies revealed by 3,260 muscle biopsies studied at the National Center of Neurology and Psychiatry (NCNP) over the past 14 years.

the data were gathered by members of a muscular-dystrophy research group sponsored by Japan's Department of Health and Welfare. Among those cases were patients with IBM, DMRV, oculopharyngeal muscular dystrophy (4), oculopharyngodistal myopathy (5, 6), limb-girdle myopathy, spinal muscular atrophy, Marinesco-Sjögren syndrome, polymyositis, and glycogenoses.

The following data for the 248 patients were recorded: age, gender, age at onset of myopathy, distribution of muscle weakness and atrophy, systemic involvement (complication), electromyographic (EMG) findings, serum creatine kinase (CK) concentration, muscle biopsy findings, final diagnosis, course of disease, and degree of disability, evaluated as activities-of-daily-living (ADL) scores (13) in relation to the disease duration.

Results

The numbers of patients in the diagnostic categories are shown in Table 15.2. There were 7 patients (2.8%) with oculopharyngeal muscular dystrophy, 23 (9.3%) with oculopharyngodistal myopathy, 114 (46.0%) with DMRV, 41 (16.5%) with IBM, and 63 (25.4%) with other myopathies, including limb-girdle myopathy, spinal muscular atrophy, polymyositis, Marinesco-Sjögren syndrome, and the glycogenoses. A striking feature was that there were large numbers of patients with DMRV and oculopharyngodistal myopathy in our patient group. The incidence of IBM, on the other hand, was quite low, and the ratio of IBM to DMRV was 1 : 3.

Table 15.2. *DMRV, IBM, and related myopathies in 248 patients*[a]

Disease	Number of patients	Percentage
Oculopharyngeal muscular dystrophy	7	2.8
Oculopharyngodistal myopathy	23	9.3
DMRV	114	46.0
IBM	41	16.5
Other myopathies (limb-girdle myopahty, spinal muscular atrophy, polymyositis, Marinesco-Sjögren syndrome, glycogenosis, and others)	63	25.4
Total	248	

[a]An analysis of 248 patients with rimmed-vacuole myopathies from 53 hospitals and institutions where members of a muscular-dystrophy research group are working.

We first described oculopharyngodistal myopathy as a distinct clinical entity (6) in 1975. This is an autosomal-dominant myopathy that is characterized clinically by slowly progressive ptosis and extraocular palsy and weakness of the masseter, facial, and bulbar muscles as well as the distal limb muscles. Symptoms usually begin in the fourth or fifth decade of life. This myopathy appears to be quite rare in Western countries (7) and is also infrequently reported in Japan (8–10). For the 23 patients with oculopharyngodistal myopathy, the male-to-female ratio was 3:1, and the age at onset averaged 41 years. Their serum CK concentrations were normal or only slightly elevated. In the early stage of the disease, the muscle biopsy findings included striking variations in fiber size, with numerous rimmed vacuoles. Later there was marked loss of muscle fibers, with endomysial fibrosis and fatty infiltration. This is a very slowly progressive myopathy, and most patients survive beyond 80 years, with only some difficulties in walking, swallowing, and phonation.

Among the 114 patients with DMRV, the inheritance pattern appeared to be autosomal-recessive for 47, autosomal-dominant for 8, and sporadic for 59. Patients with the autosomal-dominant inheritance pattern appeared to differ somewhat from those with recessive inheritance, both clinically and pathologically. However, data from the autosomal-dominant group were omitted from this study. For autosomal-recessive DMRV, the ages at onset ranged from 10 to 35 years, with a mean of 24 ± 5 years, compared with 12 to 61 years, with a mean of 30 ± 11 years, for the sporadic group (Figure 15.1). The incidence of DMRV was the same for men and women. The symptoms and distributions of muscle weakness and atrophy were similar to those in our original reports (11–13). Gradually progressive distal muscle weakness and atrophy, particularly affecting the anterior tibial group of muscles, were seen very early in the disease. Neck muscles were also affected. Serum CK concentrations usually were normal or only slightly elevated. EMG showed myopathic changes, with some neurogenic features as well. There were marked size variations in muscle fibers, with numerous rimmed vacuoles seen at biopsy, but no obvious muscle-fiber necrosis.

Figure 15.2 shows the ADL functional scores (13) for the lower limbs at various stages of the disease. For example, ADL 8 means "confined to bed," and ADL 7 means "moves using wheelchair with assistance" (13). Within 10 years after the onset of symptoms, 40% of the patients had

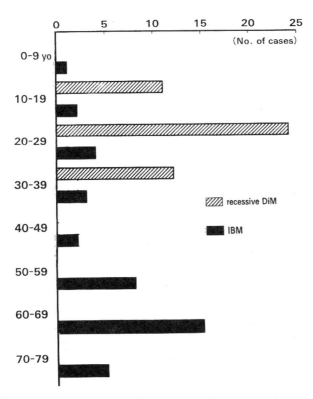

Figure 15.1. Ages at onset for 47 patients with autosomal-recessive distal myopathy with rimmed-vacuole formation (DMRV) and 41 patients with inclusion-body myositis (IBM).

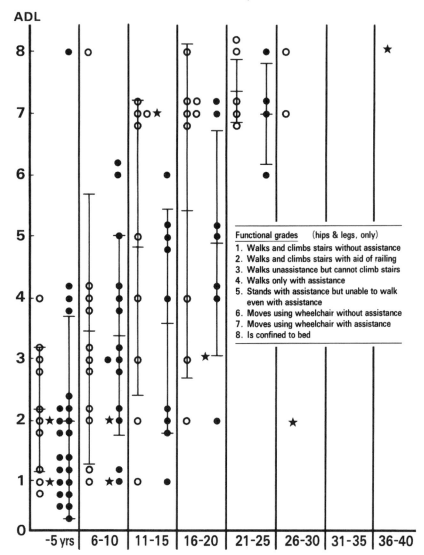

★ =autosomal dominant, ○ =autosomal recessive, ● =sporadic

Figure 15.2.   ADL scores and durations of disease for 114 patients with DMRV. ADL functional grading was limited to hips and legs. ADL 1: Walks and climbs stairs without assistance. ADL 2: Walks and climbs stairs with aid of railing. ADL 3: Walks without assistance, but cannot climb stairs. ADL 4: Walks only with assistance. ADL 5: Stands with assistance, but unable to walk even with assistance. ADL 6: Moves using wheelchair without assistance. ADL 7: Moves using wheelchair with assistance. ADL 8: Is confined to bed.

deteriorated to ADL 4 ("walks only with assistance"). Between 11 and 20 years after onset, more than 50% were severely disabled (ADL 7 or 8), and after 20 years all patients were bedridden. Thus, the prognosis in this disease is not good.

In 41 patients with IBM, the ages at onset ranged from 4 to 76 years, with a mean of 53 ± 21 years, but most of the patients became symptomatic between 50 and 70 years of age, as shown in Figure 15.1. The male-to-female ratio was 3 : 1. Muscle weakness and atrophy were generally proximal or diffuse, with some asymmetry. Only 15% of the patients had distal muscle weakness. Inflammatory changes and inclusions were seen at more than 75% of muscle biopsies. The clinical course and muscle abnormalities in IBM differed from those in DMRV.

Discussion

IBM is a nonhereditary disease with a male predominance, usually presenting with proximal muscle weakness after the age of 50 years (14–16). In Western countries, IBM is a fairly common diagnosis among the inflammatory myopathies. Lotz et al. (17) reported an IBM incidence of 28% among all inflammatory myopathies. In Japan, however, IBM is reported much less frequently. In a previous review of 3,260 muscle biopsies in our National Center of Neurology and Psychiatry there were only 5 patients with IBM among 143 patients with inflammatory myopathies, whereas there were 18 patients with DMRV. One might raise the possibility that IBM was misdiagnosed as DMRV, because rimmed-vacuole formation is common to both diseases.

Of the 248 cases of rimmed-vacuole myopathy collected from 53 hospitals in Japan, IBM accounted for only 16.5% of the cases, whereas DMRV accounted for 46%, giving a ratio of 1:3. A large-scale investigation confirmed the low incidence of IBM and the high incidence of DMRV in Japan – a striking feature of muscle disease in Japan. The different incidences of these two diseases in Japan may be related to a racial factor or some environmental factor, such as nutrition. The high incidence of autosomal-dominant oculopharyngodistal myopathy is another unusual feature in Japan; its pathologic changes seen at muscle biopsy are quite similar to those in DMRV (i.e., myopathic changes, with rimmed-vacuole formation). Clinically, distal muscle weakness, particularly anterior tibial muscle weakness, and atrophy are seen in both diseases. These findings suggest that the two diseases may have pathogenetic similarities, but molecular-genetic studies will be required to define the relationship between them.

A review of 106 patients with autosomal-recessive and sporadic forms of DMRV showed that the age at onset of DMRV was different from that for IBM. The onset of DMRV usually was in early adulthood, whereas for IBM the onset usually was after 50 years of age. The gender ratios in the two diseases were also different: There was a male predominance of 3:1 in IBM, whereas DMRV affected the two genders equally. Our review of the clinical and laboratory studies of myopathies with rimmed vacuoles has not added any new information, except regarding prognosis. For all 106 patients with DMRV, the disease took a relentlessly progressive course, and most of the patients were confined to bed within 10 years. The progressive course of DMRV was quite different from that in IBM. Some patients with IBM responded to treatment, and none showed such a rapid progressive course.

Conclusions

Our review of 248 patients with rimmed-vacuole myopathies from 53 Japanese hospitals and institutions revealed the following:

1. There were 7 patients (2.8%) with oculopharyngeal muscular dystrophy, 23 patients (9.3%) with oculopharyngodistal myopathy, 114 patients (46.0%) with DMRV, 41 patients (16.5%) with IBM, and 63 patients (25.4%) with other myopathies, which included Marinesco-Sjögren syndrome, spinal muscular atrophy, and the glycogenoses.
2. In Japan, the low incidence of IBM was in striking contrast to the high incidence of DMRV, a finding quite different from those in Western countries. Oculopharyngodistal myopathy, found in approximately 10% of our patients, is also rare in Western countries.
3. There were 106 patients with autosomal-recessive or sporadic DMRV with onset in early adulthood. The DMRV affected the two genders equally, showing a progressive downhill course, and all the patients were bedridden within 20 years of onset.
4. There were 41 patients with IBM. The age at onset was after 50 years in most patients, and the male-to-female ratio was 3:1. The distributions of weakness and atrophy were proximal or diffuse, and occasionally were asymmetrical.

References

1. Satoyoshi E, Murakami N, Takemitsu M, Nonaka I. Significance of "rimmed" vacuoles in various neuromuscular disorders. In *Advances in Neuromuscular Diseases, Nervous System, Muscles and Systemic Disorders*, Serratrice G et al. (eds). Paris, Expansion Scientifique Française, 1993, pp. 83–92.

2. Murakami N, Ihara Y, Nonaka I. Muscle fiber degeneration in distal myopathy with rimmed vacuole formation. *Acta Neuropathol* 89:29–34, 1995.

3. Murakami N, Takemitsu M, Kurashige T, Nonaka I. Significance of rimmed vacuoles in neuromuscular diseases: a comparative immunohistochemical study of inclusion body myositis and distal myopathy with rimmed vacuole formation (in Japanese). *Clin Neurol* 34:782–787, 1994.

4. Victor M, Hayes R, Adams RD. Oculopharyngeal muscular dystrophy: a familial disease of late life characterized by dysphagia and progressive ptosis of the eyelids. *N Engl J Med* 267:1267–1272, 1962.

5. Satoyoshi E, Murakami K, Kowa H, Kinoshita M, Torii J. Distal involvement of the extremities in ocular myopathy. *Am J Ophthalmol* 59:668–673, 1965.

6. Satoyoshi E, Kinoshita M. Oculopharyngodistal myopathy. Report of four families. *Arch Neurol* 34:89–92, 1977.

7. Schotland DL, Rowland LP. Muscular dystrophy; features of ocular myopathy, distal myopathy and myotonic dystrophy. *Arch Neurol* 15:678–684, 1965.

8. Ukawa G, Kurisaki H, Takatsu N, Sugita H, Toyokura Y. A case of oculopharyngodistal myopathy with striking rimmed vacuoles (in Japanese). *Neurol Med* 17:71–74, 1984.

9. Morimatsu M, Hirai S, Eto H, Yoshikawa M, Tomonaga M. A family of oculopharyngodistal myopathy (in Japanese). *Clin Neurol* 13:529–535, 1973.

10. Goto I, Hayakawa T, Miyoshi Y, Iino K, Kusunoki K. A case of oculopharyngodistal myopathy with cardiomyopathy (in Japanese). *Clin Neurol* 13:529–535, 1973.

11. Nonaka I, Sunohara N, Satoyoshi E. Familial distal myopathy with rimmed vacuole and lamellar (myeloid) body formation. *J Neurol Sci* 51:141–155, 1981.

12. Nonaka I, Sunohara N, Satoyoshi E, Terasawa K, Yonemoto K. Autosomal recessive distal muscular dystrophy: a comparative study with distal myopathy with rimmed vacuole formation. *Ann Neurol* 17:51–59, 1985.

13. Sunohara N, Nonaka I, Kamei H, Satoyoshi E. Distal myopathy with rimmed vacuole formation: a follow up study. *Brain* 112:65–83, 1989.

14. Yunis EJ, Samaha FJ. Inclusion body myositis. *Lab Invest* 25:240–248, 1971.

15. Carpenter S, Karpati G, Heller I, Eisen A. Inclusion body myositis: a distinct variety of idiopathic inflammatory myopathy. *Neurology* 28:8–17, 1978.

16. Mikol J, Engel AG. Inclusion body myositis. In *Myology*, vol. 2, Engel AG, Franzini-Amstrong (eds). New York, McGraw-Hill, 1994, pp. 1384–1398.

17. Lotz BP, Engel AG, Nishino H, Stevens JC, Lichty WJ. Inclusion body myositis. *Brain* 112:724–747, 1989.

16

Inclusion-Body Myopathies

MICHEL FARDEAU AND FERNANDO TOMÉ

The spectrum of myopathies defined by the presence of rimmed vacuoles and 15–18-nm filamentous intranuclear and/or intrasarcoplasmic inclusions has grown rapidly over the past 10 years. The great majority of cases reported since the early description by Yunis and Samaha (1) have been sporadic, and the patients have shown some clinical or histopathologic inflammatory features (2,3). There was only one family study among the early reports (4). In 1986 we briefly reported the first observation of a consanguineous family in which two siblings were affected (5). Later it became obvious that those two cases were much like the cases of vacuolar myopathies with autosomal-recessive inheritance described in the Iranian Jewish community (6). More recently, a family in which there was inclusion-body myopathy, with a postulated dominant inheritance, was reported (7).

Herein we report a series of 12 familial cases of inclusion-body myopathies. We add two sporadic cases of very early onset in which there were unusual clinical features (ophthalmoplegia) and for which it is still impossible to establish an acquired or genetic origin.

Hereditary Autosomal-Recessive Inclusion-Body Myopathy (h-AR-IBM)

Five cases involving four families fell into the h-AR-IBM category (Table 16.1). The first of those families, examined in 1981, came from Iran (Jewish community); the second was from Tunisia, the third from Belgium, and the fourth from Mexico. In three of those families there was close consanguinity between the parents.

The clinical onset was generally in early adulthood, even if slight motor difficulties had sometimes been noticed during childhood (family no. 4). The mean age at clinical onset (walking difficulties) was 20.8 years, and the mean age at diagnosis was 30 years.

The muscle involvement was bilateral, sometimes slightly asymmetrical. Proximal and distal muscles were affected, and the patients showed

Table 16.1. *AR-IBM*

Patient	Sex	Age at onset (years)	Age at diagnosis (years)	Clinical pattern	CK IU/l	EMG	Evolution	Genetics	Origin
1	F	15	28	Legs > arms P & D	375	M	Slowly progressive	Parents 1st cousins; 1 brother affected	Iran
2	M	20	25	Legs > arms, P & D	470	M ± N	Slowly progressive	Parents 1st cousins; 2 sisters affected	Tunisia
3	F	20	28	Legs > arms, P & D	334	M	Slowly progressive (loss walk 25 y)	No consanguinity; 1 sister affected	Belgium
4	M	19	29	Legs > arms, P & D	—	—	Slowly progressive	Brother of patient 5; parents 1st cousins	Mexico
5	M	30	42	Legs > arms, P & D	169	M	Slowly progressive	Brother of patient 4; parents 1st cousins	Mexico

a waddling gait and steppage. Weakness was most pronounced in pelvic-girdle muscles, with consistent and surprising sparing of quadriceps muscles. Extensors and flexors of the feet were affected. There was marked weakness of neck flexors and trunk muscles. Facial, oculomotor, and velopharyngeal muscles were unaffected. Tendon reflexes were weak or absent. There was no sign of heart involvement. Intellect was normal.

The electromyographic (EMG) findings were myogenic in four cases, and one case showed a mixed pattern. Muscle conduction velocities (MCV) were normal. Serum creatine kinase (CK) levels were moderately elevated. Disease evolution was slowly and steadily progressive. Loss of the ability to walk occurred at 25 years of age for patient 3.

Histopathology

Muscle biopsies showed, in all cases, marked variation in the sizes of muscle fibers, with a few dispersed atrophic fibers. However, the most striking feature was the presence of numerous rimmed vacuoles, sometimes with red inclusions within them by trichrome staining. There was no evidence of necrotic or inflammatory changes in the biopsy specimens. At the ultrastructural level, numerous vacuoles were filled with pseudomyelinic debris and clusters of typical 15–18-nm filaments. In only one case did a single nucleus show the presence of a filamentous inclusion (not typical of IBM).

Hereditary Autosomal-Dominant Inclusion-Body Myopathy (h-AD-IBM)

Seven cases involving four families, with pedigrees compatible with autosomal-dominant inheritance, fell into the h-AD-IBM category (Table 16.2). Transmission was either from the mother or from the father to sons or daughters.

The myopathy was expressed in adulthood: The mean age at clinical onset was 35 years, and the mean age at diagnosis was 49 years. One of the families was of Portuguese origin, the three other families were French.

The pattern of muscle involvement was diffuse, without marked selectivity. Scapulohumeral and pelvihumeral muscles were weak and atrophic, including quadriceps muscles. Distal muscles were also affected, especially foot dorsiflexors. The muscle weakness was bilateral and rather symmetrical in six cases; it was markedly asymmetrical in one case. Neck flexors were weak in all cases, and variable degrees of velopharyngeal muscle involvement were present in three of the seven cases.

Table 16.2. *AD-IBM*

Patient	Sex	Age at onset (years)	Age at diagnosis (years)	Clinical pattern	EMG	Evolution	Genetics
1	M	50	57	Upper & lower limbs, SCM, trunk muscles	M	Slowly progressive	Father of patient 2
2	M	48	50	Upper & lower limbs, SCM, trunk muscles	M	Slowly progressive	Son of patient 1
3	F	35	59	Upper & lower limbs, P & D, weakness of neck muscles	M	Slowly progressive (loss walk 64 y)	Mother of patient 4
4	M	32	39	Pelvic > scapular, diffuse weakness of neck muscles	M	Slowly progressive (loss walk 37 y)	Son of patient 3
5	M	48	67	Limb muscles, P & D, SCM, velopharynx	M	Slowly progressive	(Mother affected)
6	F	11	33	Lower & upper limbs, P & D, SCM, velopharynx	M	Slowly progressive (loss walk 25 y)	Sister of patient 7 (mother affected)
7	M	20	31	Lower & upper limbs, P & D, SCM, velopharynx	M	Slowly progressive (loss walk 27 y)	Brother of patient 6 (mother affected)

Slight facial weakness was noticed in one case. Curiously, one patient (no. 3) was also affected by Paget disease.

EMG findings were myogenic in all cases, and MCVs were within the normal range. Serum CK levels were normal or slightly elevated. Disease evolution was slowly and steadily progressive. Four patients became wheelchair-bound at ages between 25 and 64 years.

Histopathology

Muscle biopsy specimens were studied for six of the seven patients; in one case (patient no. 1), only paraffin-embedded material could be examined. Besides variations in the sizes of muscle fibers and increased number of internal nuclei, rimmed vacuoles were found at all biopsies. There was no necrosis, nor any inflammatory change. Immunocytochemical techniques revealed the presence of ubiquitin in the vacuoles in the two cases in which such studies were conducted (8). At the ultrastructural level, clusters of 15–18-nm filaments were found within the cytoplasm and in the nuclei in all biopsy specimens.

Severe, Unclassified, Sporadic Cases of Inclusion-Body Myopathy with Ophthalmoplegia

This category included two very unusual cases of inclusion-body myopathy. The first case was that of a young black girl from Central Africa who presented at 9 years of age, after a pulmonary lobectomy for recurrent bronchopulmonary infections, progressive weakness of limb-girdle muscles. At examination, she was found to have almost complete ophthalmoplegia, with discrete ptosis. Dysphagia was also observed. There was no sign of cystic fibrosis. HIV and HTLV-1 tests were negative. The disease evolution was severe, without any response to corticosteroid treatment.

The second case involved a young girl of French origin who had walking difficulties, dysphonia, and dysphagia at 16 years of age. The disease evolution was rapid, with proximal and distal muscle weakness. Marked limitations of eye movements were detected at 19 years of age, with moderate ptosis. Tests with cholinergic-receptor antibodies were negative and pharmacologic tests with anticholinesterase drugs yielded no improvement. EMG showed a myogenic pattern, without neuromuscular block. Her serum CK level was slightly elevated.

Both cases were sporadic, without any family history of neuromuscular disease.

Histopathology

In both cases there were quite unusual numbers of muscle fibers, atrophic or not, that showed typical rimmed vacuoles. There was no necrosis, nor any inflammatory change. At electron microscopy, both biopsy specimens showed abundant intracytoplasmic and intranuclear clusters of 15–18-nm filaments (Figure 16.1).

Discussion

Today, hereditary inclusion-body myopathies have been clearly delineated as genetic myopathies distinct from "classic" sporadic inclusion-body myositis (1,2,9,10). At least three main forms have been described: an autosomal-recessive form well identified in the Iranian Jewish community (6,11), an autosomal-dominant form (one reported family fitting with this mode of inheritance) (7), and the autosomal-dominant oculopharyngodistal myopathy reported in Japan (12).

Our studies have included four families belonging in the category of hereditary autosomal-recessive inclusion-body myopathy (h-AR-IBM) and four families in the category of hereditary autosomal-dominant inclusion-body myopathy (h-AD-IBM). Three of the four families in the h-AR-IBM category were mentioned in other publications: case 1 of Massa et al. (13), case 2 of Hentati et al. (14), and cases 4 and 5 of Fardeau et al. (5, 15). Clinically they share the clinical pattern described by Argov and Yarom (6) and by Sadeh et al. (11), with the unusual and surprising sparing of the quadriceps muscles contrasting with the weakness and atrophy of the distal posterior thigh muscles.

The four h-AD-IBM families have not previously been reported. Their clinical pattern was different from that for the h-AR-IBM families, with proximal and distal involvement of limb muscles, including the quadriceps. Curiously, neck flexors and velopharyngeal muscles often were markedly involved. That pattern seems to be slightly different from the pattern described by Neville et al. (7), in which scapular-girdle muscles were preferentially affected.

It is noticeable that in our series the number of cases of hereditary IBM (h-IBM) equaled the number of cases of sporadic inclusion-body myositis (s-IBM). Of course, that may be partially explainable by a recruitment bias, mainly oriented toward genetic disorders in our clinic. However, it

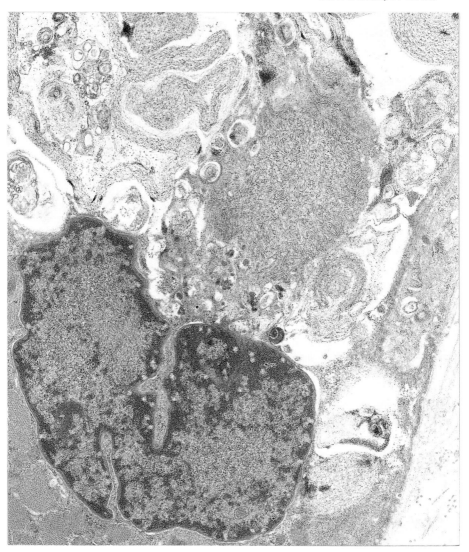

Figure 16.1. Severe sporadic case of IBM with ophthalmoplegia (case 1). Electron micrograph of a muscle fiber, transversely sectioned, showing a large collection of 15–18-nm filaments within a vacuole that also contains myelin bodies and various cytoplasmic debris. A small collection of identical filaments lies on the left portion of an indented nucleus (×12,500).

Table 16.3. *Filamentous inclusions*

Disease	Rimmed vacuoles	Cytoplasmic inclusions	Nuclear inclusions	Inflammation
s-IBM, "classic" (10 cases)	+	+	+	+
s-IBM, early onset (2 cases)	+	+	+	−
h-AD-IBM (4 cases)	+	+	+	−
h-AR-IBM (4 cases)	+	+	−	−

underlines the possibility of misdiagnosing a sporadic case as an inflammatory disease (rather than a genetic disorder), and thus it represents a serious diagnostic challenge.

In our series of cases, two unclassified cases were included. The first one has been briefly reported (16). Both were remarkable for their early onset in childhood, their unusual occurrence of ophthalmoplegia, and their evolutive severity. There were no inflammatory changes in the muscle biopsy specimens, but there were unusually large numbers of rimmed vacuoles. These cases might be compared to the oculopharyngodistal myopathy (12) or the oculopharyngeal muscular dystrophy associated with distal myopathy reported in Japan (17), both of which are characterized by the presence of rimmed vacuoles; but our cases were sporadic and of early onset, and there was no history of neuromuscular involvement in the patients' families.

The last point to be mentioned concerns the variable locations of the 15–18-nm filamentous inclusions in our series of cases (Table 16.3). The characteristic filamentous inclusions were identical in the different myopathies, but there were some differences in their locations. They were found both in the cytoplasm and in nuclei in the s-IBM cases, in the h-AD-IBM cases, and in the two severe cases with ophthalmoplegia. But in the h-AR-IBM cases they were found only in the cytoplasm of the muscle fibers. As we believe (18) that the vacuoles essentially result from nuclear abnormalities, that difference in location may only reflect variations in the frequencies of the nuclear abnormalities in these different myopathies.

References

1. Yunis E, Samaha FJ. Inclusion body myositis. *Lab Invest* 1971, 25:240–248.
2. Carpenter S, Karpati G, Heller I, Eisen A. Inclusion body myositis: a distinct variety of idiopathic inflammatory myopathy. *Neurology*, 1978, 28:8–17.

3. Ringel SP, Kenny CE, Neville HE, Giorne R, Carry MR. Spectrum of inclusion body myositis. *Arch Neurol* 1987, 44:1154–1157.

4. Eisen A, Berry K, Gibson G. Inclusion body myositis (IBM): Myopathy or neuropathy? *Neurology* 1983, 33:1109–1114.

5. Fardeau M, Tomé FMS, Chevallay M, Collin H, Lebon P, Fournier JG. Inclusion body myositis-like filamentous inclusions in several cases of hereditary neuro-muscular disorders (abstract). *Muscle Nerve* 9:5S.

6. Argov Z, Yarom R. "Rimmed vacuole myopathy" sparing the quadriceps: a unique disorder in Iranian Jews. *J. Neuro Sci* 1984, 64:33–43.

7. Neville HE, Baumbach LL, Ringel SP, Russo LS, Sujansky E, Garcia CA. Familial inclusion body myositis: evidence for autosomal dominant inheritance. *Neurology* 1992, 42:897–902.

8. Leclerc A, Tomé FMS, Fardeau M. Ubiquitin and β-amyloid protein in inclusion body myositis (IBM), familial IBM-like disorder and oculopharyngeal muscular dystrophy: an immunocytochemical study. *Neuromusc Disord* 1993, 3:283–292.

9. Salama J, Tomé FMS, Lebon P, Marie L, Delaporte P, Fardeau M. Myosite à inclusions: étude clinique, morphologique et virologique, concernant une nouvelle observation associée à une sclérodermie généralisée et à un syndrome de Klinefelter. *Rev Neurol* 1980, 136:863–878.

10. Tomé FMS, Fardeau M, Lebon P, Chevallay M. Inclusion body myositis. *Acta Neuropath (Berlin) (suppl 7)* pp. 287–291.

11. Sadeh M, Gadoth M, Hadar H, Ben-David E. Vacuolar myopathy sparing the quadriceps. *Brain* 1993, 16:217–232.

12. Satoyoshi E, Kinoshita M. Oculopharyngodistal myopathy. *Arch Neurol* 1977, 34:89–92.

13. Massa R, Weller B, Karpati G, Shoubridge E, Carpenter S. Familial inclusion body myositis among Kurdish-Iranian Jews. *Arch Neurol* 1991, 48:519–522.

14. Hentati F, Ben Hamida C, Tomé F, Oueslati S, Fardeau M, Ben Hamida M. "Familial inclusion body myositis" sparing the quadriceps with asymptomatic leukoencephalopathy in a Tunisian kindred. *Neurology (suppl 1)* 1991, 41:422.

15. Fardeau M, Askanas V, Tomé FMS, Engel KW, Alvarez RB, Chevallay M. Hereditary neuromuscular disorder with inclusion body myositis-like filamentous inclusions: clinical, pathological and tissue culture. *Neurology (suppl 1)* 1990, 40:120.

16. Tomé FMS, Leclerc A, Lopez N, Chateau D, Alvarez RB, Richardet JM, Askanas V, Fardeau M. Childhood-onset myopathy characterized by cytoplasmic and nuclear inclusions containing 16–18 nm tubulofilaments. *Neurology (suppl 2)* 1993, 43:201–202.

17. Fukuhara N, Kumamoto T, Tsubaki T, Mayuzumi T, Nitta H. Oculopharyngeal muscular dystrophy and distal myopathy. Intrafamilial difference in the onset and distribution of muscular involvement. *Acta Neurol Scand* 1982, 65:458–467.

18. Tomé FMS, Leclerc A, Villanova M, Fardeau M. Ultrastructure and immunocytochemistry of the muscle fiber nucleus in inclusion body myositis. *Muscle Nerve (suppl 1)* 1994, 17:50.

Part V
Inflammatory, Nuclear, and Mitochondrial Abnormalities in Inclusion-Body Myositis and Inclusion-Body Myopathies

17

Muscle-Fibers in IBM: Antigen-presenting Cells or Innocent Bystanders?

REINHARD HOHLFELD, ANKE BENDER, AND
ANDREW G. ENGEL

Polymyositis (PM), sporadic inclusion-body myositis (IBM), and dermatomyositis (DM) are usually classified as (idiopathic) inflammatory
myopathies (1). Recently it has been suggested that IBM is really a
degenerative disease conditioned by progressive accumulations in muscle
fibers of amyloid and various other proteins (2). According to this view,
T-cell-mediated myocytotoxicity is neither the primary nor main pathogenic event in IBM.

In this chapter, we briefly review the evidence pointing to an immunopathogenesis of IBM. We will emphasize the many parallels between
PM and IBM and discuss the various arguments suggesting that immunologic mechanisms are strongly involved in the pathogenesis of IBM
(Table 17.1).

Concepts from Immunohistochemical and Basic Immunologic Studies

Both in PM and in IBM there is a conspicuous endomysial inflammatory
exudate containing large numbers of CD8+ T cells that, along with
macrophages, surround and focally invade non-necrotic muscle fibers
(Figure 17.1) (3,4). The majority of the autoinvasive cytotoxic T cells are
activated, as indicated by their expression of HLA-DR (5). As demonstrated by immuno-electron microscopy (6), CD8+ T cells and macrophages can traverse the basal lamina, focally replace, displace, or com-
press a fiber, and ultimately replace entire segments of a muscle fiber. All
of the invaded fibers and some noninvaded fibers express increased
amounts of HLA class I antigens (7,8). By contrast, normal muscle fibers
do not express detectable amounts of HLA class I or class II antigens.

These observations are consistent with an HLA-class-I-restricted immune response mediated by CD8+ T cells. Although the target antigen(s)

Table 17.1. *Observations favoring an immunopathogenesis for IBM*

- Invasion of non-necrotic, HLA-class-I-positive muscle fibers by CD8$^+$ activated T cells
- Expression of a restricted Vβ^+ or oligoclonal TCR repertoire in IBM muscle
- Higher frequency of invaded muscle fibers than of Congo-red-positive or necrotic muscle fibers
- Association with other autoimmune diseases and autoimmune-prone HLA haplotypes

---

recognized by the T cells have not been identified in PM or IBM, some general predictions can be made on the basis of the known properties of the HLA-class-I-restricted pathway of antigen presentation (9). The antigens presented in this pathway are short (8–10-mer) peptides, mostly derived from endogenously synthesized viral proteins (or self-proteins). Because many attempts to identify viral antigens or genes in PM or IBM

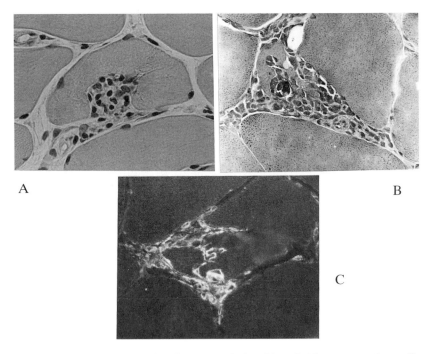

A   B

C

Figure 17.1.   Muscle fibers focally surrounded and invaded by mononuclear cells in IBM, showing early (A) and advanced (B) destruction of muscle fibers. C: Most of the invading cells are CD8$^+$ T cells, as demonstrated by immunofluorescence (A and B, ×330; C, ×360).

have failed (10–14), an autoimmune reaction against muscle self-antigens appears more likely, although the possibility that viral infections trigger an autoimmune reaction by molecular mimicry cannot be excluded.

In the HLA-class-I-restricted pathway, antigen processing occurs primarily in the cytoplasm (9). The major known pathway for cytoplasmic protein turnover involves proteasomes, which are tunnel-like multicatalytic protease assemblies (15). Before proteolysis, proteins usually are first covalently conjugated to multiple molecules of the polypeptide ubiquitin. This modification marks them for rapid ATP-dependent hydrolysis by proteasomes. Mammalian proteasomes can exhibit up to five different peptidase activities (16). The functional properties of a proteasome are determined by its subunit composition, which is regulated by cytokines. For example, interferon-γ, which enhances antigen presentation, induces the expression of certain proteasome subunits, including the HLA-encoded proteins LMP-2 and -7. The resulting proteasomes cleave proteins preferentially after hydrophobic and basic amino acid residues (16). Thus, interferon-γ favors the production of oligopeptides with hydrophobic or basic carboxy terminals. Peptides of this type are preferentially transported into the lumen of the endoplasmic reticulum by the HLA-encoded "transporter associated with antigen processing" (TAP) and bind tightly to newly synthesized HLA class I molecules. Eventually, the HLA class I–peptide complexes are transported to the cell surface, where they can be recognized by T cells.

As potential targets of cytotoxic CD8[+] T cells, muscle fibers are exceptional in that they normally do not express detectable amounts of HLA class I antigens. In the inflammatory myopathies, however, many muscle fibers express abundant HLA class I antigens (7,8). Because HLA expression can be enhanced in cultured myotubes by stimulation with interferon-γ (17,18), it is reasonable to assume that at least part of the HLA expression observed in IBM, PM, and DM is induced by locally secreted cytokines. It is likely that the cytokines influence not only HLA expression but also antigen processing by muscle fibers, favoring the presentation of self-proteins that are not normally produced in substantial amounts.

Examples of proteins that are preferentially expressed under the influence of cytokines and "immunologic stress" are the heat-shock proteins (HSPs). We found that HSPs of the 65-kDa class were strongly expressed in many muscle fibers in all inflammatory myopathies, including IBM (19). Notably, in both PM and IBM, HSP expression was increased over segments of muscle fiber invaded by T cells (19), a pattern consistent with induction by locally secreted cytokines.

In conclusion, when interpreted in the light of current immunologic concepts, several immunohistochemical studies have strongly suggested that in PM and IBM, CD8+ T cells recognize HLA-class-I-bound self-peptide(s) on the muscle-fiber surface. The most likely candidates are 8–10-mer peptides that have hydrophobic or basic carboxy-terminal residues and are derived from self-proteins.

Analysis of the T-Cell-Receptor Repertoire Expressed by Muscle-infiltrating T Cells

T cells use specific surface receptors for antigen recognition (20,21). The T-cell receptors (TCRs) are clonotypic: With few exceptions, each clone of T cells carries its own unique TCR. The TCR is a disulfide-linked heterodimer (a and β, or γ and δ). The variable (V) regions of a TCR are assembled by somatic recombinational mechanisms similar to those that assemble the variable regions of immunoglobulins. For example, the V region of the TCR β chain is encoded by three distinct genetic elements (Vβ, Dβ, and Jβ) that are separated and exist in multiple copies in germ-line DNA: The TCR β-chain gene complex on chromosome 7 incorporates approximately 60 Vβ gene segments, 2 Dβ gene segments, and 13 Jβ gene segments. During somatic recombination, an enormously diverse repertoire of distinct TCR Vβ chains is generated by (i) random combination of one particular Vβ, Dβ, and Jβ segment, (ii) junctional variability due to imprecise joining of the gene segments, and (iii) random addition of nucleotides to junctional sequences (N segments).

The spectrum of TCRs expressed by T cells in inflammatory lesions may provide important insights into immunopathologic mechanisms. For example, if an infiltrate is composed of only one clone (monoclonal) or a few clones (oligoclonal) of T cells carrying a particular TCR, one can conclude that these T cells have preferentially migrated into the lesion or have been locally stimulated to proliferate, or both. Because the TCR is used for antigen recognition, it is likely that the T cells will have been recruited or stimulated by a specific antigen (Figure 17.2). A striking example of an essentially monoclonal T-cell infiltrate was observed in a case of PM mediated by T cells expressing the $\gamma\delta$ TCR (22). In that patient's muscle, one unusual Vδ2-Jδ3/Vγ3-Jγ1 TCR recombination predominated. Parallel immunohistochemical studies confirmed that only the T cells expressing that particular TCR were autoinvasive.

If, on the other hand, the spectrum of locally expressed TCRs is extremely diverse, then the spectrum of recognized antigens must be also

ONE DOMINANT ANTIGEN:

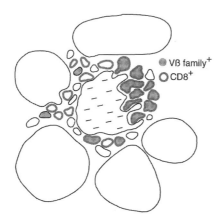

PCR --> MONO- OR OLIGOCLONAL TCRs

Figure 17.2. Model I: The autoinvasive T cells are stimulated by one predominating (auto)antigen. Most CD8+ T cells (and a few CD8− T cells) express one particular TCR Vβ family, which is detectable with anti-TCR-Vβ monoclonal antibodies. PCR amplification and sequence analysis of the expressed TCR will reveal a monoclonal or oligoclonal pattern.

diverse, or else the T cells will have been recruited in an entirely antigen-nonspecific way (Figure 17.3). A third possibility is that T cells expressing a particular TCR Vβ element will predominate in a lesion, but that these T cells will be clonally diverse, that is, will differ in the clonotypic "junctional" sequences. This situation can arise when T cells are stimulated by a "superantigen" (Figure 17.4).

Superantigens are bacterial or viral antigens that bind to HLA class II molecules and then can engage particular TCR Vβ sequences (23). Because there is only a limited number of Vβ regions, these Vβ-specific proteins can interact with a sizable percentage of all T cells. For example, toxic-shock-syndrome toxin engages nearly all T cells bearing Vβ2, a population that accounts for about 7% of the mature $\alpha\beta$ T cells in any given individual. Superantigens bind to a site on an HLA class II molecule that is outside the peptide-binding groove. Unlike conventional antigens, superantigens act on T cells as intact proteins, without the need for processing. Furthermore, superantigens bind to many alleles of HLA class II molecules; that is, they are not HLA-"restricted." Thus far, no superantigens have been discovered that bind to HLA class I molecules or are specific for the TCR Vα region (23).

MULTIPLE (OR NO) ANTIGENS:

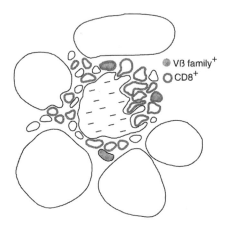

PCR --> POLYCLONAL TCRs

Figure 17.3. Model II: The autoinvasive T cells are stimulated by multiple antigens or by antigen-nonspecific mechanisms. Only few CD8$^+$ T cells react with a particular TCR Vβ-specific monoclonal antibody. PCR analysis shows a heterogeneous (polyclonal) pattern.

SUPER-ANTIGEN:

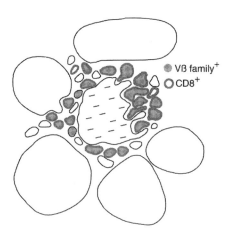

PCR --> POLYCLONAL TCRs

Figure 17.4. Model III: The autoinvasive T cells are stimulated by a superantigen. There is a striking overrepresentation of one particular TCR Vβ family. However, in contrast to the situation for model I, PCR reveals a polyclonal pattern.

Several previous studies of the $\alpha\beta$ TCR repertoire in inflammatory myopathies have focused on PM (24–26). We have combined a polymerase chain reaction (PCR) and double-fluorescence immunocytochemistry to analyze the TCR repertoire in muscle tissue from PM patients (26). One of our cases was particularly informative: PCR revealed preferential use of TCR Vα33.1, Vβ13.1, and Vβ5.1. Six of six TCR Vα33.1$^+$ and five of seven Vβ13.1$^+$ cDNA clones had identical nucleotide sequences. In contrast, the TCR Vβ5.1$^+$ clones were much more heterogeneous. Immunohistochemical analysis with TCR Vβ-specific monoclonal antibodies confirmed that Vβ13.1 and Vβ5.1 were overrepresented in the muscle lesions of that patient: 32% of all CD8$^+$ T cells were Vβ13.1$^+$, and 16% were Vβ5.1$^+$. However, about 60% of the CD8$^+$ T cells that invaded muscle fibers were Vβ13.1$^+$, whereas only 10% were Vβ5.1$^+$. Taken together, the findings from that study suggest that (i) a strikingly limited TCR repertoire is expressed in PM muscle, (ii) there is a dissociation between the TCR uses of autoinvasive and interstitial T cells, and (iii) the autoinvasive T cells are clonally expanded. This situation is consistent with the model shown in Figure 17.2.

In IBM, the TCR repertoire has been studied by immunocytochemical techniques (27) and PCR (28), but to date, no detailed analysis using a combination of both techniques has been reported. Lindberg et al. (27) compared the expressions of TCR V genes in IBM, PM, and DM using one Vα2-specific antibody and 10 different Vβ-specific monoclonal antibodies. The patterns observed in IBM, PM, and DM were similar. The most abundant TCR V elements were Vα2, Vβ3, and Vβ19. In contrast, those TCR V elements were not overexpressed in peripheral-blood lymphocytes (27). TCR sequences were not reported.

O'Hanlon et al. (28) analyzed the TCR repertoire in muscle biopsy specimens from 13 IBM patients using PCR with TCR Vα- and Vβ-family-specific primers. On average, 6 of the 22 TCR Vα and 7 of the 24 TCR Vβ families surveyed were detected per specimen. None of the Vα families was overrepresented, whereas Vβ3 and Vβ6 were detected more frequently than the other Vβ families. Sequence analyses of the expressed Vβ3 and Vβ6 receptors were carried out in three patients. In one patient, both the Vβ3 and Vβ6 sequences were exceedingly heterogeneous. This might point to a superantigen effect, as shown in Figure 17.4. However, in the two other patients, 5 of the 10 sequenced Vβ3 cDNA clones were identical. That more homogeneous pattern was similar to that observed in PM (26), indicating the presence of clonally dominant T cells recognizing a defined antigen (Figure 17.2). Clearly, further TCR repertoire studies are needed in IBM to determine whether the inflammatory T cells recognize a conventional antigen or a superantigen. It will be important to combine immunohistochemical and PCR techniques in future studies. Concerning the superantigen hypothesis (Figure 17.4), one conceptual problem is that muscle fibers do not normally express detectable levels of HLA class II antigens. It is theoretically possible, however, that HLA-class-I-binding superantigens exist. Furthermore, it is possible that the autoreactive T cells are initially stimulated by a superantigen at a different site and only later accumulate in muscle.

In conclusion, methods for analysis of TCR repertoire expressed in inflammatory lesions have been developed and greatly improved in recent years. The limited data currently available on TCR expression in IBM muscle are more consistent with T-cell stimulation by a conventional peptide antigen or superantigen than with antigen-nonspecific mechanisms.

Frequency Comparison of Congo-Red-positive; T-Cell-invaded, and Necrotic Muscle Fibers

Apart from the inflammatory changes descibed earlier, microscopic findings in IBM include rimmed vacuoles, congophilic amyloid deposits (typically near or within the vacuoles, and occasionally in nuclei), necrotic and regenerating fibers, small groups of atrophic fibers, and mitochondrial abnormalities (1,2). It is possible that IBM could be initiated or perpetuated by focal cytoplasmic or nuclear degradation, by accumulation of amyloid-related proteins, by an autoimmune attack on the muscle fibers by T cells, or by mechanisms not yet identified. Muscle-fiber destruction could result from nuclear damage, accumulation of amyloid-related proteins, invasion of fibers by autoaggressive inflammatory cells, or necrosis. In a recent study to evaluate the relative significance of those alterations, the frequencies of congophilic amyloid deposits, invasion of non-necrotic fibers by T cells, and fiber necrosis were quantitatively analyzed and compared in 31 electron-microscopy-proven cases of IBM (33).

Non-necrotic muscle fibers invaded by T cells were severalfold more frequent than fibers displaying the other pathologic alterations. Comparison of muscle samples from immunosuppressed (n = 11) and untreated (n = 20) patients revealed no significant differences in the respective frequencies of the three species of abnormal fibers. Moreover, there was no correlation between the frequency of any abnormality and disease duration or length of treatment. After long-term (mean, 68.4 months) prednisone treatment, T-cell-mediated myocytotoxicity remained the most frequent pathologic alteration in 10 of 11 patients. Neither long-term treatment nor prolonged disease duration was associated with a significant change in the median frequency for any species of abnormal fiber.

In conclusion, the much higher frequency of invaded fibers than of Congo-red-positive fibers suggests that in sporadic IBM, T-cell-mediated myocytotoxicity has greater pathologic significance than does the accumulation of congophilic deposits, pointing to the importance of an immune-mediated mechanism in the disease. However, it is clear that these observations do not establish T-cell-mediated myocytotoxicity as the only pathogenic event in sporadic IBM.

Associations of IBM with Autoimmune Diseases and HLA Antigens

IBM can be associated with a variety of other diseases, as reviewed elsewhere (1). No constant association has been recognized with malignancy, but the occurrence of IBM in a patient with Sjögren syndrome plus systemic lupus erythematosus, as well as in other patients with scleroderma, thrombocytopenia, granulomatous liver disease, sarcoidosis, and dermatomyositis, strongly suggests an association of IBM with autoimmune diseases (1). In this connection it is interesting to note that the association with other putative autoimmune diseases was one of the initial arguments suggesting that myasthenia gravis was an autoimmune disease (29).

Among other factors that can shed light on the pathogenesis of any disease is an association with specific genes. For a great number of experimental and human autoimmune diseases, the region of the major histocompatibility complex (MHC) has been established as an important locus of susceptibility (30). This is not surprising, as the MHC (HLA in humans) encodes not only the class I and class II molecules that present antigens to T cells but also many other immunologically important molecules, including complement factors, cytokines (tumor necrosis factors α and β, and critical components of the antigen-processing machinery (31)). Therefore, for any human disease, demonstration of an HLA association usually can be taken as indirect evidence that immunologic factors are involved in the pathogenesis.

In a recent study of HLA associations with IBM, 13 patients were typed for HLA class I and HLA-DR using standard serologic techniques and allele-specific oligonucleotide typing (32). IBM was found to be strongly associated with HLA-DR3 (observed in 92% of IBM patients vs. 25% in controls), HLA-DR52 (100% IBM vs. 80% controls), and HLA-B8 (75% IBM vs. 28% controls). Those findings were similar to our own (R. Hohlfeld et al., unpublished observations). Further analysis has shown that most IBM patients carry an extended haplotype that has been associated with several autoimmune diseases and is present in only 11% of the healthy caucasoid poulation (32).

In conclusion, the strong association of IBM with HLA-DR3, -DR52, and -B8 provides indirect evidence that immunologic factors are involved in the pathogenesis of IBM.

Summary and Conclusions

The combined evidence from several sources (immunohistologic studies, TCR repertoire analyses, comparisons of the frequencies of different pathologic alterations, associations with other autoimmune diseases and autoimmune-prone HLA haplotypes) suggests that immunopathologic mechanisms are strongly involved in the pathogenesis of IBM. The factors that initiate the various pathologic reactions and the manner in which the various reactions are interrelated or perpetuated in the course of IBM remain to be determined.

Acknowledgments

Our studies were supported by the Deutsche Forschungsgemeinschaft (SFB 217, C13), Wilhelm-Sander-Stiftung (94.068.1), Max-Planck-Society (R.H. and A.B.), and the National Institutes of Health (NS-6277), as well as by and a research grant from the Muscular Dystrophy Association (A.G.E.).

References

1. Mikol J, Engel AG. Inclusion body myositis. In: *Myology*, A. G. Engel AG, Franzini-Armstrong C (eds). McGraw-Hill, New York, 1994, pp. 1384–1398.
2. Askanas V, Engel WK, Mirabella M. Idiopathic inflammatory myopathies: inclusion-body myositis, polymyositis, and dermatomyositis. *Curr Opin Neurol* 7:48–456, 1994.
3. Hohlfeld R, Engel AG. The immunobiology of muscle. *Immunol Today* 15:269–274, 1994.

4. Engel AG, Hohlfeld R, Banker BQ. The polymyositis and dermatomyositis syndromes. In: *Myology*, Engel AG, Franzini-Armstrong C (eds). McGraw-Hill, New York, 1994, pp. 1335–1383.

5. Engel AG, Arahata K. Monoclonal antibody analysis of mononuclear cells in myopathies. II. Phenotypes of autoinvasive cells in polymyositis and inclusion body myositis. *Ann Neurol* 16:209–216, 1984.

6. Arahata K, Engel AG. Monoclonal antibody analysis of mononuclear cells in myopathies. III. Immunoelectron microscopy aspects of cell-mediated muscle fiber injury. *Ann Neurol* 19:112–125, 1986.

7. Karpati G, Pouliot Y, Carpenter S. Expression of immunoreactive major histocompatibility complex products in human skeletal muscles. *Ann Neurol* 23:64–72, 1988.

8. Emslie-Smith AM, Arahata K, Engel AG. Major histocompatibility complex class I antigen expression, immunolocalization of interferon subtypes, and T cell-mediated cytotoxicity in myopathies. *Hum Pathol* 20:224–231, 1989.

9. Germain RN. MHC-dependent antigen processing and peptide presentation: Providing ligands for T lymphocyte activation. *Cell* 76:287–299, 1994.

10. Leon-Monzon M, Dalakas MC. Absence of persistent infection with enteroviruses in muscles of patients with inflammatory myopathies. *Ann Neurol* 32:219–222, 1992.

11. Jongen PJH, Zoll GJ, Beaumont M, Melchers WJG, Van de Putte LBA, Galama JMD. Polymyositis and dermatomyositis: no persistence of enterovirus or encephalomyocarditis virus RNA in muscle. *Ann Rheum Dis* 52:575–578, 1993.

12. Fox SA, Finklestone E, Robbins PD, Mastaglia FL, Swanson NR. Search for persistent enterovirus infection of muscle in inflammatory myopathies. *J Neurol Sci* 125:70–76, 1994.

13. Leff RL, Love LA, Miller FW, Greenberg SJ, Klein EA, Dalakas MC, Plotz PH. Viruses in idiopathic inflammatory myopathies: absence of candidate viral genomes in muscle. *Lancet* 339:1192–1195, 1992.

14. Nishino H, Engel AG, Rima BK. Inclusion body myositis: the mumps virus hypothesis. *Ann Neurol* 25:260–264, 1989.

15. Goldberg AL. Functions of the proteasome: the lysis at the end of the tunnel. *Science* 268:522–523, 1995.

16. Ciechanover A. The ubiquitin-proteasome proteolytic pathway. *Cell* 79:13–21, 1994.

17. Goebels N, Michaelis D, Wekerle H, Hohlfeld R. Human myoblasts as antigen presenting cells. *J Immunol* 149:661–667, 1992.

18. Michaelis D, Goebels N, Hohlfeld R. Constitutive and cytokine-induced expression of human leukocyte antigens and cell adhesion molecules by human myotubes. *Am J Pathol* 143:1142–1149, 1993.

19. Hohlfeld R, Engel AG. Expression of 65-kd heat shock proteins in the inflammatory myopathies. *Ann Neurol* 32:821–823, 1992.

20. Hohlfeld R. Neurological autoimmune disease and the trimolecular complex of T-lymphocytes. *Ann Neurol* 25:531–538, 1989.

21. Moss PAH, Rosenberg WMC, Bell JI. The human T cell receptor in health and disease. *Annu Rev Immunol* 10:71–96, 1992.

22. Pluschke G, Rüegg D, Hohlfeld R, Engel AG. Autoaggressive myocytotoxic T lymphocytes expressing an unusual γ/δ T cell receptor. *J Exp Med* 176:1785–1789, 1992.

23. Scherer MT, Ignatowicz L, Winslow GM, Kappler JW, Marrack P. Super-antigens: bacterial and viral proteins that manipulate the immune system. *Annu Rev Cell Biol* 9:101–128, 1993.
24. Mantegazza R, Andreetta F, Bernasconi P, Baggi F, Oksenberg JR, Simoncini O, Mora M, Cornelio F, Steinman L. Analysis of T cell receptor repertoire of muscle-infiltrating T lymphocytes in polymyositis. *J Clin Invest* 91:2880–2886; 1993.
25. O'Hanlon TP, Dalakas MC, Plotz PH, Miller FW. Predominant TCR-*αβ* variable and joining gene expression by muscle-infiltrating lymphocytes in the idiopathic inflammatory myopathies. *J Immunol* 152:2569–2576; 1994.
26. Bender A, Ernst A, Iglesias A, Dornmair K, Wekerle H, Hohlfeld R. T cell receptor repertoire in polymyositis: clonal expansion of autoaggressive CD8$^+$ T cells. *J Exp Med* 181:1863–1868, 1995.
27. Lindberg C, Oldfors A, Tarkowski A. Restricted use of T cell receptor V genes in endomysial infiltrates of patients with inflammatory myopathies. *Eur J Immunol* 24:2659–2663, 1994.
28. O'Hanlon TP, Dalakas MC, Plotz PH, Miller FW. The *αβ* T-cell receptor repertoire in inclusion body myositis: diverse patterns of gene expression by muscle-infiltrating lymphocytes. *J Autoimmun* 7:321–333, 1994.
29. Simpson JA. Myasthenia gravis: a new hypothesis. *Scott Med J* 5:410, 1960.
30. Nepom GT, Erlich H. MHC class II molecules and autoimmunity. *Annu Rev Immunol* 9:493–526, 1991.
31. Campbell RD, Trowsdale J. Map of the human MHC. *Immunol Today* 14:349–352, 1993.
32. Garlepp MJ, Laing B, Zilko PJ, Ollier W, Mastaglia FL. HLA associations with inclusion body myositis. *Clin Exp Immunol* 98:40–45, 1994.
33. Pruitt JN, Showalter CJ, Engel AG. Sporadic inclusion body myositis: counts of different types of abnormal fibers. *Ann Neurol* 39:139–143, 1996.

18

Viruses, Immunodeficiency, and Inclusion-Body Myositis

MARINOS C. DALAKAS, ISABEL ILLA, AND
MARTA LEON-MONZON

Role of Viruses in Human Myositis: General Principles

The idea that inflammatory myopathies may have viral causes is not new.
For inclusion-body myositis (IBM) the viral hypothesis has been particularly attractive, because the vacuoles and filaments in these patients'
muscles have been thought to represent viral inclusions or even viral
particles (1–3). In considering a role for a virus in causing a chronic
inflammatory process such as IBM, one must identify in the patients'
muscle viable virus particles or detect copies of the viral genome by in
situ hybridization or an in situ polymerase chain reaction (PCR) (4–6).
Alternatively, if a "hit-and-run" phenomenon has taken place, the putative viruses will not have to continue to be present in the muscle because
they may have been cleared by the immune effector cells. In that case,
the virus would play a role by triggering an inflammatory response that
subsequently would become self-sustaining. In many PCR studies of
homogenized muscle, virus particles may have originated from the constituents of blood vessels or from the invading macrophages and lymphocytes, necessitating the use of in situ hybridization/PCR or immunocytochemistry to determine the location of the virus.

The first connection between a virus and a human muscle disease was
suggested in 1934 in a description of an ill-defined, self-limited, acute
febrile illness involving painful thoracic and abdominal muscles (epidemic pleurodynia) (7). That observation was expanded over the ensuing
years to include patients with inflammatory myopathies, because some of
them had serologic evidence of high antibody titers against enteroviruses
(8,9). The issue resurfaced when antibodies to Jo-1 antigen, a histidyl-
transfer RNA synthetase were found in up to 10% of patients with
myositis (10). A possible molecular mimicry phenomenon was proposed
because of structural homology between Jo-1 and the genomic RNA of
an animal picornavirus, the encephalomyocarditis virus. The argument
for that association was strengthened when it was reported that in situ
hybridization studies revealed enterovirus RNA within the muscle fibers

of biopsy specimens from patients with myositis (11,12). However, our very sensitive PCR studies have repeatedly failed to confirm the presence of enteroviruses in such patients' muscle biopsy specimens (13,14). Even in the muscles of patients with post-poliomyelitis syndrome, in which "red-rimmed" vacuoles and filaments similar to those seen in IBM have been observed (15), we could not amplify enteroviruses (13,16). It is unlikely, therefore, although not impossible, that replication of enteroviruses could take place within the muscles of patients with chronic inflammatory myopathies and IBM.

A connection between orthomyxoviruses and inflammatory myopathies has also been suggested because of reports that myalgia, elevated creatine kinase (CK) concentrations, or rhabdomyolysis can follow infections with influenza virus (17,18). In two cases, virus particles reportedly were revealed in muscle biopsy specimens by electron microscopy (19,20). Furthermore, the influenza B/Lee strain can infect human rhabfdomyosarcoma cell lines (21). Apart from those observations, there has been no clear evidence that such viruses are associated with the causes of sporadic myositis, including IBM.

Another group of viruses, the paramyxoviruses (mumps), were, in some early studies, implicated in the pathogenesis of IBM because the 15–20-nm microtubular filaments seen in the muscle of IBM patients resembled viral nucleocapsids (1–3). The findings in the search for mumps virus by PCR, however, have been consistently negative (22). Other viruses have also been sought by PCR in the muscles of patients with sporadic inflammatory myopathies, including IBM. Our own search for encephalomyocarditis virus, adenovirus, HIV, HTLV-I, and HTLV-II in the RNA extracted from muscle biopsy specimens from 44 patients, including 15 IBM patients, has been negative (13,14). As discussed earlier, however, the absence of virus particles from these patients' muscle fibers does not prove that IBM is not caused by a virus.

The strongest suggestion of an association between a virus and IBM, as well as other inflammatory myopathies, concerns the group of retroviruses. The first evidence that retroviruses could be associated with inflammatory myopathies was found in our studies of monkeys infected with the simian immunodeficiency virus (23,24). Shortly thereafter, we witnessed the first cases of myositis associated with human immunodeficiency virus (HIV) (25). About 3 years later, the association between myositis and infection with human T-cell lymphotropic virus type I (HTLV-I) became apparent (26). Because polymyositis has occurred during infections with at least four different retroviruses, it appears that this family of viruses offers reasonable candidates to be considered in connection with the causes of polymyositis and IBM. Consequently, the main topic of this chapter is the possible association between IBM and retrovirus infections.

Retroviruses and IBM

Animal Retroviruses

In 1986 we observed that the simian retrovirus type I (SRV-I), which is similar to the Mason Pfizer monkey virus, can, in monkeys, cause immunodeficiency, Kaposi sarcoma, and polymyositis resembling the human disease (23,24). The infected animals showed muscle weakness and wasting, and their serum creatine kinase (CK) concentrations were elevated. The pathologic changes in the muscle consisted of perivascular and interstitial inflammation, with phagocytosis and fiber necrosis. Immunocytochemical studies revealed viral antigens in endomysial lymphoid cells, but not in muscle fibers. In some muscle fibers we observed red-rimmed vacuoles, which raised the suspicion of a connection between retroviruses and IBM (24). A previously reported (24) muscle fiber with such vacuoles is shown in Figure 18.1.

Transgenic mice carrying the *bel* region of the human foamy retrovirus (HFV), which is under transcriptional control of its own long terminal repeat, expressed the transgene in striated muscle and exhibited a destructive myopathy (27). The majority of the viable muscle fibers expressed viral RNA before degenerative features developed, suggesting that HFV was directly responsible for the myopathy. It is of interest that *bel*-1 has homology with the regulatory proteins *tat* and *tax* of HIV-1 and HTLV-I, respectively.

Human Retroviruses

HIV Infection Associated with Inflammatory Myopathy and IBM

Inflammatory myopathy can sometimes be present early in an infection with HIV, but more often it occurs during the course of AIDS (28–32). In some patients it coexists with other neurologic manifestations, such as peripheral neuropathy and, rarely, dementia or myelopathy. The myopathy begins subacutely, with proximal, often symmetrical, muscle weakness with or without wasting, affecting arms and legs. The serum CK concentration can be as much as 10–15 times normal. In addition to the

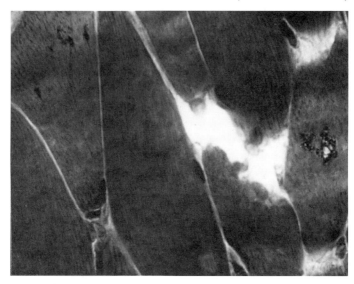

Figure 18.1.   Cross section of a muscle biopsy specimen from a monkey infected with SRV-I stained with trichrome, showing one fiber with vacuoles. Inflammation was seen in a different plane of sectioning.

classic polymyositis seen in HIV-infected patients, we have seen two patients who presented with most of the clinical and histologic features of IBM, the only exceptions being their young ages and the high (up to 10,000 IU/L) elevation of CK in one of them (33). That observation was of sufficient importance to justify the following detailed clinicopathologic description, as previously reported (33).

One of those two patients was a 37-year-old man with asymptomatic HIV-1 infection (detected 30 months prior to evaluation) and a 2.5-year history of progressive muscle weakness that began prior to anti-retrovirus treatment and affected proximal, distal, and swallowing muscles. An initial muscle biopsy was interpreted as showing inflammatory myopathy with features suggestive of IBM. Oral prednisone (60 mg/day) and zidovudine (300 mg/day) were initiated, without clinical improvement. Symptoms progressed to the point that he was unable to stand up from a chair, walk without a cane, open jars, or swallow normally. When he was admitted to the NIH Clinical Center, his major findings included weakness of the muscles selectively affected in IBM patients. These included mild facial-muscle weakness, bilateral forearm atrophy, and asymmetric weakness in the range of 4 to 4− on the Medical Research Council (MRC) scale affecting proximal muscles (neck flexors, deltoids, biceps, triceps, iliopsoas, glutei, and quadriceps) and distal muscles (wrist extensors and flexors, finger extensors and flexors, intrinsic hand musculature, tibialis anterior, and toe extensors). Findings at sensory examination were normal, as were tendon reflexes and coordination. Relevant laboratory data included the following: CK, 10,474 U/L (normal, 52–386 U/L); aldolase, 30 units (normal, 1–7 units); lactate dehydrogenase (LDH), 904 U/L (normal, 113–226 U/L); alanine aminotransferase (ALT), 143 U/L (normal, 6–42 U/L); aspartate aminotransferase (AST), 144 U/L (normal, 9–34 U/L); CD4$^+$ cell count, 208/mL; IgG, 3,130 mg/dL (normal, 523–1,482 mg/dL); IgA, 184 mg/dL (normal, 51–375 mg/dL); IgM, 216 mg/dL (normal, 37–200 mg/dL). Electromyography revealed prominent fibrillations and positive sharp waves, with many small, short-duration motor-unit potentials, as seen in IBM and other inflammatory myopathies. Findings on nerve conduction studies were normal. Muscle biopsy revealed severe endomysial inflammation, with multivacuolated (red-rimmed and non-rimmed) fibers (Figure 18.2), necrotic fibers, and wide variations in fiber sizes including large fibers and small atrophic fibers in groups, internal nuclei, and eosinophilic inclusions. Amyloid was detected in some vacuoles within myofibers.

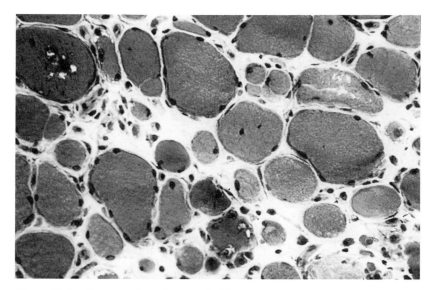

Figure 18.2. Cross section of a muscle biopsy specimen from an HIV-positive patient, demonstrating chronic myopathy, with variation of fiber size, rimmed-vacuolated fibers, and increased connective tissue. Inflammation was seen in a different plane of sectioning.

The second patient was a 37-year-old man with asymptomatic HIV-1 infection detected 99 months prior to evaluation. One year later, he developed proximal muscle weakness, myalgia, elevation of CK, and mild dysphagia while on zidovudine (AZT) treatment. Muscle biopsy findings were consistent with an inflammatory myopathy (33). Zidovudine treatment was stopped, and the pain decreased, but the weakness remained and progressed over the following 7 years to involve distal muscles. At the time of the NIH evaluation, the patient had difficulty in climbing stairs, raising off the floor, grasping, manipulating small objects, and swallowing solids. He had muscle weakness and findings typically seen in patients with sporadic IBM. There was mild facial-muscle weakness, forearm atrophy, and weakness (4 to 4+) in the proximal and distal muscles, including the neck flexors, deltoids, biceps, brachioradialis, triceps, wrist extensors, finger flexors, intrinsic hand musculature, iliopsoas, and toe extensors. Sensory functioning was normal, except for slightly decreased reactions to pinprick and vibration in the toes. Tendon reflexes were absent at the ankles. Relevant laboratory data included the following: CK, 623 U/L; aldolase, 10 units; LDH, 210 U/L; ALT, 43 U/L; AST, 52 U/L; positive anti-SS-A antibodies. The $CD4^+$ lymphocyte count was 487 cells/mL (19.1%). Serum IgG was 1,550 mg/dL, and IgA and IgM were normal. Electromyographic studies revealed mildly increased insertional activity, with scattered fibrillation potentials and positive sharp waves, along with mixed normal and large-amplitude long-duration polyphasic motor units, as seen in sporadic IBM. Findings at nerve conduction studies were normal. Muscle biopsy revealed mild endomysial inflammation, red-rimmed vacuolated fibers, occasional ragged red fibers, rare necrotic fibers, increased internal nuclei, and atrophic fibers in groups. Amyloid was detected within the myofibers.

HTLV-I

HTLV-I can cause not only a myeloneuropathy – referred to as tropical spastic paraparesis (TSP) – but also polymyositis, which can coexist with TSP or can be the only clinical manifestation of HTLV-I infection (26,34). The clinical presentation is identical with that of the sporadic polymyositis and the HIV myositis discussed earlier. In Jamaica, where HTLV-I is endemic, 7–18% of the healthy population will have positive HTLV-I antibody titers, and up to 85% of Jamaicans with polymyositis will have IgG anti-HTLV-I antibodies, indicating that the association is not due to chance.

Myositis associated with HTLV-I infection has also been seen in Haitians and, rarely, in Native Americans. We have studied five such patients born in North America, four of whom had classic polymyositis (35), and one who had IBM (33). The patient with IBM presented with proximal muscle weakness and a 3–4-year history of urinary and bowel incontinence due to the coexisting TSP. A muscle biopsy demonstrated moderate endomysial inflammation, multivacuolated (red-rimmed and non-rimmed) fibers, internal nuclei, rare nemaline rods, eosinophilic inclusions, atrophic fibers in groups, increased connective tissue, and fatty replacement. Crystal-violet and Congo-red stainings were positive for amyloid.

Pathogenesis of Retroviral IBM

The muscle biopsy specimens from the aforementioned two patients were studied with single and double immunocytochemistry in a search for various T-cell markers, MHC class I and II antigens, and viral antigens in the muscle or in the infiltrating cells. A PCR was also used to search for retrovirus integrated sequences within genomic DNA extracted from 50 mg of muscle homogenates, as described earlier (35). Amplified products were also analyzed by polyacrylamide-gel electrophoresis. The cellular infiltrates consisted mainly of CD8$^+$ cells, followed by macrophages and CD4$^+$ cells (35–37). Muscle fibers expressed MHC class I antigens and were surrounded by CD8$^+$ T cells in a pattern identical with that seen in sporadic IBM. HIV-1 or HTLV-I viral proteins were detected only in the infiltrating cells, which by double exposure were identified as macrophages. Those cells were seen within the muscle fibers, and rarely at the site of a vacuole. No viral antigens were detected within the muscle fibers. An RT-PCR in the muscle homogenate confirmed the presence of retroviral RNA. A predominance of T-cell receptors expressing the Vβ5.1 and Vβ13 gene families was detected on the inflammatory T-cell infiltrates surrounding or invading non-necrotic muscle fibers, as well as in the perimysial and perivascular spaces, suggesting that the endomysial lymphocytes had trafficked, nonspecifically, from blood vessels to all muscle compartments (38). Because retroviral proteins were not found within the myocytes, it was apparent that these viruses do not cause a persistent infection of the muscle fibers. In previous in vitro studies we had shown that human muscle is resistant to infection with HIV-1, HTLV-I, and HIV-1 or HTLV-I-infected lymphocytes (35–37). Consequently, the recruited endomysial CD8$^+$ T cells that surrounded or invaded the MHC-class-I-expressing non-necrotic muscle fibers in the previously described cases would seem not to have recognized retroviral proteins. However, we cannot exclude the possibility that endogenous peptides on the native muscle fiber may have homology with retrovirally encoded proteins and can be presented to the CD8$^+$ cells by the MHC class I antigen, in a phenomenon of molecular mimicry. The observation that the sera of patients with sporadic IBM recognize, with high frequency, the peptides of HTLV-II regulatory proteins, as discussed later, supports such a notion.

In reference to cytokines, we found that STAT (signal transducers and activators of transcription) proteins, which are induced by γ interferon, were highly expressed on the surfaces of muscle fibers even in areas remote from the inflammation (39). Because cytokines up-regulate various surface molecules in vivo and in vitro, it is possible that when secreted by the retrovirally infected endomysial macrophages, cytokines may induce MHC-I antigen expression on the muscle fibers, enhancing the ongoing immune response.

Another interesting observation was the finding of selective proliferation of T cells that bear T-cell receptor (TCR) β subunits, raising the possibility of superantigenic stimulation (40). Retroviruses are considered superantigens (41), and a superantigenic mechanism has been implicated in the progression from asymptomatic HIV-1 infection to full-blown AIDS. Because in retroviral IBM a predominance of TCR β subunits has been found in the inflammatory-cell infiltrates in all the muscle compartments, the T cells may not be clonally expanded in situ. Instead, they may have been recruited to the endomysial tissue after initial stimulation in the periphery by the retroviruses acting as superantigens. Similar superantigenic stimulation of T cells has been proposed in the immunopathogenesis of sporadic IBM, on the basis of selective amplification of specific TCR Vβ subunits within the muscle biopsy specimens by both PCR and immunocytochemistry (42,43).

Implications and Analogies between Retroviral IBM and Sporadic IBM and Sequence Homologies between Retroviral Proteins and Muscle

Because the immunopathologic characteristics of HIV-1- and HTLV-I-associated IBM were similar to those seen in retroviral IBM (44,45), it seems that a T-cell-mediated and MHC-I-restricted cytotoxic process plays a role in IBM patients, regardless of whether or not the disease is triggered by a known virus. HIV and HTLV-I persist in many extramuscular cells or tissues, but they do not seem to persist within the muscle fiber, except for rare macrophages. It is possible, however, that cytokines and lymphokines released from the activated or virus-infected endomysial inflammatory cells induce, on the surfaces of muscle fibers, the expression of antigens against which there is no self-tolerance, generating a tissue-specific autoimmune disease (4,5). Further, homologies exist between sarcolemmal proteins and retroviral sequences (46–48), which might allow circulating antibodies against the retrovirus to bind to the sarcolemma and act as muscle neoantigens, leading to further self-sensitization. Consistent with this hypothesis of molecular antigenic mimicry is the observation that some HIV-negative patients with polymyositis have circulating antibodies against ribonucleoproteins, which in turn share antigens with retroviral proteins encoded by the *gag* and *pol* genes of HIV (48).

We have explored the sharing of antigens between retroviruses and muscle by searching the sera of patients with various inflammatory myopathies, including sporadic, non-virus-related IBM, for the presence of circulating antibodies against retroviral proteins, and we have examined their muscle tissue to determine whether or not it shares retroviral sequences (49). We prepared western blots of purified retroviral proteins from HIV, HTLV-I, and HTLV-II and transferred the proteins, after electrophoresis, to nitrocellulose filters. The strips were incubated with patients' sera at 1 : 50 dilution. The sera from up to 6% of polymyositis (PM) patients and 11% of dermatomyositis (DM) patients (compared with 14% of IBM patients) recognized several proteins of the HIV and HTLV-I viral genome, including HIV p28, p19, p40, p53, and p56, and HTLV-I p24, p32, and gp41. Some sera from patients with Sjögren syndrome had similar reactivities, confirming previous observations (50,51). In reference to the HTLV-II viral antigens, however, the sera from 29% of PM patients and 17% of DM patients had antibodies to p24 or gp46, compared with 64% of sera from IBM patients that recognized gp37/40, p24, and p51 viral proteins (Figure 18.3). A search for integrated sequences in the DNA extracted from the muscle of those patients, using PCR, failed to show amplification products with the *gag* and *env* HIV primers or the *tax-rex* HTLV-I- and HTLV-I/II-specific primers, indicating an absence of retrovirus infection. The intense and frequent immunoreactivity of the serum IgG, especially from the IBM patients, with retroviral peptides may represent antibodies against an unidentified exogenous retrovirus related to HTLV-II, or

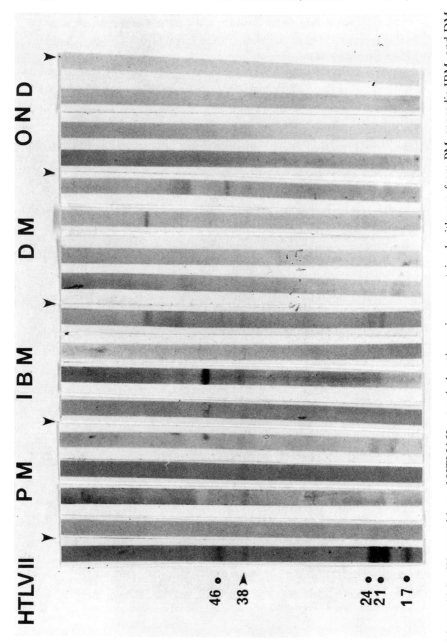

Figure 18.3.   Western blots of HTLV-II retroviral antigens immunostained with sera from PM, sporadic IBM, and DM patients. Specific retroviral proteins are recognized by the IBM patients' sera.

against endogenous retroviral sequences (52,53). Because the p24 *gag* of the HIV and the p30 *gag* antigen of the Moloney MuLV and other retroviruses share homology with antigens recognized by the anti-Sm and anti-U1 RNP antibodies (47), both of which are seen in the sera of patients with PM and IBM, the observed reactivity may be a phenomenon of molecular mimicry between endogenous muscle proteins and retroviral antigens.

Roles of Endogenous Retroviruses in Human Muscle

Retroviruses are small viruses that replicate only by reverse transcription from RNA to DNA using the retroviral-RNA-dependent DNA polymerase (reverse transcriptase), which is encoded by the viral *pol* gene (52,53). When a retrovirus infects a cell, the reverse transcriptase makes a double-strand DNA copy of the genomic RNA, which is then integrated into the host cell's DNA. The integrated proviral DNA is called provirus and is usually duplicated along with normal cellular genes when the infected cell divides (52,53). When retroviruses infect germ cells or early embryos, the retroviral genome can integrate into the host germ-line DNA, generating proviruses that are transmitted vertically in a classic Mendelian fashion by all subsequent generations. These proviruses comprise the endogenous retroviruses (ERVs) (52,53). Human ERVs (HERVs) are present in several tissues, especially syncytiotrophoblasts, placenta, and peripheral-blood mononuclear cells, in thousands of copies, accounting for up to 0.1–0.5% of human DNA. Although defective and not infectious, ERVs are not silent components of the human genome, because they are transcriptionally active and can encode proteins called HERS-I, which in certain conditions can theoretically affect immune function. Further, some ERVs, like HERV-K10, contain an open reading frame large enough to produce a full-length *pol* protein.

We have searched genomic DNA from histologically normal muscle for the presence of HERVs using specific sets of primers to detect nucleotides 1949–1968 and 2192–2211 of the *pol* gene region, which represents the most highly conserved reverse-transcriptase region in endogenous proviral DNA. These primers define the sequences coding for the conserved domains of the HERV-Ic *pol* gene. We amplified a 139-bp product which, after sequencing, demonstrated 48.9% homology with HTLV-I. Because the *pol* primers contained the nucleotide sequence unique to endogenous *pol*, and the *pol* primers from other variable regions specific for HIV or HTLV-I and other primers of the *tax/rex* or *gag* regions gave negative amplification, the *pol*-amplified product most likely represents HERV. Although the roles of HERVs in the muscle are unclear, they can encode proteins (i.e., HERS-I) expressed on the surface of the cell that during an immune response can potentially stimulate the recruitment of cytotoxic T cells with specificity for such antigenic peptides. Because the sera from patients with autoimmune diseases bind to synthetic peptides of HERV-I (53), ERVs may, under certain conditions, serve as autoantigens. Retroviral proteins have partial homologies with various self-antigens, such as ribonucleoproteins or t-RNA synthetases, which are frequent targets of autoantibodies in inflammatory myopathies, suggesting that molecular mimicry may be another mechanism of self-sensitization. Further, defective proviral DNA theoretically can become infectious, and after interaction with exogenous viruses, or in immunosuppressed patients, it has the potential to be transcribed and translated into functional gene products. These hypotheses need to be tested in further investigations.

Immunodeficiency and IBM

Because retroviruses cause immunodeficiency, it is of special interest to observe cases of IBM associated with common variable immunodeficiency (CVI). We reported (54) the occurrence of IBM in two men, ages 36 and 48 years, with long-standing CVI. Immunophenotypic analysis of their endomysial cells showed increased numbers of natural killer (NK) cells (defined as CD57+, CD56+, CD3−, CD8−, CD68−), accounting for 8.5–9.5% of the total cells, compared with a mean of 1% in sporadic IBM. NK cells were positive for intercellular cell-adhesion molecule 1, and they invaded muscle fibers negative for MHC class I antigen. In contrast to the ubiquitous endomysial expression of MHC class I antigen seen in sporadic IBM, in the cases of IBM with CVI, MHC class I antigen was absent or weakly expressed in only some of the muscle fibers surrounded by CD8+ cells. It appears, therefore, that in patients with CVI the development of IBM represents an immune myopathy mediated by NK cells in a non-MHC-class-I-restricted cytotoxicity. The description of those two cases was the first report of an inflammatory myopathy in which NK cells appeared to participate in the myocytotoxic process. Similar cases of IBM in patients with CVI have been reported by other researchers (42).

CVI is a disease of abnormal immunoregulation in which up to 20% of patients develop one or more autoimmune diseases. Because at least 20% of IBM patients may have autoimmune phenomena, the association supports the other circumstantial evidence that in some IBM patients there are signs of disturbed immunoregulation. Whether the manifestation of IBM in patients with retrovirus infection is due to immunodeficiency, or the IBM in CVI is due to infection with a putative retrovirus, remains to be determined.

References

1. Chou SM. Myxovirus-like structures in a case of human chronic polymyositis. *Science* 1967, 158:1453.
2. Chou SM. Myxovirus-like structures and accompanying nuclear changes in chronic polymyositis. *Arch Pathol* 1968, 86:649.
3. Chou SM. Inclusion body myositis: a chronic persistent mumps myositis? *Hum Pathol* 1986, 17:765.
4. Dalakas MC. Retroviral myopathies. In: Engel AG, Franzini-Armstrong C (eds), *Myology*, vol. 2. McGraw-Hill, New York, 1994, pp. 1419–1437.
5. Dalakas MC. Retroviruses and inflammatory myopathies in human and primates. *Bailliere's Clinical Neurology* 1993, 2:659–691.
6. Dalakas MC, Illa I, Leon-Monzon M. Retroviral related neuromuscular disorders. In: Hohlfeld R (ed), *Immunology of Neuromuscular Diseases*. Kluwer Academic Publishers, Lanchester, UK, 1994, pp. 255–288.
7. Sylvest E. *Epidemic Myalgia: Bernholm Disease*. Oxford University Press, 1934.
8. Tang TT, Sedmak GV, Siegesmund KA, McCreadie SR. Chronic myopathy associated with coxsackievirus type A9: a combined electron microscopical and viral isolation study. *N Engl J Med* 1975, 292:608.
9. Christensen ML, Pachman LM, Schneiderman R, et al. Prevalence of coxsackie B virus antibodies in patients with juvenile dermatomyositis. *Arthritis Rheum* 1986, 29:1365.
10. Targoff IN. Immune mechanisms of myositis. *Curr Opin Rheumatol* 1990, 2:882–888.
11. Youse GE, Isenberg DA, Mowbray JF. Detection of enterovirus specific RNA sequences in muscle biopsy specimens from patients with adult onset myositis. *Ann Rheum Dis* 1990, 49:310.
12. Rosenberg NI, Rotbart HA, Abzug MJ, et al. Evidence for a novel picornavirus in human dermatomyositis. *Ann Neurol* 1989, 26:204.
13. Leon-Monzon M, Dalakas MC. Absence of persistent infection with enteroviruses in muscles of patients with inflammatory myopathies. *Ann Neurol* 1992, 32:219–222.
14. Leff RL, Love LA, Miller FW, Greenberg SJ, Klein EA, Dalakas MC, Plotz PH. Viruses in the idiopathic inflammatory myopathies: absence of candidate viral genomes in muscle. *Lancet* 1992, 339:1192–1195.
15. Semino-Mora C, Dalakas MC. Red-rimmed vacuoles (RRV) with β-amyloid deposition in the muscles of patients with post-polio syndrome (PPS):

histopathological similarities with inclusion body myositis (IBM). *Neurology* 1996, 46:116–117.

16. Dalakas MC. Enteroviruses and human neuromuscular diseases. In: Rotbart HA (ed), *Human Enterovirus Infections*. American Society for Microbiology (ASM) Press, Washington, D.C., 1995, pp. 387–398.

17. Dietzman DE, Schaller JG, Ray CG, Reed ME. Acute myositis associated with influenza B infection. *Pediatrics* 1976, 57:255.

18. Buchta RM. Myositis and influenza. *Pediatrics* 1977, 60:761.

19. Ganboa ET, Eastwood AB, Hays AP, et al. Isolation of influenza virus from muscle in myoglobinuric polymyositis. *Neurology* 1979, 29:1323.

20. Kessler HA, Trenholme GM, Harris AA, Levin S. Acute myopathy associated with influenza A/Texas/1/77 infection: isolation of virus from a muscle biopsy specimen. *JAMA* 1980, 243:461.

21. Hays AP, Gamboa FT. Acute viral myositis. In: Engel AG, Franzini-Armstrong C (eds), *Myology*, vol. 2, McGraw-Hill, New York, 1994, pp. 1399–1418.

22. Nishino H, Engel AG, Rima BK. Inclusion body myositis: the mumps virus hypothesis. *Ann Neurol* 1989, 25:260.

23. Dalakas MC, London WT, Gravell M, Sever JL. Polymyositis in an immunodeficiency disease in monkeys induced by a type D retrovirus. *Neurology* 1986, 36:569–572.

24. Dalakas MC, Gravell M, London WT, Cunningham G, Sever JL. Morphological changes of an inflammatory myopathy in rhesus monkeys with simian acquired immunodeficiency syndrome. *Proc Soc Exp Biol Med* 1987, 185:368–376.

25. Dalakas MC, Pezeshkpour GH, Gravell M, Sever JL. Polymyositis in patients with AIDS. *JAMA* 1986, 256:2381–2383.

26. Morgan OS, Rodgers-Johnson P, Mora C, Char G. HTLV-I and polymyositis in Jamaica. *Lancet* 1989, 2:1184.

27. Bothe K, Aguzzi A, Lassmann H, Rethwilm A, Horak I. Progressive encephalopathy and myopathy in transgenic mice expressing human foamy virus genes. *Science* 1991, 253:555.

28. Dalakas MC. Polymyositis, dermatomyositis and inclusion-body myositis. *N Engl J Med* 1991, 325:1487–1498.

29. Dalakas MC, Illa I. HIV-associated myopathies. In: Pizzo A, Wilfert CM (eds), *Pediatric AIDS: The Challenge of HIV Infection in Infants, Children and Adolescents*. Williams & Wilkins, Baltimore, 1991, pp. 420–429.

30. Dalakas MC, Wichman A, Sever JL. AIDS and the nervous system. *JAMA* 1989, 261:2396–2399.

31. Dalakas MC. Inflammatory and toxic myopathies. *Curr Opin Neurol Neurosurg* 1992, 5:645–654.

32. Dalakas MC, Illa I, Pezeshkpour GH, Laukaitis JP, Cohen B, Griffin JL. Mitochondrial myopathy caused by long-term zidovudine (AZT) therapy. *N Engl J Med* 1990, 332:1098–1105.

33. Cupler EJ, Leon-Monzon ME, Miller J, Semino-Mora C, Anderson T, Dalakas MC. Inclusion-body myositis (IBM) in HIV- and HTLV-I-infected patients. *Brain* 1996; 119, 1887–1893

34. Dalakas MC, Pezeshkpour GH. Neuromuscular complications of AIDS. *Ann Neurol* 1988, 23(S):38–48.

35. Leon-Monzon M, Illa I, Dalakas MC. Polymyositis in patients infected with HTLV-I: the role of the virus in the cause of the disease. *Ann Neurol* 1994, 36:643–649.

36. Illa I, Nath A, Dalakas MC. Immunocytochemical and virological characteristics of HIV-associated inflammatory myopathies: similarities with seronegative polymyositis. *Ann Neurol* 1991, 29:474–481.
37. Leon-Monzon M, Lamperth L, Dalakas MC. Search for HIV proviral DNA and amplified sequences in the muscle biopsies of patients with HIV-polymyositis. *Muscle Nerve* 1993, 16:408–413.
38. Leon-Monzon M, Dalakas MC. Diversity of T cell receptor (TCR) gene families in the endomysial lymphocytes of patients with sporadic inclusion body myositis (s-IBM). *Neurology* 1996, 46:115.
39. Illa I, Dalakas MC. Upregulation of STAT-1 and cytokine activity in the muscles of patients with sporadic inclusion body myositis (s-IBM), but not in hereditary IBM (h-IBM). *Neurology* 1996, 46:115.
40. Herman A, Kappler JW, Marrack P, Pullen AM. Superantigens – mechanism of T cell stimulation and role in immune responses. *Ann Rev Immunol* 1991, 9:745–772.
41. Pantaleo G, Graziosi C, Fauci AS. The immunopathogenesis of human immunodeficiency virus infection. *N Engl J Med* 1993, 328:327–335.
42. Lindberg C, Oldfors A, Tarkowski A. A restricted use of T cell receptor V genes in endomysial infiltrates in patients with inflammatory myopathies. *Eur J Immunol* 1994, 24:2659–2663.
43. O'Hanlon TP, Dalakas MC, Plotz PH, Miller FW. The $\alpha\beta$ T-cell receptor repertoire in inclusion body myositis: diverse patterns of gene expression by muscle-infiltrating lymphocytes. *J Autoimmunity* 1994, 7:321–333.
44. Arahata K, Engel AG. Monoclonal antibody analysis of mononuclear cells in myopathies. I. Quantitation of subsets according to diagnosis and sites of accumulation and demonstration and counts of muscle fibers invaded by T cells. *Ann Neurol* 1984, 16:193.
45. Engel AG, Arahata K. Monoclonal antibody analysis of mononuclear cells in myopathies. II. Phenotypes of autoinvasive cells in polymyositis and inclusion body myositis. *Ann Neurol* 1984, 16:209.
46. Denman AM. Viral aetiology of polymyositis/dermatomyositis. In: Dalakas MC (ed), *Polymyositis and Dermatomyositis*. Butterworth, Stoneham, MA, 1988, pp. 97–120.
47. Query CC, Keene JD. A human autoimmune protein associated with U1RNA contains a region of homology that is cross-reactive with retroviral p30 *gag* antigens. *Cell* 1987, 51:211–220.
48. Rucheton M, Graafland H, Fanton H, Ursule L, Ferrier P, Larsen CJ. Presence of circulating antibodies against *gag*-gene MuLV proteins in patients with autoimmune connective tissue disorders. *Virology* 1985, 144:468.
49. Illa I, Leon-Monzon M, Dalakas M. Retroviral sequences in patients with polymyositis (PM), dermatomyositis (DM) and inclusion body myositis (IBM). *Neurology* 1992, 42(S):302.
50. Talal N, Dauphinee MJ, Dang H, Alexander SS, Hart DJ, Garry RF. Detection of serum antibodies to retroviral proteins in patients with primary Sjögren's syndrome (autoimmune exocrinopathy). *Arthritis Rheum* 1990, 13:774–781.
51. Green JE, Hinrichs SH, Vogel J, Jay G. Exocrinopathy resembling Sjögren's syndrome in HTLV-I tax transgenic mice. *Nature* 1989, 341:72–74.
52. Shih A, Misra R, Rush MG. Detection of multiple, novel-reverse transcriptase coding sequences in human nucleic acids: relation to primate retroviruses. *J Virol* 1989, 63:64.

53. Krieg AM, Gourley MF, Perl A. Endogenous retroviruses: potential etiologic agents in autoimmunity. *FASEB J* 1992, 6:2537–2544.
54. Dalakas MC, Illa I. Common variable immunodeficiency and inclusion body myositis: a distinct myopathy mediated by Natural Killer cells. *Ann Neurol* 1995, 38:267–269.

19

Myonuclear Abnormalities May Play a Central Role in the Pathogenesis of Muscle-Fiber Damage in Inclusion-Body Myositis

GEORGE KARPATI AND STIRLING CARPENTER

Microscopic abnormalities of myonuclei are not uncommon in neuromuscular diseases (6). In denervated muscle fibers, the nuclear/cytoplasmic volume ratio increases, and the chromatin pattern becomes coarse. In regenerating fibers, the sizes of nuclei are increased, the nuclear staining is lighter, and the nucleolus becomes prominent. These alterations presumably reflect increased transcriptional activity. To a lesser extent, similar changes ("activated" myonuclei) also occur in other types of pathologic muscle fibers, such as ragged red fibers and damaged fibers in dermatomyositis. Prominent myonuclear alterations are characteristic for a peculiar form of infantile polymyositis (20). In oculopharyngeal muscular dystrophy, the 8.5-nm-diameter myonuclear filaments are disease-specific (21).

In both sporadic inclusion-body myositis (IBM) and hereditary inclusion-body myopathy, myonuclear abnormalities not only are prominent and characteristic (5) but also probably play central roles in the pathogenesis of muscle-fiber damage (12). Nuclear abnormalities in IBM include abnormal shape, pyknosis, and peripheral crowding of the chromatin. However, the three most characteristic alterations are (5,11) (i) 15–18-nm-diameter tubular filaments, (ii) breakdown of myonuclei, and (iii) expression of a single-strand-DNA-binding protein (15).

The myonuclear tubular filaments may be so abundant as to fill most of the nuclear volume. Their chemical identity is undetermined. They are unlikely to be viral particles. According to a hypothesis to be discussed later, they could represent altered nuclear-matrix components. The role of these filaments in the pathogenesis of the nuclear breakdown is still unclear. They could perturb myonuclear function simply by a space-occupying effect and/or by a more specific mechanism. The percentage of myonuclei that contain masses of tubular filaments has not been determined; a crude estimate is 1–3%. Masses of tubular filaments are also found in rimmed vacuoles in the cytoplasm of muscle fibers, probably released from breakdown of myonuclei. The tubular filaments in the cytoplasm presumably are destined for slow degradation by the neutral-pH, ATP-dependent protease system that requires prior ubiquitinization of the degradable molecule. Possibly they may also be exocytosed, as discussed later.

Actual breakdown of a myonucleus, with discharge of its contents into the cytoplasm, is rarely observed by electron microscopy, presumably because of the rapid sequence of events involved. However, masses of tubular filaments whose shapes, sizes, and locations are reminiscent of those of myonuclei are sometimes found in cytoplasmic spaces next to whorls of cytomembranes. These cytoplasmic areas (which correspond to the so-called rimmed vacuoles seen on cryostat sections) almost certainly mark the sites of previous myonuclear breakdown. Prior to nuclear dis-integration, the nuclear membrane may show focal breaches and even vesiculation, which could be forerunners of the whorls of cytomembranes (G. Gosztonyi, personal communication).

Approximately 3–5% of the myonuclei in most cases of IBM show strong binding of any single-strand DNA without sequence specificity (15). Similar single-strand-DNA-binding sites can be identified as vacuo-lar spaces in the cytoplasm. This indicates that the vacuoles mark sites of myonuclear breakdown. The nature of the single-strand-DNA-binding protein is unclear. Although a well-characterized nuclear single-strand-DNA-binding protein, replication protein A (RP-A) (19), is markedly up-regulated in IBM myonuclei, it is unlikely to be responsible for most of the DNA binding described, because many more myonuclei show immunoreactive RP-A than single-strand-DNA binding. Abnormal sin-gle-strand-DNA binding by IBM myonuclei appears to be the earliest discernible myonuclear abnormality.

Can pathologic alterations in the nuclear matrix explain the observed myonuclear alterations in IBM? The nuclear matrix (NM), a complex cytoskeletal system of insoluble fibrous and nonfibrous proteins ("non-histone proteins"), is a key organizer of nuclear structure and function (2,4,7,8,10). Some of the NM molecules are cell-specific, whereas others are common to all cells. In structural terms, the NM determines nuclear size and shape (10), as well as the dissolution and reestablishment of the nuclear membrane during mitosis (17). The NM is also responsible for the three-dimensional organization of DNA into loops (8). As a result of these structural specifications, the NM is critically involved in essential nuclear functions that include the following (4): regulation of DNA replication (13), RNA splicing and transport, regulation of tissue-specific gene expression (by positioning genes so that they are optimally configured for interaction with transcription factors), and signal transduction from within and without the nucleus (13). Abnormalities of the NM have been observed in malignant cells by two-dimensional electrophoresis and/or with monoclonal antibodies (21). These abnormalities appear to be specific for certain types of cancer cells (i.e., prostate) and can be used for diagnosis (22).

In view of the essential roles of the NM, a putative NM perturbation in IBM could subvert many functions of myonuclei and lead to their physical breakdown. According to this supposition, a hypothetical scheme of pathogenic events in IBM can be offered (Figure 19.1). This hypothesis postulates serious perturbations of the structure and function of the NM due to still-elusive etiologic factor(s). Because in IBM the muscle fibers seem to be the only cells involved, one can theorize that the target of the etiologic agent(s) is a muscle-specific NM molecule. A putative old-age-related alteration of the NM may render the system more vulnerable to noxious agents. In hereditary inclusion-body myopathies (9), different gene defects could affect NM-related molecules, leading to their functional disturbance.

The consequences of an NM abnormality could be multiple and could explain most of the myopathologic findings in IBM, as follows:

1. Myonuclear disintegration would eventually lead to progressive myonuclear attrition. That, in turn, would bring about progressive reduction of the myofiber volume (atrophy), as is prominent in IBM muscle. Myonuclear breakdown entails the fragmentation of the nuclear membrane and may provide the nidus for the formation of the abundant whorls of cytomembranes. The strongly basic nuclear contents rich in phosphates could combine with the phospholipid pool to join the membranes that populate the rimmed vacuoles. The presence of rimmed vacuoles is obviously a handicap for the normal functioning of muscle fibers.

2. The NM abnormalities could pervert gene expression, and that could explain the apparent aberrant expression of molecules that are not normally present in extrajunctional portions of muscle fibers (i.e., β-amyloid-like material)(1). Whether such molecules contribute to muscle-fiber damage is still unclear. At the same time, one can expect that other essential genes would be underexpressed, although a specific deficiency of a molecule has not been demonstrated in IBM muscle fibers.

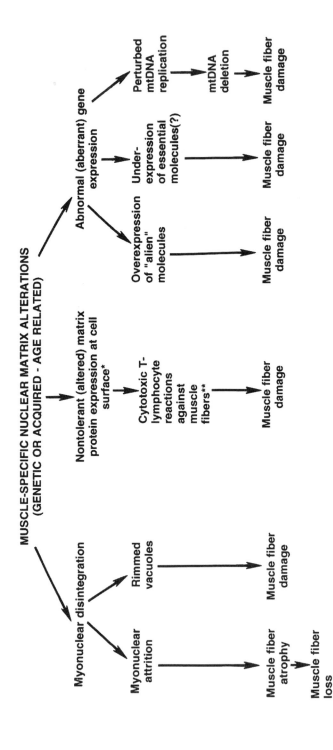

Figure 19.1. Hypothetical scheme for the pathogenic events in IBM. (Source: Griggs et al., Inclusion body myositis and myopathies, *Ann Neurol* 1995, 38:205–713.)

3. Altered nuclear gene expression could explain the excessive mitochondrial proliferation and mitochondrial-DNA (mtDNA) deletions (16), because mtDNA replication is, in part, regulated by putative nuclear gene(s)(23).
4. The basis of the inflammatory reaction (18) is still puzzling. A possibility is that an altered NM protein could be released by nuclear disintegration and subsequently exocytosed and picked up by antigen-presenting cells. That, in turn, would evoke a delayed hypersensitive response targeting muscle fibers in a nontolerized host. Some muscle-fiber damage is mediated by partial invasion of non-necrotic muscle fibers by CD8$^+$ lymphocytes and macrophages, similar to what occurs in polymyositis (11). The partially invaded muscle fibers might suffer damage by mechanical pressure from the invading cells or by their release of cytokines. The contribution of the inflammatory reaction to muscle-fiber damage is variable from muscle to muscle and from case to case. When it is strong, anti-dysimmune medication can have a modest and temporary beneficial effect (3), but such medication will not influence the basic deleterious processes that lead to progressive atrophy of muscle fibers. The lack of an inflammatory reaction in hereditary inclusion-body myopathies is also puzzling, but it does not invalidate this hypothesis.

The NM hypothesis for the pathophysiology of IBM can be tested. Techniques are available for microscopic study of NM (i.e., confocal immunocytochemistry or fluorescent in situ hybridization) (2) and for biochemical analysis (two-dimensional electrophoresis, etc.).

The NM hypothesis of IBM would also gain support if in a hereditary form of IBM the culprit molecule proved to be an NM protein. Identification of the gene whose mutation is responsible for the hereditary IBM in Iranian Jews is within reach now that positional cloning has localized the gene to chromosome 9 (14).

References

1. Askanas V, Engel WK, Alvarez RB. Enhanced detection of Congo-red-positive amyloid deposits in muscle fibers of inclusion-body myositis and brain of Alzheimer disease using fluorescence technique. *Neurology* 1993, 43:1265–1267.
2. Baskin Y. Mapping the cell's nucleus. *Science* 1995, 268:1564–1565.
3. Basta M, Dalakas MC. High dose intravenous immunoglobulin exerts its beneficial effect in patients with dermatomyositis by blocking endomysial

deposition of activated complement fragments. *J Clin Invest* 1994, 94:1729–1735.

4. Berezney R. The nuclear matrix: a heuristic model for investigating genomic organization and function in the cell nucleus (review). *J Cell Biochem* 1991, 47:109–123.

5. Carpenter S, Karpati G, Heller I, Eisen A. Inclusion body myositis: a distinct variety of idiopathic inflammatory myopathy. *Neurology* 1978, 28:8–17.

6. Carpenter S, Karpati G. *Pathology of Skeletal Muscle*. Churchill Livingstone, New York, 1984, pp. 246–271.

7. Driel RV, Humbel B, DeJong L. The nucleus: a black box being opened. *J Cell Biochem* 1991, 47:311–316.

8. Getzenberg RH, Peinta KJ, Ward WS, Coffey DS. Nuclear structure and the three-dimensional organization of DNA (review). *J Cell Biochem* 1991, 47:289–299.

9. Griggs RC, Askanas V, DiMauro S, Engel AG, Karpati G, Mendell JR, Rowland LP. Inclusion body myositis and myopathies. *Ann Neurol* 1995, 38:705–713.

10. Hoffman M. The cell's nucleus shapes up. *Science* 1993, 259:1257–1259.

11. Karpati G, Carpenter S. Pathology of the inflammatory myopathies (review). *Bailliere's Clinical Neurology* 1993, 2:527–556.

12. Karpati G, Carpenter S. Evolving concepts about inclusion body myositis. In: *Actualités Neuromusculaire: Aquisitions Récentes*, Serratrice G, Pellissier JF, Pouget J (eds). Exp. Scient. Française, Paris, 1993, pp. 93–98.

13. Leonhardt H, Page AW, Weier HU, Bestor TH. A targeting sequence directs DNA methyltransferase to sites of DNA replication in mammalian nuclei. *Cell* 1992, 71:865–873.

14. Mitrani-Rosenbaum S, Argov Z, Blumenfeld A, Seidman CE, Seidman JG. Hereditary inclusion body myopathy maps to chromosome 9p1-q1. *Hum Mol Genet* 1996, 5:159–163.

15. Nalbantoglu J, Karpati G, Carpenter S. Conspicuous accumulation of a single-stranded DNA binding protein in skeletal muscle fibers in inclusion body myositis. *Am J Pathol* 1994, 144:874–882.

16. Oldfors A, Larsson NG, Lindberg C, Holme E. Mitochondrial DNA deletions in inclusion body myositis. *Brain* 1993, 116:325–336.

17. Pfaller R, Smythe C, Newport JW. Assembly/disassembly of the nuclear envelope membrane: cell cycle-dependent binding of nuclear membrane vesicles to chromatin in vitro. *Cell* 1991, 65:209–217.

18. Sekul EA, Dalakas M. Inclusion body myositis: new concepts. *Semin Neurol* 1993, 13:256–263.

19. Seroussi E, Lavi S. Replication protein A is the major single-stranded DNA binding protein detected in mammalian cell extracts by gel retardation assays and UV cross-linking of long and short single-stranded DNA molecules. *J Biol Chem* 1993, 268:7147–7154.

20. Sripathi N, Karpati G, Carpenter S. A distinctive type of infantile inflammatory myopathy with abnormal myonuclei. *J Neurol Sci* 1996, 136:47–53.

21. Tomé FMS, Fardeau M. Nuclear inclusions in oculopharyngeal dystrophy. *Acta Neuropathol* 1980, 49:85–87.

22. Travis J. Looking for cancer in nuclear matrix proteins. *Science* 1993, 259:1258.

23. Zeviani M, Tiranti V. Inherited mendelian defects. In: *Mitochondrial DNA in Human Pathology*, DiMauro S, Wallace DC (eds). Raven Press, New York, 1993, pp. 85–95.

20

Nuclear Degeneration and Rimmed-Vacuole Formation in Neuromuscular Disorders

IKUYA NONAKA, NOBUYUKI MURAKAMI,
YUME SUZUKI, AND EIJIRO SATOYOSHI

Although nuclear changes, including central nuclei and pyknotic nuclear clumps, have occasionally been described in the literature in a variety of disorders, particularly myotonic dystrophy, very little is known about the relationship between nuclear degeneration and muscle-fiber atrophy. It is believed that the tubulofilamentous inclusions seen in inclusion-body myositis (IBM) (1), distal myopathy with rimmed-vacuole formation (DMRV) (2), and oculopharyngeal muscular dystrophy (OPMD) (3) play an important role in muscle-fiber degeneration, but the exact nature and significance of that role remain to be determined. Because muscle fibers with nuclear inclusions are almost always associated with rimmed-vacuole formation, the vacuolar change is believed to result from defective nuclear function. We therefore examined a variety of muscle biopsy specimens with rimmed vacuoles by electron microscopy, paying particular attention to their nuclei. Striking nuclear changes were seen in IBM, DMRV, and OPMD, as well as in several other diseases, including Marinesco-Sjögren syndrome, reducing-body myopathy, and hypokalemic periodic paralysis of unknown cause. Because the nuclear changes in DMRV and reducing-body myopathy have already been described (4), we concentrated on Marinesco-Sjögren syndrome.

Patients and Methods

We studied 12 patients ranging in age from 1 to 36 years who showed the clinical characteristics of Marinesco-Sjögren syndrome, which included delayed developmental milestones, congenital cataracts, cerebellar ataxia, and mental retardation. In addition, all 12 patients had progressive muscle weakness. Five patients became nonambulant at ages from

16 to 20 years because of muscle weakness. Serum creatine kinase concentrations were slightly to moderately elevated.

Two unrelated female patients with the fatal infantile form of reducing-body myopathy developed rapidly progressive generalized muscle weakness at the ages of 2 $^{10}/_{12}$ years and 2 $^{3}/_{12}$ years. Their muscle weakness and hypotonia were quite striking and involved neck and respiratory muscles. They died at the ages of 4 $^{11}/_{12}$ and 3 $^{9}/_{12}$ years from respiratory failure (4).

One female patient with hypokalemic periodic paralysis had unusual progressive muscle weakness from the early infantile stage (9). She had a mildly elevated serum creatine kinase concentration of 230 U/L (normal, < 150 U/L).

In all patients, the biceps brachii muscle was biopsied and frozen in isopentane cooled by liquid nitrogen for histochemical and immunohistochemical examination. Serial frozen sections were stained with hematoxylin and eosin (H&E), modified Gomori trichrome and various histochemical methods. To determine whether or not the rimmed vacuoles in other diseases featured the same process of protein degradation seen in IBM, DMRV, and OPMD, we applied antibodies against β-amyloid protein ($A\beta$, against the NH2 terminal and COOH terminal of β-amyloid precursor protein (βPPN and βPPC), and against τ protein to eight biopsy specimens from five patients with Marinesco-Sjögren syndrome, two patients with reducing-body myopathy, and one patient with periodic paralysis who had prominent rimmed-vacuole formation (10). To determine if there was fragmentation of nuclear DNA, the 3'-OH ends of double- or single-strand DNA were labeled with Apop Tag (Oncor Inc.) and examined after diaminobenzidine (DAB) staining. For electron-microscopic examination, small pieces of the biopsy specimens were fixed in cacodylate-buffered 2% glutaraldehyde solution for 2 hours, postfixed in 1% osmium tetraoxide, and embedded in epoxy resin after dehydration. Ultrathin sections were double stained with uranyl acetate and lead nitrate.

Results

Marinesco-Sjögren Syndrome

In all muscle biopsy specimens there were myopathic changes consisting of variations in the sizes of both type-1 and type-2 fibers and interstitial fibrosis (7,8). Rimmed vacuoles were identified in 1–18% of the fibers, especially those from younger patients less than 6 years of age. In advanced-stage disease, muscle fibers were largely replaced by connective tissue and fatty tissue. There were some ragged red fibers in five biopsy specimens. The most striking changes were in the nuclei, which were enlarged or pyknotic, occasionally with fragmented nucleoplasm (Figure 20.1). In two younger patients, almost 10% of myonuclei were abnormal. The nuclear changes were almost always associated with rimmed-vacuole formation. Immunohistochemical examination with anti-Aβ, anti-βPP, and anti-τ-protein antibodies showed positive immunoreactivities in the fibers with rimmed vacuoles. The overall findings were similar to those seen in DMRV and IBM (10,12). In two of five muscle specimens from younger patients with striking nuclear changes, 15 and 7 myonuclei stained positively with the Tunel method, indicating nuclear DNA fragmentation (data not shown); the other three muscle specimens had a few equivocally positive myonuclei. None of the control specimens had positively stained myonuclei, but the nuclei of a few lymphocytes showed positive staining.

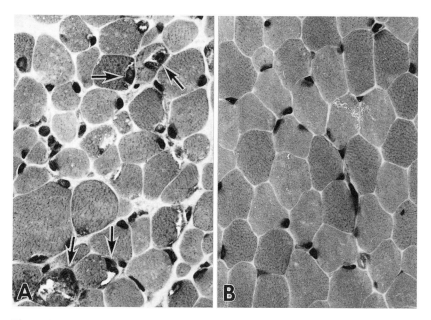

Figure 20.1. In addition to variations in fiber size, there are numerous enlarged and fragmented nuclei (arrows). Most fibers with degenerating nuclei are vacuo-lated, forming "rimmed vacuoles." These specimens are from a 2-year-old boy with Marinesco-Sjögren syndrome (A) and a healthy boy of the same age (B) (H&E, ×600).

At electron microscopy, the most outstanding findings were nuclear changes. Even in muscle fibers with normal myofibrillar organization there were numerous degenerating myonuclei. A dense membranous structure (13) around the nucleus was the most common early change, and that structure probably originated via dissociation of the nuclear membrane from the shrunken nucleoplasm (Figure 20.2). In the more advanced stages, the nuclei were pyknotic and contained fine granular inclusions and myelin figures (Figure 20.3). The amounts of chromatin granules were markedly decreased. In the final stages, the entire nucleoplasm was densely pyknotic and shrunken, leaving the dense nuclear membrane. Myofibrils near the degenerating nuclei were almost always abnormal, with numerous autophagic vacuoles and myelin figures (Figure 20.4). Those nuclear changes were found more frequently in the younger patients, and only rarely in adults.

Reducing-Body Myopathy

Because the clinical and pathologic findings have already been reported in detail (4), only a brief description will be given here. In addition to the variations in fiber size, in almost all the fibers there were eosinophilic

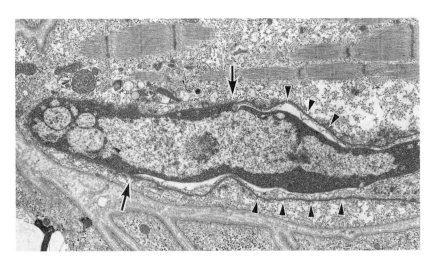

Figure 20.2. Early nuclear changes seen in Marinesco-Sjögren syndrome. A dense membranous structure (arrowheads) connects to nuclear membrane (arrows), suggesting dissociation of the nuclear membrane from the shrunken nucleoplasm. Decreased amounts of chromatin granules were condensed at the periphery of the nucleoplasm (×10,000).

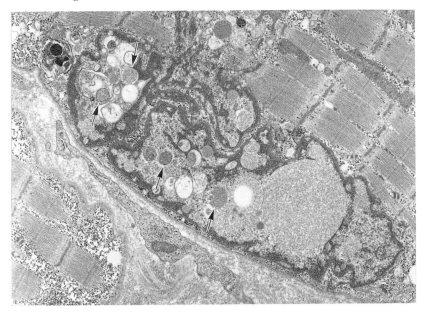

Figure 20.3. A typical degenerated myonucleus seen in Marinesco-Sjögren syndrome. Note indented nuclear membrane, numerous fine granular inclusions (arrows), and a small amount of condensed chromatin granules at the periphery of the nucleus (×11,000).

amorphous inclusions that stained very intensely with menadione-linked α-glycerophosphate dehydrogenase (MAG) – the histochemical characteristic of a reducing body. In the severely damaged fibers, the myonuclei were pyknotic and shrunken, and the cytoplasm contained rimmed vacuoles with increased acid-phosphatase activity. The immunohistochemical reactivities to anti-Aβ, anti-βPP, and anti-τ-protein antibodies were similar to those seen in DMRV and Marinesco-Sjögren syndrome. At electron microscopy, the reducing bodies were perinuclear or in the vicinity of nuclei. Occasionally the nuclei were shrunken and pyknotic. Myofibrils were disorganized, with numerous autophagic vacuoles and myelin figures (Figure 20.5).

Periodic Paralysis with Rapid Muscle Weakness

The striking pathologic abnormalities included nuclear fragmentation and myofibrillar degeneration, with rimmed-vacuole formation. There were moderate variations in fiber size, with a few necrotic fibers. Tu-

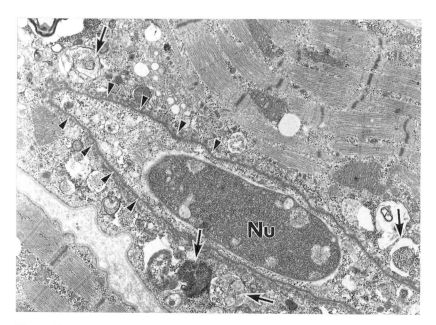

Figure 20.4. In the advanced stage of Marinesco-Sjögren syndrome the myonucleus (Nu) is shrunken and condensed, leaving a dense membranous structure (arrowheads). In the vicinity of the degenerated nucleus, myofibrils are disorganized, with numerous autophagic vacuoles (arrows) (×14,000).

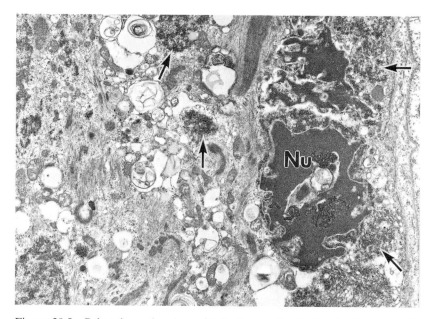

Figure 20.5. Pyknotic nucleoplasm (Nu), dispersed reducing bodies (arrows), degenerated myofibrils, and numerous autophagic vacuoles in reducing-body myopathy (×10,000).

bular aggregates were not found. Nuclear fragmentation was confirmed by electron microscopy. Fragmented nuclei occasionally contained crystalline inclusions. Myofibrils in the vicinity of the degenerated myonuclei were disorganized, with numerous autophagic vacuoles (Figure 20.6).

Discussion

The presence of nuclear and cytoplasmic inclusions consisting of tubulofilamentous structures measuring 16–19 nm in diameter is a diagnostic finding in IBM and is also commonly seen in DMRV (2). In both diseases, at muscle biopsy, rimmed-vacuole formation is always associated with structural abnormalities. These two structural changes strongly suggest that the nuclear changes may be playing important roles in inducing myofibrillar degeneration and vacuole formation. Therefore, we reviewed the muscle biopsy studies in our files in which there were large numbers of rimmed vacuoles, which are thought to be responsible for the degeneration of muscle fibers. In addition to IBM and DMRV, striking

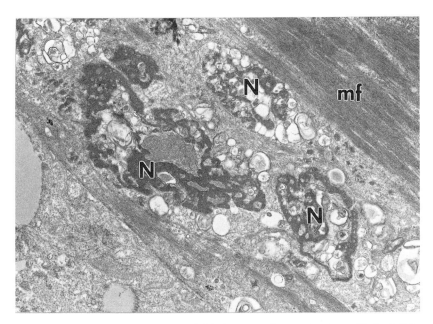

Figure 20.6   Fragmentated myonuclei (N) among disorganized myofibrils (mf) in a female patient with an unusual form of periodic paralysis with progressive weakness (X 10,000).

nuclear changes were found in all 12 patients with Marinesco-Sjögren syndrome, 2 patients with reducing-body myopathy, and 1 patient with an unusual form of periodic paralysis.

In addition to congenital cataracts, mental retardation, and cerebellar ataxia, progressive muscle weakness is a common feature in Marinesco-Sjögren syndrome (5–7). Because rimmed-vacuole formation, with minimal muscle-fiber necrosis and regeneration (7,8), is the most prominent finding, muscle degeneration associated with vacuole formation is thought to be the primary pathologic process in this syndrome. A dense membranous structure around the nucleus, reported to be the characteristic ultrastructural change in this syndrome (13), probably is an early structural alteration resulting from dissociation of the nuclear membrane from the shrunken nucleoplasm. The nuclear change is progressive, leading to almost complete loss of chromatin granules (14).

Nuclear damage probably is responsible for defective protein synthesis, which results in degeneration of myofibrils and intracytoplasmic organelles. The damaged organelles are then scavenged by autophagosomes and form myelin figures (i.e., the rimmed vacuoles). There is little doubt that this nuclear change is closely related to apoptosis, because the nuclear DNA is fragmented in degenerating muscle fibers, as shown by the Tunel method, and electron micrographs have shown the characteristic findings of apoptosis and chromatin condensation, followed by complete loss of nucleoplasm. Therefore, this syndrome appears to be the ideal disease in which to study the relationship between apoptosis and muscle degeneration.

Condensed and karyolytic nuclei in two patients with reducing-body myopathy, and fragmented nuclei in a patient with an unusual form of periodic paralysis, are additional nuclear changes leading to myofibrillar degeneration. Although we failed to demonstrate evidence of nuclear DNA fragmentation by immunohistochemistry, the ultrastructural findings are strongly suggestive of apoptosis. Although the nuclear abnormalities differ from one disease to another, all these diseases may have similar pathogenetic mechanisms of muscle degeneration.

Whether or not the nuclear changes are of primary importance, the processes of protein degradation resulting in rimmed-vacuole formation may not differ significantly from one disease to another. In IBM, DMRV, OPMD, and the three diseases discussed here, the rimmed vacuoles were acid-phosphatase-positive and had Aβ, βPP, and τ-protein deposits (12).

References

1. Carpenter S, Karpati G, Heller I, Eisen A. Inclusion body myositis: a distinct variety of idiopathic inflammatory myopathy. *Neurology* 1978, 28:8–17.
2. Nonaka I, Sunohara N, Ishiura S, Satoyoshi E. Familial distal myopathy with rimmed vacuole and lamellar (myeloid) body formation. *J Neurol Sci* 1981, 51:141–155.
3. Tomé FMS, Fardeau M. Nuclear inclusion in oculopharyngeal dystrophy. *Acta Neuropathol (Berlin)* 1980, 49:85–87.
4. Kiyomoto BH, Murakami N, Kobayashi Y, Nihei K, Tanaka T, Takeshita K, Nonaka I. Fatal reducing body myopathy: ultrastructural and immunohistochemical observations. *J Neurol Sci* 1995, 128:58–65.
5. Marinesco G, Draganesco S, Vasiliu D. Nouvelle maladie familiale caractériseé [ar une cataracte congénitale et un arrêt du développement somato-neuropsychique]. *L' Encéphale* 1932, 26:97–109.
6. Sjögren T. Hereditary congenital spinocerebellar ataxia accompanied by congenital cataract and oligophrenia. *Confin Neurol* 1950, 10:293–308.
7. Komiyama A, Nonaka I, Hirayama K. Muscle pathology in Marinesco-Sjögren syndrome. *J Neurol Sci* 1989, 89:103–113.
8. Goto Y, Komiyama A, Tanabe Y, Katafuchi Y, Ohtaki E, Nonaka I. Myopathy in Marinesco-Sjögren syndrome: an ultrastructural study. *Acta Neuropathol* 1990, 80:123–128.
9. Obo Y, Suzuki Y, Nonaka I. A girl with hypokalemic periodic paralysis and progressive muscle weakness with myonuclear degeneration and myopathic change (in Japanese). *No to Hattatsu (Tokyo)* 1987, 19:519–521.
10. Murakami N, Ihara Y, Nonaka I. Muscle fiber degeneration in distal myopathy with rimmed vacuole formation. *Acta Neuropathol* 1995, 89:29–34.
11. Gavrieli Y, Sherman Y, Ben-Sasson SA. Identification of programmed cell death in situ via specific labeling of nuclear DNA fragmentation. *J Cell Biol* 1992, 119:493–501.
12. Askanas V, Engel WK. New advances in inclusion-body myositis. *Curr Opin Rheumatol* 1993, 5:732–741.
13. Sewry CA, Voit T, Dubowitz V. Myopathy with unique ultrastructural feature in Marinesco-Sjögren syndrome. *Ann Neurol* 1988, 24:576–580.
14. Suzuki Y, Murakami N, Goto Y, Orimo S, Komiyama A, Kuroina Y, Nonaka I. Apoptotic nuclear degeneration in Marimesco-Sjögren syndrome. *Acta Neuropathol* 1997 (in press).

21

Mitochondrial Alterations in Sporadic Inclusion-Body Myositis

ANDERS OLDFORS, ALI-REZA MOSLEMI,
ELISABETH HOLME, AND CHRISTOPHER
LINDBERG

Morphologic Changes of Mitochondria and Partial Cytochrome-c-oxidase Deficiency Are Consistent Findings in Sporadic Inclusion-Body Myositis

Ragged red fibers are muscle fibers that have accumulations of mitochondria with abnormal ultrastructure. Their occurrence in muscle biopsies has been regarded as an indication of mitochondrial disease. They are abundant in disorders such as Kearns-Sayre syndrome, PEO (progressive external ophthalmoplegia), MERRF (myoclonus epilepsy with ragged red fibers), MELAS (myoclonus epilepsy, lactic acidosis, and stroke-like episodes), and many other mitochondrial diseases due to mitochondrial DNA (mtDNA) mutations (40).

Ragged red fibers are also frequently encountered in sporadic inclusion-body myositis (s-IBM) (3,5,30). In 1975, Carpenter el al. (4) suggested that mitochondria and muscle-cell nuclei may be primarily affected in s-IBM. That hypothesis was based on the finding of ultrastructural changes in the mitochondria and nuclei. The ultrastructural abnormalities of the mitochondria in s-IBM are not specific, because the same types of changes, such as paracrystalline inclusions (Figure 21.1), can be seen in a variety of mitochondrial myopathies (26).

Enzyme histochemical analysis has demonstrated that the mitochondria in ragged red fibers in s-IBM show deficient enzyme activity. Partial cytochrome c oxidase (COX) deficiency is a consistent finding that presents as segments of muscle fibers with low COX activity (Figure 21.2) (26,27,30). Ragged red fibers, as well as other muscle fibers, can show COX deficiency. The frequency of COX deficient muscle fibers in s-IBM varies and can exceed 10% (27,30).

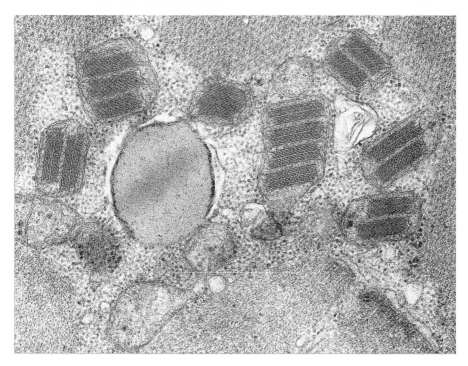

Figure 21.1. Electron micrograph showing paracrystalline inclusions in mitochondria in s-IBM.

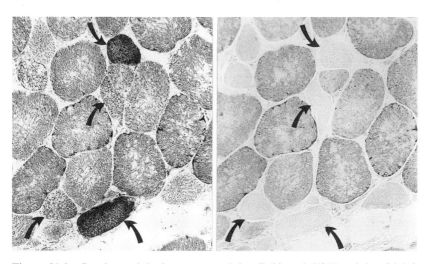

Figure 21.2. Succinate dehydrogenase staining (left) and COX staining (right) of skeletal muscle in a case of s-IBM showing multiple muscle fibers with COX deficient mitochondria (arrows).

COX Deficiency in Muscle Fibers in s-IBM Is Caused by mtDNA Deletions

Human mtDNA is a 16.6-kb circular molecule that encodes 13 peptides, including cytochrome b and subunits of the respiratory chain enzymes NADH dehydrogenase, COX, and ATP synthase. In addition, all tRNAs and the rRNAs necessary for synthesis of those peptides are encoded by mtDNA. Some mitochondrial diseases are due to single large deletions of mtDNA (12,31,42,45). These deletions usually remove several tRNA genes, in addition to one or several protein encoding genes, resulting in impaired synthesis of all mtDNA encoded proteins (11,23). In disorders due to mtDNA deletions there is always heteroplasmy, with a mixture of mutant and wild-type mtDNAs. The phenotypic expression of disease is partially dependent on the proportions and distributions of wild-type and deleted mtDNAs in the tissue (20,25). In muscle tissue, accumulation of deleted mtDNA in muscle fiber-segments with low levels of wild-type mtDNA is associated with COX deficiency in these fiber segments (10,19,20,25,34). A mixture of cells with normal and deficient COX activities can be observed in tissues other than muscle in diseases due to mtDNA deletions (42).

In situ hybridization demonstrated that COX deficient ragged red fibers in s-IBM patients had accumulated mtDNA with deletions and showed reduced amounts of wild-type mtDNA (26). By using a probe corresponding to transcripts of the NADH-dehydrogenase subunit 4 gene, which is located in a deletion prone region of mtDNA, it was demonstrated that many COX deficient muscle fiber segments showed lower levels of mtDNA transcripts than surrounding muscle fibers. The same COX deficient fiber segments showed accumulation of mtDNA transcripts when a probe corresponding to the NADH-dehydrogenase subunit 2 gene was used. Those COX-deficient fibers thus had accumulated transcripts of mtDNA with a deletion including at least the NADH-dehydrogenase subunit-4 gene but not the NADH-dehydrogenase subunit-2 gene.

There Are Multiple mtDNA Deletions in s-IBM

To address the question of which types of mtDNA deletions are present in s-IBM, muscle mtDNA has been studied by Southern analysis and by analysis of mtDNA after amplification with a polymerase chain reaction (PCR). The strategy to detect rearranged mtDNA by PCR analysis involves the use of multiple primer pairs (Figure 21.3). In each set of primer

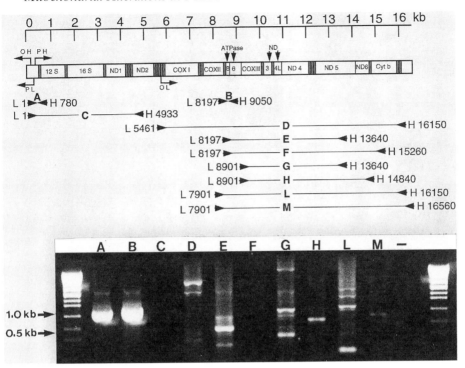

Figure 21.3. PCR analysis of mtDNA in s-IBM. Top: Linearized map of mtDNA showing the genes for NADH-dehydrogenase (ND) subunits 1 to 6, COX subunits I to III, ATP synthase (ATPase) subunits 6 and 8, and cytochrome b (Cyt b). The filled boxes represent tRNA genes. 12S and 16S represent the genes for rRNA. The origins of replication for the heavy (OH) and the light (OL) strands and the promoters of transcription for the heavy (PH) and light (PL) strands are indicated by arrows. The primer pairs used for PCR analysis are indicated (A to M). The L primers constitute parts of the light strand, and the H primers constitute parts of the heavy strand. Primer pairs A and B are used to amplify wild-type mtDNA. The widely separated primer pairs C to M are used to amplify mtDNA with deletions. The sequences of the primers are numbered according to the Cambridge mtDNA sequence (1), with nucleotide sequences (5′-3′) given within parenthesis: L 1 (1–20), L5461 (5461–5480), L7901 (7901–7920), L8197 (8197–8216), L8901 (8901–8920), H780 (780–761), H4933 (4933–4914), H9050 (9050–9031), H13640 (13640–13621), H14840 (14840–14821), H15260 (15260–15241), H16150 (16150–16131), and H16560 (16560–16541). The lower part of the figure illustrates the findings at PCR analysis in one s-IBM patient. The primer pairs used are indicated above each lane. The dash indicates control PCR without addition of DNA. The bands in lanes D to L are amplified fragments of mtDNA with deletions.

pairs the primers hybridize to mtDNA sequences that are widely separated by several thousand base pairs. If there is a large deletion in the region between the primers, the size of the amplified fragment will be considerably shorter and more efficiently amplified than a fragment of normal mtDNA. With the use of that strategy, many short fragments corresponding to deleted mtDNA are detected in s-IBM patients (Figure 21.3). PCR analysis of muscle tissue from 20 s-IBM patients showed multiple mtDNA deletions in all patients (27). Each patient showed many different deletions, but individual deletions appeared not to be equally abundant in the different patients. One deletion, called the "common deletion" because it is present in about one third of all patients with Kearns-Sayre syndrome/PEO (33), was seen in all 20 s-IBM cases. Multiple mtDNA deletions may be detected in about 45% of the s-IBM patients by Southern analysis (32). However, the major mtDNA molocule was of normal size in all cases. Those findings show that there are low levels of multiple mtDNA deletions in s-IBM.

There Is Clonal Expansion of Deleted mtDNA in Ragged Red Fibers in s-IBM

To investigate whether there is a mixed population of mtDNA molecules with deletions or only one type of deletion in each COX deficient ragged red fiber, two different methods have been employed: PCR analysis of isolated single muscle fiber segments, and mapping of the deletions by in situ hybridization using multiple mtDNA probes on consecutive tissue sections (27).

When muscle sections are stained for both succinate dehydrogenase and COX activity, fibers with accumulations of COX-deficient mitochondria are easy to detect, because they exhibit a dark-blue color, in contrast to surrounding normal brown fibers (34). These fibers can be dissected with a sharp needle and further analyzed by PCR (27,37). With the use of several primer pairs in PCR analysis, as described earlier, but on DNA from single, isolated muscle fiber segments, it can be demonstrated that only one deletion is detected in each COX deficient fiber in s-IBM (27). Deletion breakpoints can be analyzed by direct sequencing of the PCR fragments, further strengthening the hypothesis of a monoclonal population of deleted mtDNA in each COX-deficient fiber. In some of these fiber segments, wild-type mtDNA is not detected.

By in situ hybridization, the distribution of multiple deletions in muscle tissue can be mapped (27). When different mtDNA probes are used on consecutive sections the hybridization signal will vary between different COX deficient muscle fibers in s-IBM (Figure 21.4). Some COX deficient fibers will show accumulation of mtDNA transcripts using a probe corresponding to the NADH-dehydrogenase subunit-4 gene, but low levels of mRNA using a probe corresponding to the NADH-dehydrogenase subunit-6 gene. Adjacent fibers may show a reverse pattern (Figure 21.4). This hybridization pattern indicates that each COX deficient fiber contains mtDNA with only one type of deletion.

Thus the findings from single fiber PCR analysis and *in situ* hybridization analysis indicate that there is clonal expansion of mtDNA with different deletions in individual COX deficient ragged red fibers, in s-IBM. In addition to clonal expansion of multiple mtDNA deletions, duplications and depletion of mtDNA in muscle fiber segments have been reported in s-IBM (13).

Deletion Breakpoints Usually Are Flanked by Direct Nucleotide Repeats

Insight into the pathogenesis of mtDNA deletions in mitochondrial disorders has been gained by analyzing the deletion breakpoints. In Kearns-Sayre syndrome and PEO the deletions usually are flanked by direct nucleotide repeats. It has been speculated that mtDNA deletions may occur during replication by slipped mispairing of directly repeated sequences (18,36).

Analysis of deletion breakpoints in s-IBM has been performed by sequencing of the multiple deletions found by PCR analysis (21). These studies have shown that the deletions usually are flanked by direct repeats. In most cases, one copy of the repeats has been totally or partly deleted. In this respect the deletions in s-IBM do not differ from those in other conditions with mtDNA deletions. However, there are certain hot spot regions of mtDNA that are involved in deletion break-points in s-IBM. Except for the "common deletion," the deletion breakpoint regions in s-IBM appear to be different from those in diseases due to single large-scale deletions (21).

Other Conditions With Multiple mtDNA Deletions in Muscle

Multiple mtDNA deletions are normal findings in muscle and some other tissues in elderly individuals (2,7,8,47). It has been shown that there is an age-related increase in the amount of mutated mtDNA, but COX-

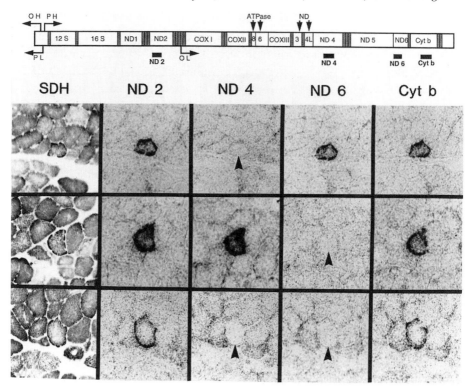

Figure 21.4. In situ hybridization of mtDNA transcripts using four different mtDNA probes (ND 2, ND 4, ND 6, and Cyt b). Top: Linearized map of mtDNA and the probes (abbreviations as in Figure 21.3). SDH is enzyme histochemical staining of succinate dehydrogenase. Three different adjacent ragged red fibers are illustrated. In one there is a deletion of the ND 4 gene (upper row), in the second there is a deletion of the ND 6 gene (middle row), and in the third there is a deletion of both the ND 4 and ND 6 genes (lower row). Accumulation of mtDNA transcripts is evident in all three fibers using the ND 2 and Cyt b probes. The hybridization signals with the probes corresponding to deleted parts of mtDNA are reduced in the ragged red fibers, as compared with surrounding fibers, indicating low levels of wild-type mtDNA in the ragged red fibers.

deficient muscle fibers are only occasionally observed in normal individuals in old age (15,26,30). Multiple mtDNA deletions have also been observed in a number of diseases, that have been associated with the occurrence of ragged red fibers. Among these are autosomal dominant PEO (adPEO) (35,39,44,46) and other familial and sporadic disorders with or without PEO (6,14,15,24,28,29,43). In late-onset mitochondrial myopathy, there appears to be clonal expansion of mtDNA with deletions in ragged red fibers, as in s-IBM (15). We studied a family with adPEO with multiple mtDNA deletions and found that in each COX-deficient fiber segment there was accumulation of mtDNA with only one type of deletion, indicating clonal propagation of deleted mtDNA in individual fibers (22).

Various Mechanisms May Account for the Accumulation of mtDNA with Deletions in s-IBM

The distributions in muscle of mtDNAs with multiple deletions appear to be similar in s-IBM and adPEO (22,27). In addition, the hot spot regions for deletion break-points appear to be very similar in s-IBM and adPEO (21). Because of the heredity of adPEO, a nuclear factor has been suggested to be involved in the development of multiple mtDNA deletions, although this factor has not been identified. Linkage analysis has identified a locus on chromosome 10 associated with multiple mtDNA deletions in a Finnish family (38). An additional locus on chromosome 3 was identified in Italian families with adPEO, indicating genetic heterogeneity (16). A nuclear factor, that might account for many of the abnormally expressed proteins associated with rimmed vacuoles in muscle in s-IBM has been discussed (9). Such a factor might also be involved in the development of multiple mtDNA deletions in s-IBM.

Damage of mtDNA by oxygen radicals has been discussed in aging and also in adPEO (38). That might be a common factor, involved in the development of multiple mtDNA deletions in adPEO and in s-IBM. In adPEO and s-IBM a nuclear factor could be involved by either increasing the formation of oxygen radicals or by impairing their removal.

Mutant mtDNA has a replicative advantage compared to wild-type mtDNA in certain situations (11), which may explain the clonal expansion of mtDNA with deletions.

Clinical Importance of mtDNA Deletions in s-IBM

Although the appearance of multiple mtDNA deletions in s-IBM most probably is a secondary phenomenon, it may have clinical importance. Patients with mitochondrial myopathies due to point mutations or deletions of mtDNA show various muscular symptoms, such as muscle weakness, muscle fatigue, exercise induced muscle pain, and muscle cramps (41). The major symptom in s-IBM patients is muscle weakness. There are several possible explanations for muscle weakness in s-IBM, such as endomysial fibrosis, segmental muscle fiber degeneration and necrosis, and polyneuropathy in some cases (17). The role of the mitochondrial changes is difficult to evaluate. Even if the total amount of deleted mtDNA is low, the selective distribution to certain fiber segments probably is of importance for the clinical symptoms. It has previously been shown that the distribution of deleted and wild-type mtDNAs in muscle tissue is important for the phenotypic expression of disease (20,25). In late-onset mitochondrial myopathy with multiple mtDNA deletions, the main abnormality in muscle is the mitochondrial changes, and the proportion of COX-deficient muscle fiber segments is similar to what is found in many patients with s-IBM (15,27). In late-onset mitochondrial myopathy, the patients show mild to moderate proximal muscle weakness and fatigue. Consequently, the mitochondrial alterations may be responsible for a significant part of the clinical symptoms also in some patients with s-IBM. The search for factors leading to generation of multiple mtDNA deletions may be of importance both for understanding the pathogenesis and for designing treatment for s-IBM.

Acknowledgments

This study was supported by grants from the Swedish Medical Research Council (Projects 07122 and 10823).

References

1. Anderson S, Bankier AT, Barrell BG, de Bruijn MHL, Coulson AR, Drouin J, Eperon IC, Nierlich DP, Roe BA, Sanger F, Schreier PH, Smith AJH, Staden R, Young IG. Sequence and organization of the human mitochondrial genome. Nature 290:457–465, 1981.
2. Baumer A, Zhang CF, Linnane AW, Nagley P. Age-related human mtDNA deletions: a heterogeneous set of deletions arising at a single pair of directly repeated sequences. Am J Hum Genet 54:618–630, 1994.
3. Carpenter S, Karpati G. Pathology of Skeletal Muscle. ed. Churchill Livingstone, New York, 1984.
4. Carpenter S, Karpati G, Eisen A. A morphologic study in polymyositis: clues to pathogenesis of different types. In: Bradley WG (ed), Recent Advances in Myology. Excerpta Medica, Amsterdam, 1975, pp. 374–379.
5. Carpenter S, Karpati G, Heller I, Eisen A. Inclusion body myositis: a distinct variety of idiopathic inflammatory myopathy. Neurology 28:8–17, 1978.
6. Casademont J, Barrientos A, Cardellach F, Rötig A, Grau JM, Montoya J, Beltran B, Cervantes F, Rozman C, Estivill X, Urbanomarquez A, Nunes V. Multiple deletions of mtDNA in two brothers with sideroblastic anemia and mitochondrial myopathy and in their asymptomatic mother. Hum Mol Genet 3:1945–1949, 1994.

7. Cortopassi GA, Arnheim N. Detection of a specific mitochondrial DNA deletion in tissues of older humans. Nucleic Acids Res 18:6927–6933, 1990.
8. Cortopassi GA, Shibata D, Soong N-W, Arenheim M. A pattern of accumulation of a somatic deletion of mitochondrial DNA in aging human muscle. Proc Natl Acad Sci USA 89:7370–7374, 1992.
9. Griggs RC, Askanas V, DiMauro S, Engel A, Karpati G, Mendell JR, Rowland LP. Inclusion body myositis and myopathies. Ann Neurol 38:705–713, 1995.
10. Hammans SR, Sweeney MG, Wicks DAG, Morgan-Hughes JA, Harding AE. A molecular genetic study of focal histochemical defects in mitochondrial encephalomyopathies. Brain 115:343–365, 1992.
11. Hayashi JI, Ohta S, Kikuchi A, Takemitsu M, Goto Y, Nonaka I. Introduction of disease-related mitochondrial DNA deletions into HeLa cells lacking mitochondrial DNA results in mitochondrial dysfunction. Proc Natl Acad Sci USA 88:10614–10618, 1991.
12. Holt IJ, Harding AE, Morgan-Hughes JA. Deletions of muscle mitochondrial DNA in patients with mitochondrial myopathies. Nature 331:717–719, 1988.
13. Horwath R, Karpati G, Fu K, Genge A, Shoubridge EA. Mitochondrial DNA abnormalities in inclusion body myositis. Presented at Euromitt III, Chantilly, France, 1995.
14. Johns DR, Threlkeld AB, Miller NR, Hurko O. Multiple mitochondrial DNA deletions in myo-neuro-gastrointestinal encephalopathy syndrome. Am J Ophthalmol 115:108–109, 1993.
15. Johnston W, Karpati G, Carpenter S, Arnold D, Shoubridge EA. Late-onset mitochondrial myopathy. Ann Neurol 37:16–23, 1995.
16. Kaukonen JA, Amati P, Suomalainen A, Rötig A, Piscaglia MG, Salvi F, Weissenbach J, Fratta G, Comi G, Peltonen L, Zelviani M. An autosomal locus predisposing to multiple deletions of mtDNA on chromosome 3p. Am J Hum Genet 58:763–769, 1996.
17. Lindberg C, Oldfors A, Hedström A. Inclusion body myositis - peripheral nerve involvement. Combined morphological and electrophysiological studies on peripheral nerves. J Neurol Sci 99:327–338, 1990.
18. Mita S, Rizzuto R, Moraes CT, Shanske S, Arnaudo E, Fabrizi GM, Koga Y, DiMauro S, Schon EA. Recombination via flanking direct repeats is a major cause of large-scale deletions of human mitochondrial DNA. Nucleic Acids Res 18:561–567, 1990.
19. Mita S, Schmidt B, Schon EA, DiMauro S, Bonilla E. Detection of "deleted" mitochondrial genomes in cytochrome-c oxidase-deficient muscle fibers of a patient with Kearns-Sayre syndrome. Proc Natl Acad Sci U S A 86:9509–9513, 1989.
20. Moraes CT, Sciacco M, Ricci E, Tengan CH, Hao H, Bonilla E, Schon EA, DiMauro S. Phenotype-genotype correlations in skeletal muscle of patients with mtDNA deletions. Muscle Nerve Suppl 3:S150–S153, 1995.
21. Moslemi A-R, Lindberg C, Oldfors A. Analysis of mitochondrial DNA deletions in inclusion body myositis. Hum Mutat In press:1997.
22. Moslemi AR, Melberg A, Holme E, Oldfors A. Clonal expansion of mitochondrial DNA with multiple deletions in autosomal dominant progressive external ophthalmoplegia. Ann Neurol 40:707–713, 1996.
23. Nakase H, Moraes CT, Rizzuto R, Lombes A, DiMauro S, Schon EA. Transcription and translation of deleted mitochondrial genomes in Kearns-

Sayre syndrome: implications for pathogenesis. Am J Hum Genet 46:418–427, 1990.

24. Ohno K, Tanaka M, Sahashi K, Ibi T, Sato W, Yamamoto T, Takahashi A, Ozawa T. Mitochondrial DNA deletions in inherited recurrent myoglobinuria. Ann Neurol 29:364–369, 1991.

25. Oldfors A, Larsson N-G, Holme E, Tulinius M, Kadenbach B, Droste M. Mitochondrial DNA deletions and cytochrome-c oxidase deficiency in muscle fibres. J Neurol Sci 110:169–177, 1992.

26. Oldfors A, Larsson N-G, Lindberg C, Holme E. Mitochondrial DNA deletions in inclusion body myositis. Brain 116:325–336, 1993.

27. Oldfors A, Moslemi AR, Fyhr IM, Holme E, Larsson N-G, Lindberg C. Mitochondrial DNA deletions in muscle fibers in inclusion body myositis. J Neuropathol Exp Neurol 54:581–587, 1995.

28. Otsuka M, Niijima K, Mizuno Y, Yoshida M, Kagawa Y, Ohta S. Marked decrease of mitochondrial DNA with multiple deletions in a patient with familial mitochondrial myopathy. Biochem Biophys Res Commun 167:680–685, 1990.

29. Prelle A, Moggio M, Checcarelli N, Comi G, Bresolin N, Battistel A, Bordoni A, Scarlato G. Multiple deletions of mitochondrial DNA in a patient with periodic attacks of paralysis. J Neurol Sci 117:24–27, 1993.

30. Rifai Z, Welle S, Kamp C, Thornton CA. Ragged red fibers in normal aging and inflammatory myopathy. Ann Neurol 37:24–29, 1995.

31. Rötig A, Bourgeron T, Chretien D, Rustin P, Münnich A. Spectrum of mitochondrial DNA rearrangements in the Pearson marrow-pancreas syndrome. Hum Mol Genet 4:1327–1330, 1995.

32. Santorelli FM, Sciacco M, Tanji K, Shanske S, Vu TH, Golzi V, Griggs RC, Mendell JR, Hays AP, Bertorini TE, Pestronk A, Bonilla E, DiMauro S. Multiple mitochondrial DNA deletions in sporadic inclusion body myositis: a study of 56 patients. Ann Neurol 39:789–795, 1996.

33. Schon EA, Rizzuto R, Moraes CT, Nakase H, Zeviani M, DiMauro S. A direct repeat is a hotspot for large-scale deletion of human mitochondrial DNA. Science 244:346–349, 1989.

34. Sciacco M, Bonilla E, Schon EA, DiMauro S, Moraes CT. Distribution of wild-type and common deletion forms of mtDNA in normal and respiration-deficient muscle fibers from patients with mitochondrial myopathy. Hum Mol Genet 3:13–19, 1994.

35. Servidei S, Zeviani M, Manfredi G, Ricci E, Silvestri G, Bertini E, Gellera C, DiMauro S, DiDonato S, Tonali P. Dominantly inherited mitochondrial myopathy with multiple deletions of mitochondrial DNA – clinical, morphologic, and biochemical studies. Neurology 41:1053–1059, 1991.

36. Shoffner JM, Lott MT, Voljavec AS, Soueidan SA, Costigan DA, Wallace DC. Spontaneous Kearns-Sayre/chronic external ophthalmoplegia plus syndrome associated with a mitochondrial DNA deletion: a slip-replication model and metabolic therapy. Proc Natl Acad Sci U S A 86:7952–7956, 1989.

37. Shoubridge EA, Karpati G, Hastings KE. Deletion mutants are functionally dominant over wild-type mitochondrial genomes in skeletal muscle fiber segments in mitochondrial disease. Cell 62:43–49, 1990.

38. Suomalainen A, Kaukonen J, Amati P, Timonen R, Haltia M, Weissenbach J, Zeviani M, Somer H, Peltonen L. An autosomal locus predisposing to deletions of mitochondrial DNA. Nat Genet 9:146–151, 1995.

39. Suomalainen A, Majander A, Haltia M, Somer H, Lönnqvist J, Savontaus ML, Peltonen L. Multiple deletions of mitochondrial DNA in several tissues of a patient with severe retarded depression and familial progressive external ophthalmoplegia. J Clin Invest 90:61–66, 1992.

40. Tulinius M, Holme E, Kristiansson B, Larsson N-G, Oldfors A. Mitochondrial encephalomyopathies in children. I Biochemical and morphological investigations. J Pediatr 119:242–250, 1991.

41. Tulinius M, Holme E, Kristiansson B, Larsson N-G, Oldfors A. Mitochondrial encephalomyopathies in children. II Clinical manifestations and syndromes. J Pediatr 119:251–259, 1991.

42. Tulinius MH, Oldfors A, Holme E, Larsson N-G, Houshmand M, Fahleson P, Sigström L, Kristiansson B. Atypical presentation of multisystem disorders in two girls with mitochondrial DNA deletions. Eur J Pediatr 154:35–42, 1995.

43. Uncini A, Servidei S, Silvestri G, Manfredi G, Sabatelli M, DiMuzio A, Ricci E, Mirabella M, DiMauro S, Tonali P. Ophthalmoplegia, demyelinating neuropathy, leukoencephalophathy, myopathy, and gastrointestinal dysfunction with multiple deletions of mitochondrial DNA: a mitochondrial multisystem disorder in search of a name. Muscle Nerve 17:667–674, 1994.

44. Zeviani M, Bresolin N, Gellera C, Bordoni A, Pannacci M, Amati P, Moggio M, Servidei S, Scarlato G, DiDonato S. Nucleus-driven multiple large-scale deletions of the human mitochondrial genome: a new autosomal dominant disease. Am J Hum Genet 47:904–914, 1990.

45. Zeviani M, Moraes CT, DiMauro S, Nakase H, Bonilla E, Schon EA, Rowland LP. Deletions of mitochondrial DNA in Kearns-Sayre syndrome. Neurology 38:1339–1346, 1988.

46. Zeviani M, Servidei S, Gellera C, Bertini E, DiMauro S, DiDonato S. An autosomal dominant disorder with multiple deletions of mitochondrial DNA starting at the D-loop region. Nature 339:309–311, 1989.

47. Zhang C, Baumer A, Maxwell RJ, Linnane AW, Nagley P. Multiple mitochondrial DNA deletions in an elderly human individual. FEBS Lett 297:34–38, 1992.

22

Mitochondrial DNA Analysis in Muscle of Patients with Sporadic Inclusion-Body Myositis and Hereditary Inclusion-Body Myopathy

CLAUDE DESNUELLE, VÉRONIQUE PAQUIS, RACHEL PAUL, W. KING ENGEL, ANNE SAUNIÈRES, RENATE B. ALVAREZ, AND VALERIE ASKANAS

Ragged red fibers (RRFs) (1), which can be identified in morphologic studies of muscle biopsy specimens by Gomori trichrome staining (2), with increased succinic dehydrogenase (SDH) staining and often negative cytochrome-c-oxidase (COX) staining, are important markers for a group of heterogeneous diseases called mitochondrial myopathies (MMs) (3). Such conditions usually are associated with deficiencies in the activities of mitochondrial oxidative-phosphorylation enzymes. In many patients with MMs, demonstration of sporadic or maternally inherited mutations in the mitochondrial DNA (mtDNA) is possible (4). In some families, a defect in the nuclear genome is suggested by the pattern of inheritance. However, RRFs, respiratory-chain enzyme deficiencies, or genetic alterations are not specific for primary mitochondrial disease and could result from different insults: mtDNA mutation can be induced by zidovudine treatment (5); a 5-kb deletion is frequently detected in aged patients and is called the "common deletion" (4); respiratory-chain enzyme deficiencies can be associated with neurodegenerative disorders such as Parkinson disease (6) or with aging (7,8); RRFs can be observed in muscle biopsy specimens from older patients or patients with inflammatory myopathies (9,10).

Morphologic mitochondrial changes are seen in inclusion-body myositis (IBM) muscle, and the question of a pathogenic involvement of mtDNA was raised when in situ hybridization studies demonstrated deleted mtDNA in COX-deficient fibers in IBM patients (12,13). Sporadic inclusion-body myositis (s-IBM) is the most common muscle disease among patients aged 50 years and older. s-IBM patients manifest distal and proximal muscle weakness, with prominent involvement of the quadriceps. The light-microscopic features of s-IBM include various degrees of mononuclear-cell inflammation (varying from abundant in the early stages to little or none in the later stages), muscle fibers with irregular rimmed vacuoles, and atrophic muscle fibers (12,13). The presence of paired helical filaments in the vacuolated muscle fibers is the ultrastructural diagnostic criterion for IBM (13). The term "hereditary inclusion-body myopathy" (h-IBM) is used to designate patients with myopathies of autosomal-recessive or dominant inheritance, various clinical features, and no inflammation seen at muscle biopsy (12,13). Their vacuolated muscle fibers and paired helical filaments are identical with those present in s-IBM (12,13). Moreover, in the vacuolated muscle fibers in both s-IBM and h-IBM there are accumulations of ubiquitin, β-amyloid precursor protein, a_1-antichymotrypsin, hyperphosphorylated τ protein, and prion protein, suggesting similar pathogenic mechanisms (reviews: 12,13). In s-IBM patients, the presence of RRFs has been reported to be more frequent than in age-matched normal controls or in patients with other inflammatory myopathies (9). The causes of mitochondrial abnormalities in IBM are not known, and mtDNA has not been studied in h-IBM, which occurs earlier in life than s-IBM and differs by its lack of inflammation.

In the study reported here, using molecular-genetic analysis of mtDNA extracted from muscle biopsy specimens, the proportion of deleted mtDNA was found to be very low and to be present in only few patients with s-IBM. No mtDNA abnormality was detected in patients with h-IBM.

Materials and Methods

Patients

Seven patients with s-IBM (ages 37–78 years; mean, 66.8) and 9 patients with h-IBM (ages 34–53 years; mean, 41.4) were investigated, and all met the clinical and morphologic diagnostic criteria for s-IBM or h-IBM (12). Eight of the h-IBM patients had an autosomal-recessive genealogy, 7 being Iranian Jews. One, not of Iranian Jewish origin, had an autosomal-dominant genealogy (Table 22.1). The control samples were 7 muscle biopsy specimens, 6 from patients with no mitochondrial disorder: 3 patients with amyotrophic lateral sclerosis (ages 29–53 years), 1 with vacuolar myopathy (16 years old), 1 with facial dystonia (65 years old), and 1 with neuropathy (53 years old). One muscle specimen was from an

Table 22.1. *Characteristics of our s-IBM and h-IBM populations*

s-IBM patients (7)			h-IBM patients (9)			
No.	Age	Sex	No.	Age	Sex	Family
1	37	M	8	44	M	Iranian Jews, autosomal-recessive
2	73	M	9	34	F	Iranian Jews, autosomal-recessive
3	71	F	10	36	M	Iranian Jews, autosomal-recessive
4	77	F	11	39	M	Iranian Jews, autosomal-recessive
5	78	F	12	39	M	Iranian Jews, autosomal-recessive
6	55	M	13	53	M	Iranian Jews, autosomal-recessive
7	61	M	14	45	M	Iranian Jews, autosomal-recessive
			15	45	M	Not Iranian Jews, autosomal-recessive (brother affected)
			16	50	F	Autosomal-dominant (mother + daughter affected)

18-year-old patient with ocular myopathy. Muscle samples were obtained, with informed consent, by open muscle biopsy from either the deltoid muscle or the vastus lateralis muscle and were immediately frozen in isopentane chilled in liquid nitrogen. One part of each sample was used for histochemistry. Ultrathin sections were taken and conserved at −80°C until used for the molecular analysis.

mtDNA Analysis

Total DNA was extracted from 15 thick cryostat sections (40 μm) of frozen muscle using a standard procedure, with proteinase-K digestion followed by phenol-chloroform extraction (14).

For Southern-blot analysis, 5 μg of total DNA was digested with the restriction enzyme *Pvu* II (nt 2656), electrophoresed in an 0.8% agarose gel and transferred on nylon membranes, as previously described (14). The filter was hybridized with the mtDNA ^{32}P-labeled probe (pGT10/12.2) containing a 14,032-bp *Eco*RI mtDNA insert cloned into pBB3 vector (15). The nylon filters were prehybridized, hybridized, washed, and exposed according to the supplier's protocol (Amersham, UK).

A polymerase chain reaction (PCR) was performed (16) with 100 ng of total DNA. A set of primers encompassing the region of the "common deletion" (nt 8470–13446) was used for amplification [5′-GGTATACTACGGTCAATGCTC-3′ (nt 8155–8176) and 5′-GGATCCTATTGGTGCGGG-3′ (nt 14263–14246)]. The amplification reaction was performed in a thermal cycler (GenAmp PCR system 480, Perkin-Elmer) with one cycle of denaturation for 1 minute at 94°C and 30 cycles of annealing for 1 minute at 57°C and 20 seconds at 72°C. PCR products were then electrophoresed on a 1.5% agarose gel. PCR products were expected to be detected if the "common deletion" was present, because with this procedure only small fragments less than 0.5 kb will be amplified.

A large-fragment PCR using the "Expand Long PCR System" (Boehringer Mannheim) was carried out on 250 ng of total DNA, as described elsewhere (17). This technique allows amplification of wild-type and deleted mtDNA in patients by use of a set of primers within the mtDNA noncoding region and a part of the tRNA Phe coding sequence [5'-CCCACAGTTTATGTAGCTTACCTCCTCA-3' (nt 571–598) and 5'-TTGATTGCTGTACTTGCTTGTAAGCATG-3' (nt 16220–16193)]. Amplification reactions were performed in a GenAmp PCR System 480 (Perkin-Elmer): one cycle of 4 minutes at 93°C 30 cycles of 10 seconds at 93°C, 30 seconds at 62°C, and 13 minutes at 68°C (during the 10 last cycles, 20 seconds per cycle were added for the extension step), followed by a 10-minute hold at 72°C. PCR products were analyzed on 0.6–0.8% standard agarose gel (Biorad).

Results

RRFs and COX-deficient Muscle Fibers

In 6 of the 7 specimens from patients with s-IBM, few fibers harbored the morphologic hallmark of a mitochondrial alteration. Fewer than 1% of the muscle fibers were RRF- and/or SDH-hyperreactive, and only about 50% of those fibers were COX-negative. In patient no. 5, aged 78 years, the proportion was higher. No clear correlation was found between the prevalence of morphologic mitochondrial involvement and either age or the degree of inflammation.

In the group with autosomal-recessive h-IBM, as in the patient with the autosomal-dominant form and in controls with no MM, occasional RRFs were seen, but no COX-negative muscle fibres were observed.

mtDNA Analysis

The search for mtDNA deletions was conducted using three different techniques. With one exception (the muscle specimen from the patient with an MM), no deletion was detected in the control muscle specimens.

No mtDNA deletions were observed by Southern-blot analysis when technical standard conditions were used (exposure time for the autoradiograms, 6 hours). The standard conditions described allow the detection of pathogenic deletions in MMs. Figure 22.1 shows an example of the patterns obtained for patients no. 5, 6, 7, and 12 and from the control muscle specimen from the patient with ocular myopathy. The normal 16.5-kb mtDNA was present in all cases. Deleted mtDNA was evident in the lane corresponding to the ocular-myopathy control specimen, demonstrating a heteroplasmic deletion in that patient. An additional band indicating a very small amount of deleted mtDNA was observed in the lane corresponding to patient no. 5. Figure 22.2 shows data obtained when autoradiograms were overexposed for 3 days. In cases no. 1, 2, and 8, very small amounts of additional bands associated with the normal 16.5-kb mtDNA were detected, thus showing multiple deletions in those patients using this technique. The PCR method, using primers emcompassing the "common deletion," was unable to detect such deletions in any patients (data not shown). The large-fragment PCR (Figure 22.3) clearly demonstrated the presence of an approximately 9-kb deletion in patient no. 5. Slight indications of an approximately 8-kb deletion were seen in patients no. 2 and 7. No accurate quantitative estimation of deleted mtDNA can be made using this procedure.

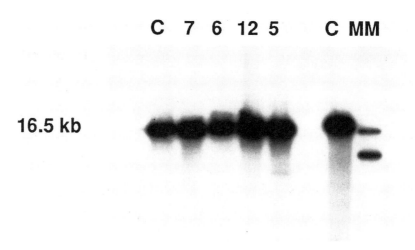

Figure 22.1. Southern-blot analysis: Total DNA extracted from thin sections of frozen muscle hybridized with a ^{32}P-labeled mtDNA probe in patients 7, 6, 12, and 5 (corresponding to the numbered lanes), control muscle with no mitochondrial disease (lanes C), and control muscle from a patient with ocular myopathy (MM). Exposure time for the autoradiogram was 6 hours.

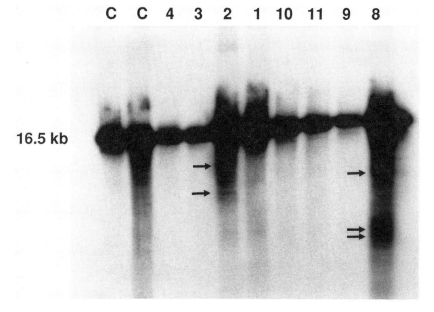

Figure 22.2. Southern-blot analysis, as in Figure 22.1, except with overexposure of the autoradiogram for 3 days, for patients 4, 3, 2, 1, 10, 11, 9, and 8 (corresponding to the numbered lanes) and control muscle from patient with no mitochondrial disease (lanes C).

As shown in Table 22.2, deleted mtDNA was detected by Southern-blot analysis in patients 1, 2, 5, 7, and 8 (4 of 7 patients with s-IBM and 1 of 9 patients with h-IBM). If the findings from large-fragment PCR analysis are considered, deleted mtDNA was revealed only in patients 2, 5, and 7 (3 of 7 patients with s-IBM and none of 9 patients with h-IBM). When present, the deletion was not the "common deletion."

Discussion

In this study we have compared s-IBM and h-IBM, which have the same ultrastructural criteria (reviews: 12,13), but differ in regard to age at onset (>50 years for s-IBM), the lack of inflammation in h-IBM, and other features (12,13,18). Molecular analysis revealed differences in the two populations. We confirmed the presence of heteroplasmic mtDNA deletions in s-IBM patients (detected in 3 of 7 patients), with the percentage of deleted mtDNA very low when it was present in an individual. The patient with a detectable deletion shown by the standard technique was

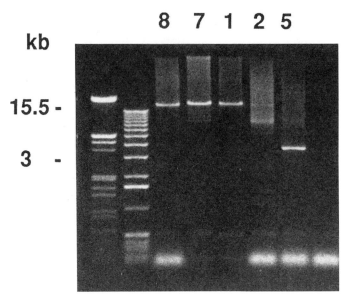

Figure 22.3. Large-fragment PCR for amplification of deleted mtDNA for patients 8, 7, 1, 2, and 5, with molecular-weigh markers (lanes on the left); 250 ng of total DNA extracted from thin sections of frozen muscle was used (see Materials and Methods section); 15.5-kb product was obtained from wild mtDNA; shorter fragment was amplified from patients bearing a deleted mitochondrial population.

aged 78 years. Our strategy did not demonstrate the presence of the "common deletion" in all patients tested. No mtDNA deletion was found in the 9 patients with h-IBM.

Mitochondrial dysfunction has been proposed as a pathogenic mechanism in several neurodegenerative disorders, including aging. A study by Oldfors et al. (11) suggested that muscle fibers with deficient COX activity were more frequent in patients with s-IBM than in age-matched normal controls, and in situ hybridization studies of those fibers detected mtDNA deletions. It was hypothesized that mtDNA deletions could be caused by highly reactive oxygen radicals arising as by-products of a malfunction in the respiratory chain, but no evidence of a mitochondrial oxidative phosphorylation defect in IBM is known. Recently, Oldfors et al. (19) extended their studies to 20 patients with s-IBM. In that population, COX-negative fibers were present at frequencies ranging from 0.5% to 5% in the muscle biopsy specimens, and PCR analysis of isolated COX-deficient muscle fibers showed the presence of deleted mtDNA in each fiber, identified as the "common deletion," flanked by direct repeats, mostly in regenerative

Table 22.2. *Numbers of mtDNA deletions in s-IBM and h-IBM patients detected using Southern-blot analysis and large-fragment PCR*

	s-IBM			h-IBM	
Patient no.	Southern blot	Large-fragment PCR	Patient no.	Southern blot	Large-fragment PCR
1	del[a]	no del	8	del	no del
2	del	del	9	no del	no del
3	no del	no del	10	no del	no del
4	no del	no del	11	no del	no del
5	del	del	12	no del	no del
6	no del	no del	13	no del	no del
7	del	del	14	no del	no del
			15	no del	no del
			16	no del	no del

[a] del, deletion.
Findings with Southern-blot analysis are from overexposed gels (see Materials and Methods section).

segments. In our series of patients, we did not detect the "common deletion," but we did find large deletions up to 8 kb in patients more than 60 years of age. Similarly, in 7 of 30 patients with s-IBM, mtDNA deletions were reported by Santorelli et al. (20) using Southern-blot analysis of total DNA extracted from muscle biopsy specimens, but the "common deletion" was not evidenced by mapping the deleted region by PCR.

It must be pointed out that in morphologic analysis of MMs, the mitochondrial abnormalities are known to be segmental when observed on longitudinal section. That might explain the discrepancy in the molecular data obtained from IBM patients, that is, the differences between the DNA studied from isolated COX-negative ultrathin sections of muscle fibers and the DNA extracted from all the fibers included in the section. If in a local area of a muscle fiber the activity of the COX enzyme is decreased, it could be expected that in COX-negative sections the proportion of altered mtDNA would be higher than in other "normal" areas of the fiber. The methods used in our study, chosen for assessment of pathogenic deletions in MM, could not detect the deletions when very few segments were affected. This consideration will raise the question of the pathogenic significance of an mtDNA deletion if minor parts of some fiber sections in the muscle are affected. Oldfors et al. (19) advocated the hypothesis that in IBM, mtDNA deletion would result during muscle regeneration from satellite cells after segmental muscle-fibers necrosis. Numerous studies have demonstrated in various tissues, accumulations of mtDNA deletions occurring during replication in the human aging process (21). The role of ischemia or of an immune-mediated toxicity has been considered as a possibility to explain the increased numbers of RRFs observed in inflammatory myopathies, including IBM (9,11). We demonstrated mitochondrial-enzyme dysfunction in Polymyalgia rheumatica without giant-cell arteritis (10), and in those patients, multiple deletions in mtDNA were observed with the same techniques used in the study reported here. It has recently been demonstrated in muscle (22) that high amounts of deleted mtDNA are necessary to induce a biochemical phenotype (and presumably a clinical phenotype). Thus it does not seem possible that the low amounts found here could be responsible for a pathogenic influence in the disease process.

There are many morphologic similarities between s-IBM and h-IBM, suggesting similar pathogenic mechanisms (12). The pathogenic significance of mtDNA remains unclear in the disease process of s-IBM, and it has been suggested that mtDNA deletions could be caused by regeneration, aging, or inflammation. We found no deletions in h-IBM, and when mtDNA deletions were present in s-IBM, the proportion of mutant DNA was very low, associated with inflammation in the form of s-IBM that affected the oldest patients. Although the causes of the mtDNA deletions remain unknown in IBM, our findings suggest that in s-IBM, additional factors may be added to the generally accepted insults that can cause deletions in mtDNA, thus favoring the hypothesis of a secondary process that could be environmental (affecting inflammation, aging, or regeneration) or could be triggered by an alteration in the nuclear genome controlling the stability of the mtDNA.

Acknowledgment

Supported in part by the Association Française contre les Myopathies (AFM).

References

1. Engel WK. "Ragged-red fibers" in ophthalmoplegia syndromes and their differential diagnosis. Presented at the Second International Congress on Muscle Diseases, 1971

2. Engel WK, Cunningham GG. Rapid examination of muscle tissue and improved trichrome method for fresh-frozen biopsy sections. *Neurology* 13:919–923, 1963.

3. Shoffner JM, Wallace DC. Oxidative phosphorylation diseases. Disorders of two genomes. *Adv Hum Genet* 19:267–330, 1990.

4. DiMauro S, Moraes CT. Mitochondrial encephalomyopathies. *Arch Neurol* 50:1197–1208, 1993.

5. Dalakas MC, Illa I, Pezeshkpour GH. Mitochondrial myopathy caused by long-term zidovudine therapy. *N Engl J Med* 322:1098–1105, 1990.

6. Blin O, Desnuelle C, Rascol O, Borg M, Azulay JP, Pellissier JF, Montastruc JL, Serratrice G. Mitochondrial respiratory failure in skeletal muscle from patients with Parkinson's disease and multi-system atrophy. *J Neurol Sci* 125:95–101, 1994.

7. Trounce I, Byrne E, Marzuki S. Decline in skeletal muscle mitochondrial respiratory chain function: possible factor in aging. *Lancet* 1:637–639, 1989.

8. Johnston W, Karpati G, Carpenter S, Arnold D, Shoubridge EA. Late-onset mitochondrial myopathy. *Ann Neurol* 37:16–23, 1995.

9. Rifai Z, Welle S, Kamp C, Thornton CA. Ragged-red fibers in normal aging and inflammatory myopathy. *Ann Neurol* 37:24–29 1995.

10. Harlé JR, Pellissier JF, Disdier P, Figarella-Branger D, Weiller PJ, Desnuelle C. Polymyalgia rheumatica and mitochondrial myopathy: clinicopathologic and biochemical studies. *Am J Med* 92:167–172, 1992.

11. Oldfors A, Larsson NG, Lindberg C, Holme E. Mitochondrial DNA deletions in inclusion-body myositis. *Brain* 116:325–336, 1993.

12. Askanas V, Engel WK. New advances in inclusion-body myositis. *Curr Opin Rheumatol* 5:732–741, 1993.

13. Askanas V, Engel WK, Mirabella M. Idiopathic inflammatory myopathies: inclusion-body myositis, polymyositis and dermatomyositis. *Curr Opin Neurol* 7:448–456, 1994.

14. Davis GL, Dibner MD, Battey JF. *Basic Methods in Molecular Biology.* Elsevier, New York, 1986.

15. Luftalla G, Blanc H, Bertolotti R. Shuttling of integrated vectors from mammalian cells to *E. coli* is mediated by head-to-tail mutimeric inserts. *Somat Cell Genet* 11:223–238, 1985.

16. Inis MA, Gerfand DH, Sninsky JJ, White TJ. *PCR Protocols.* Academic Press, San Diego, 1990.

17. Paul R, Santucci S, Saunières A, Desnuelle C, Paquis V. Rapid mapping of mitochondrial DNA deletions by large fragments PCR. *Trends Genet* 12:131–132, 1996.

18. Mirabella M, Askanas V, Bilak M, Alvarez R, Engel WK. Abnormal accumulation of phophorylated neurofilament heavy-chain in s-IBM. Difference between s-IBM and h-IBM. *Neurology* 45(S4):A209, 1995 (abstract).

19. Oldfors A, Moslemi AR, Fyhr IM, Holme E, Larsson NG, Lindberg C. Mitochondrial DNA deletions in muscle fibers in inclusion body myositis. *J Neuropathol Exp Neurol* 54:581–587, 1995.

20. Santorelli FM, Sciacco M, Shanske S, Griggs RC, Mendell JR, Bonilla E, DiMauro S. Mitochondrial DNA deletions in patients with inclusion-body myositis. *Neurology* 44(S2):A131, 1994 (abstract).

21. Baumer S, Zhang C, Linnane AW, Nagley P. Age-related human mtDNA deletions: a heterogeneous set of deletions arising at a single pair of directly repeated sequences. *Am J Hum Genet* 54:618–630, 1994.

22. Sciacco M, Bonilla E, Schon E, DiMauro S, Moraes CT. Distribution of wild-type and deleted ("common deletion") mtDNA in normal and respiration-deficient muscle fibers from patients with mitochondrial myopathy. *Hum Mol Genet* 3:13–19, 1994.

Part VI
Treatment

23

Evaluation of Treatment for Sporadic Inclusion-Body Myositis

ROBERT C. GRIGGS AND MICHAEL R. ROSE

Inclusion-body myositis (IBM) has been recognized for 25 years as a distinctive, pathologically defined disease. Early descriptions of the disorder noted its resistance to the usual treatment for inflammatory myopathies. Indeed, in the minds of many neuromuscular-disease specialists, a patient with a corticosteroid-resistant inflammatory myopathy is assumed to have IBM, unless proved otherwise. Nonetheless, there have been continuing anecdotal reports and studies of small numbers of cases that have suggested a beneficial response to corticosteroids. Similar information is available regarding other putative treatments. In this chapter we (a) review the published studies on the results of treatment, (b) consider the inherent challenges to discovering a treatment for IBM, (c) argue the necessity for a natural-history study of IBM, and (d) list the treatments that have been effective for dealing with the complications and coincidental conditions occurring in IBM.

Assessment of Responses to Treatment for IBM

Clinical Response. In most of the retrospective studies and single-case reports, the assessments of clinical responses to treatment have been qualitative, and it has not been clear whether those have been the patients' or the therapists' subjective assessments. In some instances, Medical Research Council (MRC) grades of muscle strength have been quoted. In prospective trials, strength-testing regimens have included standard or expanded MRC scores and quantitative myometry scores. A few prospective studies have used functional rating scores, and one added a dysphagia score (1). "Improvement" has had a variety of meanings (specified in Table 23.2, when known). A "partial response" has meant any response short of full recovery and thus could imply a functional gain or no functional improvement at all. Leff et al. (2) and Lindberg et al. (1) introduced the concept of "stabilization" as a treatment outcome, implying that lack of any worsening of the weakness during the treatment trial represents a treatment effect. Because natural-history data on IBM are lacking, that may be a unjustifiable assumption. Preliminary data from our ongoing natural-history study of IBM show that quantitative myometry scores can remain unchanged over at least a 6-month period, a period of time longer than many of the reported treatment trials.

Laboratory Response. Several reports have remarked on "improvement" as evidenced by a decline in creatine kinase (CK) with treatment, often with rebound when the treatment, such as prednisone (1,3,4), was reduced or discontinued. Those declines in CK levels did not correlate with clinical responses.

Histologic Response. Barohn et al. (4) showed that although the inflammation seen in muscle biopsy specimens decreased significantly following 8 weeks of corticosteroid treatment, that was not matched by any clinical response. Furthermore, the numbers of vacuoles and amyloid deposits increased significantly during the treatment (4). Lindberg et al. (1) did not find any clear pattern of changes in the inflammatory infiltrates following immunosuppressive treatment.

Predictors of Response

Leff et al. (2) found that muscle appearances at magnetic-resonance imaging (MRI) were not predictive of treatment responses. In one prospective trial of corticosteroid treatment, responders had higher CK levels on entry than did nonresponders (2). In that same trial, three of four responders to corticosteroids had large areas of inflammation (2). Three patients who showed rapid responses to corticosteroid treatment had extensive inflammatory infiltrates (5; Y. Harati, personal communication)

Summary of Past Treatments for IBM

The agents and approaches that have been tried are listed in Table 23.1.

Prednisone

Worldwide, 112 patients have been described in 15 retrospective reports of corticosteroid treatment for IBM, with 6 of those reports describing

Table 23.1 *Immunosuppressive agents and therapeutic procedures used for IBM*

Prednisone (and other corticosteroids)
Cyclophosphamide
Chlorambucil
Azathioprine
Methotrexate
Cyclosporin
Total-body irradiation
Leukapheresis
Plasma exchange
Intravenous immunoglobulin

single cases (Table 23.2). Carpenter et al. (6) described four patients, one of whom had been reported earlier (7). The cases reported in abstracts by Harati et al. (5) and Levin et al. (8) have not been further elaborated in print (personal communication). Fourteen of the 25 retrospective cases described by Leff et al. (2) had previously been reported as part of a larger retrospective study of treatment for the inflammatory myopathies (9). The 14 cases reported by Joffe et al. (10) were part of a larger series of 113 patients with inflammatory myopathies. Many of the patients reported retrospectively in those various studies had undergone trials of corticosteroids without any appreciation of the diagnosis of IBM, which became evident only as a result of their failure to respond to treatment. Prednisone was given at maximum dosages of 20–100 mg daily, with subsequent reductions of dosages or alternate-day dosing for maintenance treatment. The overall periods of treatment ranged from 2 weeks to 2 years. The reports generally do not clearly state the lengths of time that the maximum dosages were given, nor how the dosage taperings were carried out. Of the 112 patients, 77 patients either showed no response to corticosteroid treatment or continued to deteriorate despite treatment. One patient was said to show "slight improvement" on an unspecified dosage and duration of corticosteroid treatment (11), and 2 of 13 patients in one series (12) showed transient "benefit." Four patients remained stable for a mean follow-up of 36 months (12). Twenty-three patients showed partial responses (10) or improvement (2,5,8,13), with one of those improving to "normal" and being maintained in that state for 24 months of follow-up (13). In another report of a good response to corticosteroid treatment, a second patient was mentioned who refused corticosteroid

Table 23.2

Corticosteroid	No. Treated	Assessment	Agent/Max. dosage/Total duration	Response
Chou (37), 1967	1 retrospective	qualitative	prednisone/not specified/2 wk	none
Carpenter et al. (7), 1970	1 retrospective	qualitative	methylprednisone/32 mg qd/2 mo	none
Sato et al. (38), 1971	1 retrospective	qualitative	prednisone/50 mg ad/3 mo	none
Yunis and Samaha (39), 1971	1 retrospective	qualitative	prednisone/60 mg qd/8 wk	none
Hughes and Esiri (11), 1975	1 retrospective	qualitative	prednisone/not specified/not	slight improvement
Carpenter et al. (6), 1978	3 retrospective	qualitative	1 prednisone/60 mg qd/1 mo	worsened
			1 prednisone/60 mg qd/3 wk, then	none
			100 mg/qod/3 mo	
			1 prednisone/5 mg qd/years	none
Danon et al. (40), 1982	6 retrospective	qualitative	prednisone/"high dosage"/not specified	none
Harati et al. (5), 1986	3 retrospective	qualitative, MRC grades	prednisone/100 mg qd/not specified	3 of 3 improved in days, improved MRC grades in months
Levin et al. (8), 1986	1 retrospective	qualitative	prednisone/high dosage/not specified	improved, with maintained improvement at 6-mo follow-up

Study	Design	Outcome measures	Treatment	Results
Calabrese et al. (41) 1987	3 retrospective	qualitative	prednisone/40–60 mg qd/3 mo–4 yr	none
Cohen et al. (13), (1989)	10 retrospective	qualitative, CK	prednisone/50–60 mg qd/not specified	1 improved to normal, maintained at 24-mo FU
Lotz et al. (42), 1989	29 retrospective	qualitative	prednisone/40 mg qd/3 mo minimum	25 at 2-yr FU all deteriorated
Sayers et al. (12), 1992	13 retrospective	strength testing, functional rating	prednisone/not specified/not	4 stable, 2 transient benefit
Leff et al. (2), 1993	25 retrospective	qualitative	prednisone/>40 mg qd/1 mo	10 improved
Joffe et al. (10), 1993	14 retrospective	qualitative, strength testing	prednisone/>0.75 mg/kg/qd/4 wk	8 partial (PR) response.
Lindberg et al. (1), 1994	16 prospective, open	MRC grading, dysphagia score, hand-held myometry	prednisone/20–60 mg qd/>2 mo	2 not assessed, 4 had stabilization or brief improvement
Barohn et al. (4), 1995	8 prospective, open label	Expanded MRC score, CK, functional rating score	prednisone/100 mg qd/4 wk, then 100 mg qod/6-24 mo	All worsened by 6–24 mo

treatment but nevertheless experienced a spontaneous 90% improve-ment in strength (8). The patient treated with corticosteroids sub-sequently deteriorated, and the one who experienced spontaneous remission was lost to follow-up after 1 year (K. Levin, personal com-munication). In one report, improvement was seen in three cases and occurred within days, with slower improvements in MRC grades over subsequent months (5). Those three cases showed marked inflammatory infiltrates at muscle biopsy (Y. Harati, personal communication).

There have been two prospective, open-label trials of prednisone (1,4). Five of the six cases first reported in abstract (9b) have sub-sequently been published (4; C. Lindberg, personal communication). In the first study (1), 4 of 16 patients showed transient improvements or stabilization of disease on corticosteroid treatment: in one case, no quantitative testing was performed; in a second patient, improvement was confined to the knee extensors; in a third case, although there was no clinical deterioration, quantitative myometry showed a steady de-cline throughout the 41 months of treatment (1); the fourth patient showed a remarkable but short-term improvement, with a mean 19% gain in strength in all tested muscles (1). By contrast, the second pro-spective trial of corticosteroid treatment (4) found continuing deterio-ration in all 8 patients.

In summary, in only rare instances has there been any evidence that corticosteroids have produced sustained, quantitatively demonstrated *improvement*. At best, "stabilization," usually for a matter of months, has sometimes been reported. In the rare instances in which improvement was reported, the studies were uncontrolled; it was also unclear whether or not coincidental corticosteroid-responsive diseases were present. At least 25–30% of patients might be expected to have coincidental diseases (obstructive lung disease, polymyalgia, osteoarthritis, etc.) that would improve with corticosteroid treatment.

Cytotoxic Treatments

All of the reported patients treated with cytotoxic agents had failed treatment trials with corticosteroids. In many cases the cytotoxic treat-ment was in addition to corticosteroid treatment (Table 23.3).

Cyclophosphamide. Of 11 patients with refractory inflammatory myopathy treated with cyclophosphamide, 2 had IBM (14). One patient received only one course of treatment, which caused severe nausea and vomiting, and the other patient received the planned seven courses. Neither showed any response.

Chlorambucil. Two patients who failed to respond to intravenous cyclophosphamide also failed to respond to a trial of chlorambucil (14). Another patient who had failed to respond to previous trials of prednisone, both alone and in combination with methotrexate, azathioprine, and cyclophosphamide, improved in terms of function and quantitative muscle strength during the first 15 months of treatment with chlorambucil. The treatment was continued for a 3-year period, but without further improvement. Withdrawal of the chlorambucil after 3 years had not resulted in any deterioration at the time of the report (15).

Azathioprine. In a retrospective study, 3 of 15 patients treated with azathioprine showed minor improvements but the rest deteriorated (2). Azathioprine was given with methotrexate in one arm of a prospective, open, randomized crossover study. Of 9 patients, 2 showed minor improvements, and 4 stabilized during the 6-month study period (2). Azathioprine was one of three additional immunosuppressants given in combination with prednisone to 15 patients; individual outcomes were not detailed, but in that group 1 patient stabilized, and 5 experienced short-term benefits (12). Seven patients given azathioprine at 150 mg/day for an unspecified period showed no response (1).

Methotrexate. Three patients experienced long-term remission while on methotrexate (12). Two of 9 patients improved and a further 4 patients became stabilized when treated with methotrexate in combination with azathioprine (2). Six of the 10 patients reported by Joffe et al. (10) did not respond to methotrexate at all, and the rest showed partial responses. Of the 12 patients reported by Leff et al. (2), 3 patients showed minor responses, and 1 become stabilized.

Cyclosporin. This was one of the drugs added to prednisone for treatment of 15 patients, with some receiving azathioprine or methotrexate as alternatives; individual outcomes were not detailed, but 6 patients either became stable or had short-term benefits (12). In a prospective trial in 6 patients, 2 had to withdraw at 4 weeks because of side effects, and the rest showed no benefit (1).

Table 23.3

Cytotoxic Treatment	No. Treated	Assessment	Agent/Max. Dosage/Total Duration	Response
Cronin et al. (14), 1989	2 prospective	MRC grade, self-reporting for 1	cyclophosphamide/$0.75\,\mathrm{g}\,\mathrm{m}^{-2}/\mathrm{mo}^{-1}$ titrated to leukopenia; 1 and 7 courses chlorambucil/not specified/not specified	none
Sayers et al. (12), 1992	15 retrospective	qualitative, strength testing, functional rating	methotrexate/not specified/not specified; azathioprine/not specified/not specified; cyclosporin/not specified/not specified	none (patients not individually, identified), 1 stable, 5 short-term benefit, 3 long-term remission (all these were on methotrexate)
Leff et al. (2), 1993	retrospective	qualitative	15 azathioprine/$>75\,\mathrm{mg/d}/>8\,\mathrm{wk}$ 12 methotrexate/$>5\,\mathrm{mg/wk}/>8\,\mathrm{wk}$	3 minor improvement 3 minor improvement, 1 stabilized
			3 chlorambucil, cyclophosphamide, or apheresis/not specified/not specified	cyclophosphamide & apheresis "each of some benefit once"
Leff et al. (2), 1993	11 prospective randomized crossover, open	strength testing, ADL assessment	oral azathioprine ($0.3\,\mathrm{mg}\,\mathrm{kg}^{-1}/\mathrm{d}^{-1}$) plus methotrexate ($0.3\,\mathrm{mg}\,\mathrm{kg}^{-1}/\mathrm{wk}^{-1}$) for 6 mo	2 of 9 minor improvements, 4 of 9 stabilized
			intravenous biweekly methotrexate given with leucovorin 'rescue' ($0.5\,\mathrm{g/m^2}$ in 1 hr every 2 wk), 6 mo maximum	1 of 10 improved, 7 of 10 stabilized

Joffe et al. (10), 1993	10	qualitative, strength testing	methotrexate/>5 mg/wk/>8 wk	6 none, 4 PR
Lindberg et al. (1), 1994	7 prospective, open	MRC grading dysphagia score, hand-held myometry	azathioprine/150 mg/d/ not specified	none
Lindberg et al. (1), 1994	6 prospective, open	MRC grading, dysphagia score, hand-held myometry	cyclosporin/5 mg/kg^{-1}/d^{-1} (adjusted to serum concentration of 125–175 ng/mL)/up to 24 mo	none
Jongen et al. (15), 1995	1 prospective	qualitative, myometry	chlorambucil/0.1 mg/kg^{-1}/d^{-1}/3 yr	improved for first 15 months, then static

Total-Body Irradiation

Four patients have been treated with whole-body irradiation (16,17). An initial report (17) suggested partial improvement in one patient. That improvement was subjective and was not substantiated by objective measures; the patient subsequently deteriorated (16). The other three patients showed no subjective improvement and continued to deteriorate despite treatment (16).

Plasma Exchange

No controlled trials of plasma exchange have been conducted, but two patients were inadvertently included in a randomized trial of plasma exchange as treatment for dermatomyositis and polymyositis; no benefit was noted (18).

Leukapheresis

The patient reported by Dau (19) showed a partial response to leukapheresis that was not maintained. Another patient showed a partial response to apheresis on one occasion, but no further details were given (2).

Intravenous Immunoglobulin

Five prospective trials of intravenous immunoglobulin (IVIG) have been reported. The two patients reported by Lindberg et al. (1) received low-dosage IVIG (400 mg $\cdot$ Kg^{-1} $\cdot$ mo^{-1}) on a long-term for coexisting common variable immune deficiency and were also treated with corticosteroids and cyclosporin A. Neither the low-dosage IVIG nor occasional 10-fold dosage increases had any effect on their muscle weakness. Three of four patients responded to high-dose IVIG (total dose 2 g/kg) in one prospective open-label trial (20), but in another similar trial (21) there was no response in nine patients. In five patients treated with IVIG for periods of up to 6 months, myometry showed improvement in some muscle groups in some patients, but no functional improvements occurred (22,23). A recent placebo-controlled, double-blind crossover trial (24) showed no significant difference in MRC scores between the treated and untreated groups, but two patients showed significant functional improvements, and when individual muscle scores were analyzed, some showed improvements during IVIG treatment. Those were all upper-limb muscles which had lesser degrees of weakness at the beginning of treatment.

IBM Associated with Connective-Tissue Disease

There have been seven single-case reports in the English literature (3,25–30) of IBM associated with connective-tissue disease, and it seems reasonable to consider the responses to treatment in this group separately. All patients were treated with corticosteroids, and in five cases (3,25–28) with additional immunotherapy, either initially or subsequently. One patient (25) had a brief course of plasma exchange. In two cases the corticosteroid trial was without benefit (25,28), and in another two cases only slight improvement was seen (29,30). In one case (3) there was minor functional improvement, without an objective increase in muscle strength, after 3 months of treatment. During corticosteroid tapering, that patient had an exacerbation of her systemic lupus erythematosus, with resolution of her rash and systemic malaise and an increase in muscle strength 1 month after her prednisone dosage was increased. Another patient (25) had no initial response to prednisone. That patient subsequently developed fever, rash, and increasing muscle weakness associated with muscle tenderness. An increased dosage of prednisone with azathioprine resulted in resolution of the systemic symptoms and improvement in muscle strength, but not to previous levels. A brief course of plasma exchange did not produce additional improvement. The patient reported by Lane et al. (27) showed corticosteroid responsiveness in regard to muscle function that paralleled systemic improvement, followed by relapse in both symptom categories when corticosteroids were reduced. Thus, in those cases where there was a corticosteroid response in terms of improved muscle strength, this appears to have been related more to the response of the associated connective-tissue disease, which may have been responsible per se for a component of the muscle weakness, particularly as muscle tenderness was a feature of the weakness in one case (25).

In conclusion, the literature shows little evidence that immunotherapy is efficacious for patients with IBM. Reports of major improvement or normalization have been rare, and in even fewer instances (13,15) has the follow-up been sufficiently long to qualify any improvement as "sustained." Anecdotally, many specialists can recall patients whose initial responses to treatment were promising but were not maintained. Reports of stabilization during relatively brief periods of treatment may reflect the natural history of the disease, as discussed later. There remains the possibility that, for example, corticosteroids may worsen some aspects of the disease (4). There have been no large, randomized, prospective treatment trials.

Developing a Treatment for IBM

It is disappointing that thus far no treatment for any muscle disease has been widely accepted as being of proven benefit [e.g., by the U.S. Food and Drug Administration (FDA)]. This lack reflects the state of experimental therapeutics in the field, because several agents have been shown to be effective for various disorders. Demonstration that a treatment for IBM is effective will require showing a change in the course of the disease. Because the course of IBM has not yet been clearly defined, it is difficult to know what will be required of a trial to show that a treatment works. The possible outcomes of treatment for any disease are illustrated in Figure 23.1, and each can be identified if the disease's natural history of progressive decline has been established:

(a)   A rapid improvement in the patient, with a return to normal. Any study that shows such a "Lazarus effect" requires only a small number of patients to prove efficacy if the disease under study is ho-

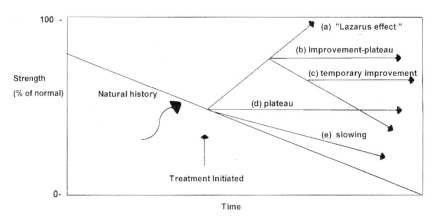

Figure 23.1. Hypothetical responses to a treatment for IBM. The (natural-history) course of untreated IBM as quantitated by muscle strength (*y* axis) is assumed to show a linear decline with time (*x* axis). Five potential improvements with treatment are illustrated: (a) Lazarus effect; return to normal; (b) limited improvement to a stable plateau; (c) temporary improvement, with subsequent decline; (d) plateau, without subsequent decline; (e) a slowing of the rate of progressive decline.

mogeneous. Such a response is seen in some patients with myasthenia gravis. However, for myasthenia gravis, which responds with a return to normal in some, but not all, patients, and in which spontaneous remissions sometimes occur, it was initially difficult to prove efficacy. Only if IBM is a homogeneous disorder will such a response to any treatment be likely to occur in all patients.

(b) A prompt improvement, followed by a plateau. Depending on the degree of improvement, a treatment effect might be readily detectable. Without knowing the natural history of the disease, however, it would be difficult to detect even a moderate improvement. Detection of a subsequent plateau is likely to require a lengthy follow-up. Such an improvement (4%) was reported among patients with Duchenne dystrophy who were treated with prednisone (31,32), with the plateau lasting 3–4 years.

(c) Improvement, with a subsequent decline, would, as in (b), be rapidly detectable only if the improvement was major. Subsequent long-term follow-up would not clarify matters.

(d) Plateau. Here there is no improvement, and the duration of study needed to detect a benefit will depend entirely on the reproducibility of the testing conditions and the rate of decline, defined by the natural history. In practice, such plateau effects have been difficult to detect in any disease, and such studies invariably require large numbers of patients.

(e) Slowing of progression. Detection of a change in patients' rates of decline will require the same information as in (d), but in addition will require much larger numbers of patients and a much longer period of follow-up. For example, such a response has been reported for patients with amyotrophic lateral sclerosis (ALS). ALS is rapidly progressive, in comparison with IBM, and its study still requires large numbers of patients to detect such a response (W. Bradley, personal communication).

To epitomize: Only a relatively rapid return to normal or a major improvement is likely to be easily detected in a slowly progressive disorder such as IBM.

Defining the Natural History

The natural history of IBM is unknown. Determining the natural history is of great importance for characterizing the disease and its possible responses to contemplated treatments. It is not known at present whether the disease causes decline in a linear fashion, occurs in bursts of worsening with intermittent plateaus, or has an overall decline punctuated by periods of actual improvement. Natural-history studies could also provide information that would allow estimation of the time of onset of the disease for patients who are first seen late in the course of the disease, assuming that the disease has a linear progression.

Quantitation of the natural history in a number of patients with IBM will be essential to address the question whether or not IBM progresses at the same rate in all patients. Unless the disease progresses at comparable rates in all patients, it will be difficult to design a reasonably sized trial to compare groups of subjects. Natural- history data may prove to be essential for treatment trials in individual patients, because if the course is variable from patient to patient, it may be impractical to show a treatment response by group means.

In preliminary studies of the natural history of IBM, we have been interested in characterizing muscle strength by quantitative myometry and muscle wasting by studies of the following:

- total-body muscle mass (calculated on the basis of urinary creatinine excretion)
- lean body mass, assessed by dual-energy x-ray absorptiometry (DEXA) and whole-body ^{40}K counts

Our preliminary findings at 6 months regarding muscle strength, muscle mass, and lean body mass indicate that thus far there have been no significant detectable changes in those parameters in a group of 10 patients.

Strategies for Treatment Trials in IBM

The randomized controlled trial has dominated the literature of experimental therapeutics. Randomized controlled trials require large numbers of patients and are designed to exclude atypical cases; they therefore involve the potential problem of ending up with homogenized groups in order to get enough patients to complete a study. The requirement of a large number of patients makes it difficult to study an uncommon disease like IBM and mandates the cooperation of multiple research centers, with consequent diffusion of responsibility. A large trial involves the risks of variations in quality control and methodologic inconsistencies.

Should alternatives to the large randomized controlled trial be considered in the effort to develop new treatments for IBM? We believe so. First, it is intuitively obvious that a large trial cannot be justified unless there is clinical evidence or at least a theoretical rationale favoring a trial of a possible treatment. Second, exclusive reliance on randomized controlled trials involving large numbers of patients ignores much of what clinicians have learned in practice with regard to other inflammatory myopathies (i.e., the responses of patients to a treatment tend to be variable). Moreover, we have an instructive example from the treatment of another disease: plasma exchange in Guillain-Barré syndrome. We now know that although plasma exchange will be effective (i.e., statistically beneficial) in a population of patients, only a proportion of those patients will respond rapidly and recover. Some patients will experience adverse effects and have life-threatening complications, some patients will have one or two relapses, and some patients will not benefit at all.

What alternative, specific clinical-trial methods should be considered? There are at least three possible approaches: (a) natural-history-controlled trials, (b) the *n*-of-1 trial, and (c) blind luck or serendipity. As Oates and Wood (33) pointed out, "in circumstances in which therapeutic outcomes are qualitative (eg, complete cures in an illness that has been uniform and rapidly fatal), randomized controlled trials may not be required."

The *n*-of-1 trial is in some ways preferable to a randomized controlled trial for evaluating a treatment in a given patient. After all is said and done, it is how my patient's condition has benefited (or worsened) that matters (33). Is my patient one of the 90% who improved dramatically or the 10% who did not? There is great disdain for the *n*-of-1 trial among unsophisticated scientists. As Guyatt et al. (34) have pointed out, the *n*-of-1 trial features the same randomization, double blinding, and comparable measures of outcome as the randomized controlled trial. Until a large-scale study can document that an agent is effective, the use of *n*-of-1 trials may be worth considering. It is also increasingly important for clinicians to support the involvement of their patients in large-scale randomized controlled trials. For a disease such as IBM, the numbers of drug-naive patients who can be studied in methodologically sound, FDA-approvable, randomized controlled trials are so small that is incumbent upon clinicians to try to make their patients available to those centers involved in studying the disease.

Future Treatments

Our current knowledge of the pathophysiology of IBM, though rapidly expanding, does not yet suggest any alternative therapeutic strategy apart from immunosuppressive treatment. The apparent poor outcomes from immunotherapy to date do not necessarily mean that immunologic mechanisms do not play a part in the pathophysiology of IBM. In this respect, the immune mechanisms of IBM may resemble those seen in type 1 diabetes mellitus, multiple sclerosis, or chronic organ rejection. In those situations, more prolonged immunosuppression or novel immuno-suppressant or immune-modulating treatments may be required.

Treatments for Complicating and Coincidental Conditions in IBM

Patients with IBM often are elderly and frequently are subject to respi-ratory, cardiac, or other systemic diseases. Involvement of systems other than skeletal muscle seldom, if ever, occurs in IBM per se. Specifically, symptomatic respiratory-muscle weakness and cardiac disease do not occur. Thus, the presence of respiratory symptoms or cardiac failure indicates the presence of coincidental disease. Because more than 25% of patients over the age of 65 have obstructive pulmonary disease, respi-ratory symptoms often relate to obstructive disease rather than restrictive disease. The one exception to this rule is that patients with IBM occasion-ally may develop cricopharyngeal achalasia. Patients with crico-pharyngeal achalasia often have aspiration and if there is associated pulmonary disease, they can develop infections. Aspiration by itself, without cough impairment, or structural pulmonary disease, rarely causes pulmonary infections. Cardiac disease does not occur in IBM. The occur-rence of palpitations, arrhythmias, or symptoms of heart failure invari-ably implies the presence of coincidental disease.

Finally, the muscle weakness is virtually always painless in IBM. If there is pain in association with weakness, the diagnosis should be reevaluated. If the diagnosis of IBM is correct, a second disease should be sought. Polymyalgia rheumatica (present in 2–5% of elderly patients) is frequent and occasionally is the reason for a "dramatic" response to corticosteroids in patients with IBM (R. Griggs, unpublished data). In general, corticosteroids are not indicated for polymyalgia rheumatica; a nonsteroidal anti-inflammatory agent such as enteric coated aspirin is the appropriate treatment unless there is biopsy evidence of giant-cell arteri-tis. Pain in patients with IBM should be treated with a similar strategy.

There are certain manifestations of IBM for which a patient can derive major benefit from specific treatment. Dysphagia resulting from crico-pharyngeal achalasia will respond in many instances (at least in other diseases) to cricopharyngeal myotomy. The caveat here is that there have been no large studies of this procedure in IBM (35,36). Aspiration of oropharyngeal material is frequent in patients with cricopharyngeal acha-lasia; aspiration does not improve following cricopharyngeal myotomy. If pulmonary function and glottic control are adequate, respiratory infec-tion will not be a problem, despite recurrent aspiration.

Distal anterior-compartment leg weakness is a typical manifestation of IBM. Lightweight ankle-foot orthoses (AFOs) frequently are helpful in counteracting this foot-drop. Patients with severe quadriceps weakness may, however, have difficulty with even the lightest of AFOs.

There have been several reports of autoimmune disease in association with IBM. If these disorders are associated with pain or other neuromus-cular manifestations, these autoimmune-disease manifestations may re-spond promptly to corticosteroids or other immunosuppressive treat-ments. In general, however, patients with IBM do much better without corticosteroids. If they are on corticosteroids, it is particularly important to maintain adequate exercise. Treatment of pain with adequate analge-sia is often helpful in restoring muscle function in such patients.

Acknowledgments

This work was supported in part by the Gilbert and Beatrice Bloch Family Foundation, by NIH grant R01 NS22099-09, and by the Clinical Research Center (M01-RR0044). M.R. was a visiting fellow supported by the W.A. Young Charitable Trust, The Muscular Dystrophy Association of Great Britain, The King Edward's Hospital Fund, London, The Guar-antors of Brain, The Mercer's Company, and Sanofi Winthrop UK.

References

1. Lindberg C, Persson LI, Bjorkander J, Oldfors A. Inclusion-body myosi-tis: clinical, morphological, physiological and laboratory findings in 18 cases. *Acta Neurol Scand* 89:123–131, 1994.
2. Leff RL, Miller FW, Hicks J, Fraser DD, Plotz PH. The treatment of inclu-sion-body myositis: a retrospective review and a randomised prospective trial of immunosuppressive therapy. *Medicine* 72:225–235, 1993.
3. Yood RA, Smith TW. Inclusion-body myositis and systemic lupus erythe-matosus. *J Rheumatol* 12:568–570, 1985.

4. Barohn RJ, Amato AA, Sahenk Z, Kissel JT, Mendell JR. Inclusion-body myositis: explanation for poor response to immunosuppressive therapy. *Neurology* 45:1302–1304, 1995.

5. Harati Y, Niakan E, Kolimas R, Goodman JC. Response to corticosteroid in inclusion-body myositis. *Muscle Nerve (suppl)* 9:216, 1986 (abstract).

6. Carpenter S, Karpati G, Heller I, Eisen A. Inclusion-body myositis: a distinct variety of idiopathic inflammatory myopathy. *Neurology* 28:8–17, 1978.

7. Carpenter S, Karpati G, Wolfe L. Virus-like filaments and phospholipid accumulation in skeletal muscle. Study of a histochemically distinct chronic myopathy. *Neurology* 20:889–903, 1970.

8. Levin K, Mitsumoto H, Agamanolis D. Steroid resposiveness and clinical variability in inclusion-body myositis. *Muscle Nerve* 9:217, 1986 (abstract).

9a. Love LA, Leff RL, Fraser DD, et al. A new approach to the classification of idiopathic inflammatory myopathy: myositis-specific autoantibodies define useful homogeneous patient groups. *Medicine* 70:360–374; 1991.

9b. Lindberg C, Persson L, Oldfors A, Soederstroem T, Hedstroem A, Bjoerkander J. Inclusion body myositis - association with immunodeficiency. *J Neurol Sci* 98(suppl):178, 1990.

10. Joffe MM, Love LA, Leff RL, Fraser DD, Targoff IN, Hicks JE, Plotz PH, Miller FW. Drug therapy of the idiopathic inflammatory myopathies: predictors of response to prednisone, azathioprine, and methotrexate and a comparison of their efficacy. *Am J Med* 94:379–387, 1993.

11. Hughes JT, Esiri MM. Ultrastructural studies in human polymyositis. *J Neurol Sci* 25:347–360, 1975.

12. Sayers ME, Chou SM, Calabrese LH. Inclusion-body myositis: analysis of 32 cases. *J Rheumatol* 19:1385–1389, 1992.

13. Cohen MR, Sulaiman AR, Garancis JC, Wortmann RL. Clinical heterogeneity and treatment response in inclusion-body myositis. *Arthritis Rheum* 32:734–740, 1989.

14. Cronin ME, Miller FW, Hicks JE, Dalakas M, Plotz PH. The failure of intravenous cyclophosphamide therapy in refractory idiopathic inflammatory myopathy. *J Rheumatol* 16:1225–1228, 1989.

15. Jongen PJH, Terlaak HJ, Vandeputte LBA. Inclusion-body myositis responding to long-term chlorambucil treatment. *J Rheumatol* 22:576–578, 1995.

16. Kelly JJ Jr, Madoc-Jones H, Adelman LS, Andres PL, Munsat TL. Total-body irradiation not effective in inclusion-body myositis. *Neurology* 36:1264–1266, 1986.

17. Kelly JJ, Madoc-Jones H, Adelman L, Munsat TL. Treatment of refractory polymyositis with total-body irradiation. *Neurology (suppl 1)* 34:80, 1984 (abstract).

18. Miller FW, Leitman SF, Cronin ME, Hicks JE, Leff RL, Wesley R, Fraser DD, Dalakas M, Plotz PH. Controlled trial of plasma exchange and leukapheresis in polymyositis and dermatomyositis. *N Engl J Med* 326:1380–1384, 1992.

19. Dau PC. Leukocytapheresis in inclusion-body myositis. *J Clin Apheresis* 3:167–170, 1987.

20. Soueidan SA, Dalakas M. Treatment of inclusion-body myositis with high-dose intravenous immunoglobulin. *Neurology* 43:876–879, 1993.

21. Amato AA, Barohn RJ, Jackson CE, Papert EJ, Sahenk Z, Kissel JT. Inclusion-body myositis: treatment with intravenous immunoglobulin. *Neurology* 44:1516–1518, 1994.

22. Mastaglia FL, Zilko P, Laing B, Churchyard A. Immunoglobulin therapy in patients with inflammatory myopathies. *Aust NZ J Med* (*suppl 2*) 21:607, 1991.

23. Mastaglia FL, Laing BA, Zilko P. Treatment of inflammatory myopathies. In: *Inflammatory Myopathies*, Mastaglia FL (ed). Bailliere Tindall, London, 1993, pp. 717–740.

24. Dalakas MC, Dambrosia JM, Sekul EA, Cupler EJ, Sivakumar K. 1995. The efficacy of high-dose intravenous immunoglobulin (IVIg) in patients with inclusion-body myositis (IBM). *Neurology* (*suppl 4*) 45:1745, 1995 (abstract).

25. Chad D, Good P, Adelman L, Bradley WG, Mills J. Inclusion-body myositis associated with Sjögren's syndrome. *Arch Neurol* 39:186–188, 1982.

26. Gutmann L, Govindan S, Riggs JE, Schochet SS Jr. Inclusion-body myositis and Sjögren's syndrome. *Arch Neurol* 42:1021–1022, 1985.

27. Lane RJ, Fulthorpe JJ, Hudgson P. Inclusion-body myositis: a case with associated collagen vascular disease responding to treatment. *J Neurol Neurosurg Psychiatry* 48:270–273, 1985.

28. Danon MJ, Perurena OH, Ronan S, Manaligod JR. Inclusion-body myositis associated with systemic sarcoidosis. *Can J Neurol Sci* 13:334–336, 1986.

29. Khraishi MM, Jay V, Keystone EC. Inclusion-body myositis in association with vitamin B_{12} deficiency and Sjögren's syndrome. *J Rheumatol* 19:306–309, 1992.

30. Soden M, Boundy K, Burrow D, Blumbergs P, Ahern M. Inclusion-body myositis in association with rheumatoid arthritis. *J Rheumatol* 21:344–346, 1994.

31. Fenichel GM, Mendell JR, Moxley RT, Griggs RC, Brooke MH, Miller JP, Pestronk A, Robinson J, King W, Signore L, Pandye S, Schierbecker J, Wilson B. A comparison of daily and alternate-day prednisone therapy in the treatment of Duchenne muscular dystrophy. *Arch Neurol* 48:575–579, 1991.

32. Mendell JR, Moxley RT, Griggs RC, Brooke MH, Fenichel GM, Miller JP, King W, Signore L, Pandya S, Florence J, Schierbecker J, Robison J, Kaiser K, Mandel S, Arkfen C, Gilder B. Randomised double blind six month trial of prednisone in Duchenne's muscular dystrophy. *N Engl J Med* 320:1592–1597, 1989.

33. Oates JJ, Wood AJ. Regulation of discovery and drug development. *N Engl J Med* 320:311–312, 1989.

34. Guyatt G, Sackett D, Taylor W, Chong J, Roberts R, Pugsley S. Determining optimal therapy; randomised trials in individual patients. *N Engl J Med* 314:889–892, 1986.

35. Danon MJ, Friedman M. Inclusion-body myositis associated with progressive dysphagia: treatment with cricopharyngeal myotomy. *Can J Neurol Sci* 16:436–438, 1989.

36. Verma A, Bradley WG, Adesina AM, Sofferman R, Pendlebury WW. Inclusion-body myositis with cricopharyngeus muscle involvement and severe dysphagia. *Muscle Nerve* 14:470–473, 1991.

37. Chou SM. Myxovirus-like structures in a case of human chronic polymyositis. *Science* 158:1453–1455, 1967.

38. Sato T, Walker DL, Peters HA, Reese HA, Chou SM. Chronic myositis and myxovirus-like inclusion: electronmicroscopic and viral studies. *Arch Neurol* 24:409–418, 1971.
39. Yunis EJ, Samaha FJ. Inclusion-body myositis. *Lab Invest* 25:240–248, 1971.
40. Danon MJ, Reyes MG, Perurena OH, Masdeu JC, Manaligod JR. Inclusion-body myositis. A corticosteroid-resistant idiopathic inflammatory myopathy. *Arch Neurol* 39:760–764, 1982.
41. Calabrese LH, Mitsumoto H, Chou SM. Inclusion-body myositis presenting as treatment-resistant polymyositis. *Arthritis Rheum* 30:397–403, 1987.
42. Lotz BP, Engel AG, Nishino H, Stevens JC, Litchy WJ. Inclusion-body myositis. Observations in 40 patients. *Brain* 112:727–747, 1989.

24

Treatment of Inclusion-Body Myositis and Hereditary Inclusion-Body Myopathy with Reference to Pathogenic Mechanisms: Personal Experience.

W. KING ENGEL AND VALERIE ASKANAS

Defining the Patients Being Treated – Diagnostic Aspects

Discussing treatment of a disease "entity" implies the entity can be defined by results of "adequate" diagnostic procedures and that the treating physician is familiar with their interpretation.

For sporadic inclusion-body myositis (s-IBM), the pivotal diagnostic point is the muscle biopsy showing muscle-fiber vacuoles having characteristic features: (a) light microscopy–amyloid (1) (detectable by fluorescence-enhanced Congo-red [2] or by crystal-violet staining); (b) immunocytochemistry – SMI-31 and SMI-310 positivity (3–6); (c) electron microscopy – 15–21 nm diameter paired-helical filaments (PHFs), and 6–10 nm diameter amyloid-like fibrils (4–6). Treatment-literature cases diagnosed before 1994 did not address the now-pivotal criteria (a) and (b), and some not (c). Other supportive biopsy features (3–6) are: (a) the vacuoles stained by Engel-Gomori trichrome often show a red rim and contain loose red and some green material; (b) a lymphocytic mononuclear inflammatory-cell response (although patients taking a glucocorticoid may lack lymphocytes in the biopsy); and (c) a few necrotic-phagocytosed muscle fibers and "regen-degen" (regenerating-degenerating) fibers (the regen-degen fibers are often alkaline-phosphatase-positive [7,8]).

A usual, supportive or not-distracting, biopsy feature of s-IBM and h-IBM is the presence of small angular muscle fibers that are often dark with NADH tetrazolium-reductase (NADH-TR) and pan-esterase stainings, like those typical of an ordinary denervation disease (4–6); we interpret such muscle fibers as denervated. That denervation can be, hypothetically, the result of neurogenous or myogenous (8,9) de-innervation of the muscle fiber. Virtually all s-IBM biopsies have at least a few small angular muscle fibers. In some hereditary IBM (h-IBM) muscle biopsies, these denervated fibers are the major feature, and in others they may be the only abnormality in the biopsy of a patient in an h-IBM family (4–6; unpublished observations).

The accumulations of various proteins within IBM muscle fibers (which include the same proteins abnormally accumulated in the brains of Alzheimer-disease patients [4–6]) is partly due to upregulation of the mRNAs of some of them (4–6); but the accumulations might also involve a yet-unanalyzed component of impaired catabolism. In s-IBM and h-IBM we could not find evidence of DNA-fragmentation ("apoptosis") by the TUNEL technique (12).

Within the muscle-fiber vacuoles of s-IBM, HTLV1-IBM, and h-IBM there are easily recognized large and small membranous whorls. These imply impaired lysosomal catabolism of the accumulated glycolipids and glycoproteins (and possibly lipoproteins), similar to what one sees in acid maltase deficiency and other lysosomal-enzyme disorders [cf. 10]. We consider that these vacuoles result from an "endodissolution." ("Endodissolution" is a term we introduced [11] to describe the formation of vacuoles within muscle fibers that are not undergoing ordinary necrosis; the endodissolution is presumably caused by focally excessive lytic processes producing the vacuoles. Disorders of different etiologies manifesting endodissolution include acid-maltase deficiency [10], muscle carnitine deficiency [11], and dermatomyositis.)

In later stages, the s-IBM muscle can contain a variable number of non-diagnostic "increase-decrease" muscle fibers, in which the oxidative-enzyme reactions (NADH-TR, succinate dehydrogenase, or cytochrome oxidase) display, within an individual muscle fiber, foci of increased staining intermixed with foci of absent staining (unpublished observations).

Not evident in s-IBM biopsies (4–6) are: (a) perifascicular accentuation of disease (which is typical of dermatomyositis [13]); and (b) prominent alkaline-phosphatase staining of perimysial connective-tissue regions, which is probably based on enzymatic activity of activated fibroblasts (typical of dermatomyositis, polymyositis, and lupus myositis [7,8]).

The electromyogram (EMG) of s-IBM is not of specific diagnostic value. It can show a pattern of BSAPs (*b*rief-duration, *s*mall-amplitude, overly *a*bundant, motor-unit action-*p*otentials), or BSAPPs (with *p*olyphasics). BSAPs and BSAPPs indicate fractionated motor-units, which can occur on the basis of damage to individual(a) distal axonal twigs (neuropathy), (b) post-synaptic junctions (junctionopathy), or (c) muscle fibers in their vast non-junctional regions (myopathy) (14,15). BSAPs are not exclusively diagnostic of "myopathy," as erroneously assumed recently (16). There is nonesuch animal as a diagnostic "myopathic EMG" (14,15). The EMG in s-IBM virtually always shows some positive waves and/or fibrillations (17; WKE, unpublished), which are indicative of recently denervated muscle-fibers, resulting, hypothetically, from a neurogenous or a myogenous de-innervation mechanism. ("Myogenous de-innervation" is a term introduced by one of us [9] to describe impaired influence of the lower motor neuron on a muscle fiber due to a muscle-fiber disorder located at the post-synaptic region of the neuromuscular junction or between that junction and a surviving more distal part of the muscle fiber.) A few fasciculations occur in occasional s-IBM patients. Sometimes the s-IBM patient's EMG shows only fibrillations, positive-waves, and a few fasciculations, without BSAPs, leading to a misdiagnosis of amyotrophic lateral sclerosis.

Age of onset is not an absolutely rigid diagnostic criterion of s-IBM. Although the onset of s-IBM is usually after age 50, we have two atypical patients with early-adult onset, viz. at ages 21 and 18 (the 21-year old had weakness beginning $1\frac{1}{2}$ years after "Russian flu"). They both had lymphocytic inflammation evident in their initial biopsies. However, in biopsies 15 years later they had SMI-31 positivity and, unlike s-IBM (but like autosomal-recessive h-IBM), they (a) lacked SMI-310 positivity and(b) had their muscle-fiber amyloid in the form of small plaques instead of the squiggles typical of s-IBM. Their lack of the full s-IBM cellular phenotype may be due to an absence of a "cellular aging" milieu that is present in the usual s-IBM beginning over age 50.

The milieu of cellular aging in s-IBM. A possible basis for some of the differences between typical s-IBM and autosomal-recessive h-IBM (for example, in s-IBM there is SMI-310 immunoreactivity of the accumulated paired helical filaments and a greater amount of congophilic amyloid) is that in s-IBM the pathogenic factors occur in a milieu modified by the "normal aging" process within the muscle fiber. The clinical onset of s-IBM is usually age 50–70, i.e. 35–55 years later than that of h-IBM (4–6).

Hereditary inclusion-body myopathy (h-IBM) is discussed in more detail elsewhere (4–6). In general, there are similar (but not absolutely identical) vacuolated muscle fibers in the muscle biopsy; however, there is no lymphocytic inflammatory reaction. The clinical onset is earlier, usually age 15–30. There are several forms of h-IBM: (a) autosomal-recessive type-1a (R1a-IBM), that locus the mutation originally localized to chromosome 9 p1-q1 (18) and recently confirmed (Middleton, Christodoulou, Askanas, Engel et al., [18a]; (b) autosomal-recessive type-2 (R2-IBM) not on chromosome 9 (Middleton [18a]); and (c) autosomal-dominant (D-IBM), of various geographic foci, chromosome(s) unlocalized.

HTLV1 Inclusion-Body Myositis (HTLV1-IBM) is discussed below in regard to pathogenesis.

Pathogenesis – What pathologic process is one attempting to treat?

Interesting questions of pathogenesis include the following. (a) What is the cell-biology basis of the myoselectivity of s-IBM and of h-IBM? Why is the quadriceps early-involved in s-IBM and late-involved ("spared") in chromosome 9 p1-q1 linked autosomal-recessive h-IBM? (b) Is the distal muscle weakness mainly neurogenic? (c) Regarding muscle fibers of a particular muscle predisposed to be affected (or spared), e.g., quadriceps in s-IBM vs. h-IBM, in what way are they sufficiently different from fibers of conversely affected muscles in their biochemical composition, including (i) their array of surface and internal receptors, and (ii) their expressed and inducible transcription factors? (d) And, of course, what are the essential pathogeneses, and how are they similar and different in s-IBM versus h-IBM (see hypotheses below)? This information should hasten the formulation of definitive treatment and prevention.

Hypothetical Pathogeneses of h-IBM and s-IBM

Concerning h-IBM and s-IBM, our current hypothetical pathogeneses are explained below and shown in Fig. 24.1.

The essence is that a cascade of aberrant transcriptions is initiated. In h-IBM the cascade is consequent to the gene mutation, in s-IBM it results from muscle-fiber infestation by the putative causative virus-x, and in HTLV1-IBM it is initiated by the HTLV1 virus (whose p19 protein was recently localized to muscle-fiber plasmalemma [19]). Steps common to the pathogenesis of h-IBM, s-IBM, and HTLV1-IBM are initiated by the hypothetical "IBM transcription factor" (TF_{IBM}). In regard to what might be an early-step pathologic increase of transcription in all three types of IBM, we elsewhere discuss our experimental results of transferred, highly overexpressed βAPP-gene in cultured normal human muscle fibers and the consequent appearance of several pathologic features of IBM (6); those results support our concept of a key role of overexpressed-βAPP in the pathogenic cascade of the IBMs.

Pathologic aspects seen in s-IBM and HTLV1-IBM but not h-IBM (such as the CD8+ lymphocyte infiltration) can be one of the indirect re-

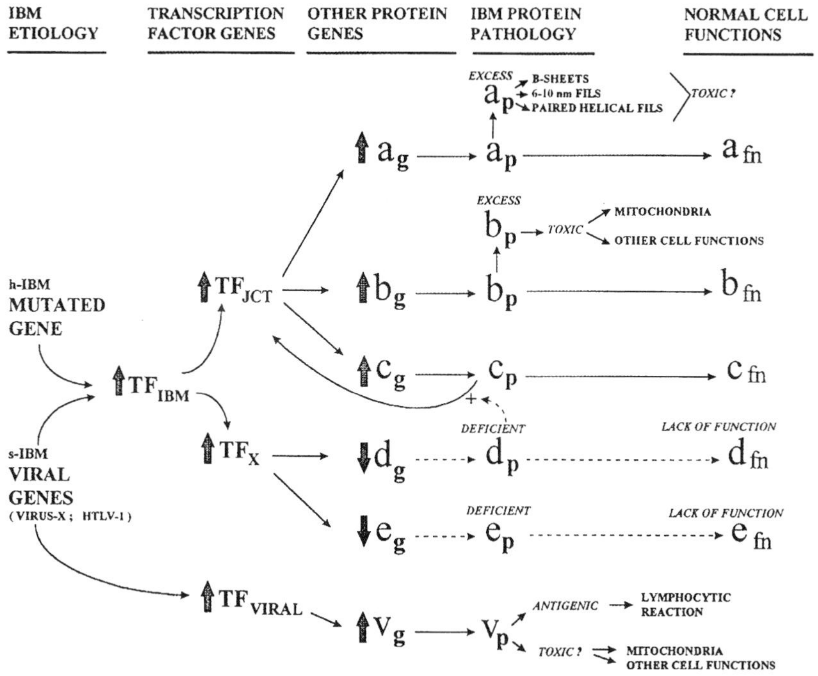

Figure 24.1. Hypothetical pathogeneses of h-IBM and s-IBM.

a, b, c, Putative genes _g), corresponding proteins (_p), and normal-functions d, e (_fn), abnormalities of which are involved in the pathogenesis of both hereditary inclusion-body myopathy (h-IBM) and sporadic inclusion-body myositis (s-IBM).

TF_{IBM} The initially-increased putative "IBM transcription-factor" is common to the pathogenesis of h-IBM, s-IBM, and HTLV1-IBM. In h-IBM, TF_{IBM} is upregulated as a result of the genetic mutation. In s-IBM, upregulation of TF_{IBM} results from a putative viral infestation of the muscle fiber. In HTLV1, TF_{IBM} is upregulated by a virus-provoked protein, for example Tax, produced within the muscle fiber. A central role of the upregulated protein βAPP in the IBM pathogenic cascade has been proposed (4–6), making it a candidate to be the TF_{IBM}.

TF_{JCT} Putative "junctionalization transcription-factor" (4–6), whose own transcription is increased (promoted) by TF_{IBM}. TF_{JCT} upregulates (promotes) genes of "junctional proteins" a_p, b_p, c_p (for example, βAPP, prion and nAChR) in extra-junctional nuclei of the muscle fiber, i.e., "protein-junctionalization" of the extra-junctional regions (4–6). TF_{JCT} might activate, or actually be, the hypothetical normal "junctionalizing master-gene" that becomes repressed in normal non-junctional nuclei (see Fig. 21.4). The TF_{JCT} might also suppress the gene of a putative "junctional proteins suppression factor" (Fig. 24.4).

TF_X Another putative transcription-factor, whose own transcription is increased (promoted) by TF_{IBM}. TF_X downregulates genes d_g and e_g governing yet-unidentified proteins d_p and e_p required for the normal muscle-fiber functions d_{fn} and e_{fn}.

a_p An a_p protein (for example, βAPP or prion), when excessive, can form sults of a putative "viral transcription factor" (TF_{VIRAL}) "foreignizing" the muscle fibers (see below). In HTLV1-IBM at least one TF_{VIRAL} might be the viral protein Tax, because it is known to modulate transcription of host-cell genes, at least partly through the NF-κB mechanism of genes containing κB sites in their upstream promotor regions, and partly through interacting with cellular Rel proteins (20). In HTLV1-IBM, cellular Tax could also activate TF_{IBM}. In s-IBM patients, evidence of definite viral protein, RNA, or DNA within muscle fibers has not yet been established. Intriguing, though, are these findings: (a) s-IBM in patients who previously had poliomyelitis (one of our patients and [21]); (b) s-IBM in HIV patients (one of ours and one of Dalakas et al. [22,23]); (c) s-IBM in HTLV1 antigen- and antibody-positive patients (one of ours from an HTLV1-endemic

---

pathologic β-sheets and 6–10 nm filaments. Prion can also contributes to the paired helical filaments (4–6).

b_p When excessive, b_p protein is toxic to mitochondria and/or other cell functions. (Mitochondrial abnormalities are much more evident in s-IBM and HTLV1-IBM, and they are absent or minimal in the h-IBM's.) Thus, mitochondrial abnormalities must be attributed (a) to b_p acting in the "aging milieu", or (b) to v_p.

c_p Excess of c_p protein can also act as a transcription factor to facilitate (promote) expression of TF_{JCT}.

d_p Decrease of this normally-inhibitory protein allows overexpression of c_p protein.

e_p Decrease of e_p protein impairs normal cell-function e_{fn}. This putative decrease could be a very important aspect of the cytopathogenesis, but might be very difficult to identify because excess of a protein in a muscle fiber is much easier to determine than a decrease.

b_{fn} or e_{fn} Either increase of a b_{fn} function or decrease of an e_{fn} function could 1–1 by modulating translation, post-translation changes, or catabolism of tau 1–1 lead to the demonstrated accumulation of hyperphosphorylated tau in paired helical filaments (4–6). (Note:

our studies to date have failed to identify increased transcription of tau mRNA in IBM muscle fibers, or at normal neuromuscular junctions [4–6]). For example, tau catabolism could be impaired by formation of nitrotyrosines on it (28), or by its abnormal phosphorylation (4–6), or its glycation. The accumulation of membranous whorls in the IBM vacuolated muscle fibers (see above) could also be attributed to decrease of a catabolic function.

TF_{VIRAL} In s-IBM (but not h-IBM), TF_{VIRAL} is a putative virus-induced transcription-factor, which upregulates (promotes) transcription of normal or altered (see above) viral genes V_g that are integrated in the s-IBM muscle-fiber genome, resulting in translation of viral proteins (V_p) within the muscle fiber. In HTLV1-IBM, TF_{VIRAL} is a viral protein (or proteins), possibly Tax (see above).

V_p These putatively-present foreign proteins in the muscle-fiber of s-IBM are antigenic, resulting in the CD8+ lymphocytic attack on muscle fibers as a pathogenic mechanism additive to the altered mechanisms consequent to upregulated TF_{IBM} (discussed above). The V_p viral proteins might also be toxic to mitochondria and/or other muscle-cell functions.

region of northeastern Iran (see below), and of Dalakas et al. [22,23]); (d) reovirus-like particles in cultured muscle fibers of a patient with a chronic vacuolar (s-IBM) myopathy (24);(e) ability of measles virus to infect normal human muscle in culture (25); (f) ability of HTLV1 retrovirus to experimentally infect animal muscle; and (g) ability of c-particles, presumably of Rous sarcoma retrovirus, to proliferate in cultured chick striated muscle (26,27).

Although viral protein or nucleic acid has not yet been detected within s-IBM muscle fibers, this does not exclude the possibility that an intramyofiber viral infestation is the etiologic and pathogenic mechanism. First, the putative IBM-virus might be one not yet sought in s-IBM muscle, or a yet unknown one. A retrovirus, or non-retrovirus, might have left a few inauspicious pieces of its related DNA integrated into the muscle-cell nuclear genome (or, less likely, the mitochondrial genome), but those might not be the sequences thus far studied utilizing the sequence-specific technique of PCR. (Possibly the putative viral DNA fragments could be truncated, spliced, or scrambled, and/or have a different transcription start-site; consequently (i) the virus-related DNA might not be detected by the usual PCR, and (ii) its protein would not be a usual viral protein.) The putative viral DNA is transcribed and translated within the muscle fiber to produce proteins that are: (i) antigenic, "foreignizing" the muscle fiber when co-expressed with MHC-I molecules (s-IBM and HTLV1-IBM muscle fibers are known to pathologically express MHC-I on their plasmalemma [23, 39, 40]) and thereby instigating an attack by CD8+ cytotoxic T-lymphocytes; (ii) toxic, e.g., to mitochondria; and (iii) able to act as transcription factors to pathologically up- and down-regulate various normal genes of the muscle fiber. These mechanisms are discussed in more detail below in regard to HTLV1-IBM (see Figs. 24.2, 24.3).

Hypothetical Pathogenesis of HTLV1 Inclusion-Body Myositis (HTLV1-IBM).

The patient we studied was a 55-year-old Muslim from Mashhad, Iran, an endemic region of HTLV1. He had 1 ½ years of typical progressive s-IBM weakness (19). Muscle biopsy by histochemistry and electron microscopy was typical of s-IBM; but in addition HTLV1 p19 protein was expressed on the plasmalemma of several slightly small muscle fibers (some containing vacuoles) (19). His blood was positive for HTLV1 by Elisa, immunoblot, and PCR, and his spinal-fluid was positive by Elisa and immunoblot. He denied risk factors of promiscuity, i.v. drugs, and blood transfusions; he

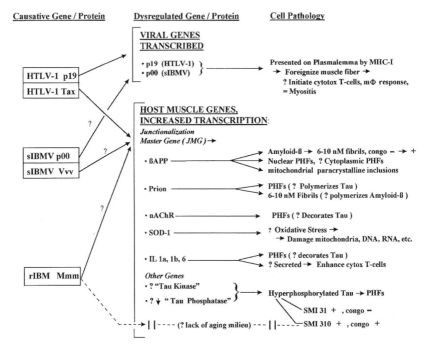

Figure 24.2.

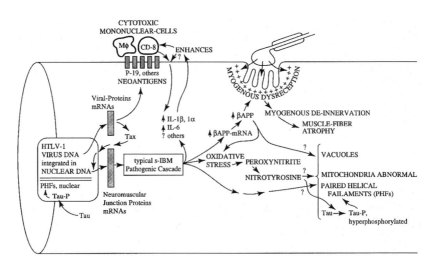

Figure 24.3.

might have acquired HTLV1-virus as an infant, through his mother's milk, as reportedly occurs in other HTLV1-endemic regions. He did not have clinical evidence of spinal cord abnormality. His wife was HTLV1 positive, without neuromuscular abnormality (she might have acquired HTLV1 in infancy from her mother's milk or sexually from her husband).

Our demonstration of HTLV1 p19 protein immunohistochemically at the plasmalemma of this patient's muscle fibers is the first evidence of an HTLV1 viral component as part of the muscle fibers themselves (previous studies have been negative for muscle fibers, localizing viral components only in macrophages [22,23]). Our current concepts of the pathogenesis of HTLV1-IBM are presented in Figs. 24.2 and 24.3.

In Fig. 24.2, the following are hypothetical: **s-IBMV**, the virus causing s-IBM; **s-IBM p00**, a protein of the putative virus of s-IBM; **s-IBMV Vvv**, a protein of the s-IBM virus capable of modulating transcription of host-cell genes; **Junctionalization Master Gene,** a gene protein product that acts as a transcription factor upregulating many (all?) of the proteins upregulated at the post-synaptic region of the human neuromuscular junction.

In Fig. 24.3, our positive laboratory findings include: p19 on plasmalemma of muscle fibers (19); increased IL-1β, IL-1α, and IL-6 (29); increased βAPP and βAPP-mRNA in non-junctional cytoplasm (4-6); increase of other junctional proteins in non-junctional cytoplasm (4-6); increased markers of oxidative stress, namely SOD1 protein and gene (28,30,31), nitric oxide synthetases (28), and nitrotyrosine (especially on PHFs) (28); hyperphosphorylated tau (4-6); and myogenous dysreception, as concluded from our finding that human muscle fibers overexpressing adenovirus-transferred βAPP gene are not able to be innervated by cocultured fetal rat spinal cord (in contrast to excellent innervation of uninfected-control cultured fibers) (32). This "myogenous dysreception" is proposed to cause "myogenous deinnervation" in the IBMs (conceivably, such myogenous dysreception could occur through the overexpressed-βAPP suppressing the production or reactivity of muscle-fiber agrin, MUSK, rapsyn, laminin-B2 (s-laminin), or syntropin-beta-subunit).

Autocrine and paracrine effects of the cytokines produced by IBM muscle fibers, – e.g., IL-1α, IL-1β, and IL-6 (29) – can act through adjacent CD8+ lymphocytes and macrophages to enhance their production of destruction cytokines, which in turn can enhance expression of the myogenous cytokines, creating a destructive positive feedback loop. This phenomenon might paracrinely damage adjacent muscle fibers even if they are not infected by the putative s-IBM virus or by HTLV1. (Because Tax can deregulate genes for cytokine receptors (20) it might do so within muscle fibers, making the fibers more sensitive to toxic cytokines.) Lymphocyte cytokines can also enhance MHC-I expression by muscle fibers (33). As noted above, Tax activates host-cell genes having NF-κB response elements in their upstream promoter regions (20).

On the basis of our findings, cellular oxidative-stress has recently been proposed to have a significant pathogenic role in s-IBM (6,28,30,31).

Hypothetical Junctionalization of Non-Junctional Nuclei in the IBM's.

The junction refers the neuromuscular junction (NMJ). To explain the "ectopic" production of junctional proteins by non-junctional nuclei in IBM-vacuolated muscle fibers, we formulated the concept of "junctionalization" of non-junctional nuclei (4–6). The concept is diagrammed in Fig. 24.4. In normal adult innervated human muscle fibers, certain proteins and their mRNAs are accumulated exclusively at the post-synaptic neuromuscular junction – for example, nicotinic acetylcholine receptor, APP, cellular prion, and superoxide dismutase 1 (4–5,28,30,31). These accumulations presumably result from the junctional nuclei uniquely expressing the genes of these proteins, whereas non-junctional nuclei of innervated mature-fibers do not (although non-junctional nuclei do so in uninnervated generating or regeneration muscle fibers). However, in IBM vacuolated muscle fibers, these "junctional proteins" and their mRNAs are overexpressed in multiple regions along the fiber, some at long distances away from the NMJ, a phenomenon attributed to "junctionalization" of non-junctional nuclei, i.e., those nuclei are de-repressed in regard to genes of certain junctional proteins. This junctionalization possibly can be attributed to: (a) direct upregulation of a "junctionalizing master gene" in the non-junctional nuclei, or (b) inhibition of a putative "junctional-protein-suppression-factor" (Fig. 24.4). Either mechanism could be activated directly or indirectly by (i) the genetic defect(s) of the h-IBMs, (ii) a viral factor in HTLV1-IBM, or (iii) a proposed viral factor in s-IBM. In s-IBM, the "aging milieu" of the muscle fiber may be contributory.

Treatment of Pathologic Components or Mechanisms.

The pathologic components or mechanisms that might be treatable in s-IBM, autosomal-recessive Persian-Jewish h-IBM (the most frequent form of AR_1-IBM), and HTLV1-IBM are summarized in Table 24.1.

A major question in s-IBM is the mechanism whereby the CD8+ cytotoxic T-lymphocytic inflammatory cells attack the muscle fibers. Pos-

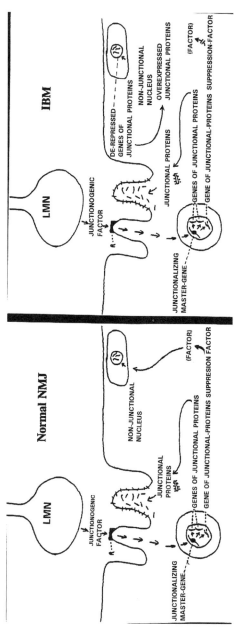

Figure 24.4.

Table 24.1. *Pathologic components and treatments*

Pathologic components	s-IBM	HTLV1 IBM	AR_1 h-IBM	Component/mechanism-directed treatment
a. Lymphocytic inflammatory	+	+	0	Immunosuppression (prednisone, IVIG, oral cyclophosphamide, etc.)
b. "Non-inflammatory" myopathy				
Necrosis	+	+	+	?
Vacuoles, formation of:	+	+	+	?
Membranous whorls	+	+	+	Prednisone?
PHFs, SMI 31-positive:	+	+	+	?
SMI-310-positive	+	+	0	?
Congophilia	+	+	0	?
6–10 nm filaments	+	+	+	?
Mitochondria	+	+	0 ?	CoQ, carnitine; Prednisone? (cf. Rx of muscle carnitine deficiency)
COX-deficiency	+	+	0	
Other abnormalities	+	+	0	
Dysreceptional junctionopathy	+?	+?	+?	?
c. Denervation atrophy	+	+	++	?
myogenous (dysreception) ?				
neurogenous?				
d. Virus	+?	+	0	Anti-retroviral agents?

sibly CD8+ lymphocytes (a) are behaving normally to attack s-IBM muscle fibers made antigenically "foreign" by a viral infestation, as we suspect in HTLV1-IBM (discussed above; see Figs. 24.1–24.3 and their explanations), or (b) are malprogrammed (e.g., by a virus in them or in macrophages) such that they attack normal muscle fibers, which become bystander victims. Although CD8+ lymphocytes may play an important pathogenic role in the early involvement of a given muscle, CD8+ lymphocytes probably do not play the major role in the later stages that involve vacuolar degeneration, when various immunosuppression treatments produce little or no benefit. Furthermore, in h-IBM CD8+ lymphocytes do not play any role, because they are not present.

In s-IBM, might immunosuppression treatment be a detrimental aspect if there is a viral cause (see above)? The answer is not known, but two points may be relevant: (a) immuno-suppression can provide long-term benefit (> 10 years) to the dysimmune aspect of HTLV1-associated myelopathy (34, case 1; WKE, current observations of case 1); and (b) individual s-IBM patients, and individual muscles, may have different amounts of the two putative arms of the pathogenesis, namely, the dysimmune aspect and the vacuolar degeneration (see Figs. 24.1–24.3).

We consider that most s-IBM patients have some benefit from treatment, and all deserve a trial of treatments.

Our Treatments and Doses Currently Used

1. Prednisone. Prednisone is converted in the liver to its active form prednisolone.

High-dose prednisone schedule - This is used for acute and/or severe neuromuscular disorders, and for some of the s-IBM patients. Prednisone 80–100 mg is given high-single-dose alternate-day (written as "80/0" or "100/0" ("__/__" representing the two doses in each pair of days) for 3–4 weeks, and then gradually reduced by 5 mg every 2–4 weeks, as tolerated (33–35). In some of our s-IBM patients whose disease has responded, the dosage cannot be reduced below 50/0 or 40/0 without the weakness reappearing. In other s-IBM patients, if there is concern about greater susceptibility to side effects, or if the patient is small, the dosage can begin as 60/0 or 50/0. If the patient does not benefit after two months of high-single-dose alternate-day prednisone treatment, the dose can be rapidly reduced to 10/0, 10/0, 5/0, 5/0, and then 0/0 (= discontinued).

Low-dose schedule. We can also use an ascending dosage of 10/0, 10/0, 15/0, 15/0, 20/0, 20/0. Then we either maintain the dosage at 20/0 or, if there is no improvement after one month, increase it gradually in the same manner to 30/0 or 40/0 and maintain. This schedule produces fewer side effects and sometimes satisfactory improvement. (If it is not beneficial, and there are no significant side effects, the low-dose schedule prednisone can be raised to 60/0 or 80/0 to try to find a beneficial dosage.) The s-IBM patients who are older and/or obese are more likely to be susceptible to prednisone-provoked hypertension or diabetes mellitus, and therefore handle better the low-dose schedule.

Obligatory adjuncts we use with every oral prednisone treatment (19,20). Diet of: no caffeine (including no herbal teas or other herbal preparations; and no adrenergic stimulants, such as weight-loss pills [e.g. "fen-phen"] or "ephedra"); "no" salt (as close to "no" as possible); and "no" fat (as close to "no" as possible). As an antiacid, calcium compound (without magnesium) 1 gm 3–4 times daily, between meals and at bedtime (2 "Tums" = 1 gm calcium carbonate); or if the calcium alone causes constipation, the patient can use the form with magnesium (e.g., Mylanta tablets). Potassium (e.g., as K-Dur), the daily mEq K^+ being the same as the average prednisone dose in mg (e.g. K^+ 10 mEq daily if the prednisone dose is 20 mg single-dose alternate-day). Monitoring the serum for a low level of potassium will not detect early total-body potassium deficiency because the tissues will give up potassium to maintain serum levels; therefore we routinely give potassium prophylactically (caution is needed if the patient is taking a potassium-sparing diuretic). A histamine H_2-receptor antagonist is used only as needed, not routinely. To help prevent osteoporosis, some clinicians suggest routine use of daily calcitriol (1,25-dihydroxyvitamin D_3) (38). Alternatively, calcitonin or alendronate can be considered. For postmenopausal women, estrogen and progesterone should be considered.

Monitoring for side-effects of prednisone. Every 4–8 weeks one should monitor fasting (or 2-hour post-prandial) glucose, hemoglobin A1C (elevation of this glycated hemoglobin indicates diabetes mellitus or impending diabetes), and blood-pressure, in addition to review of symptoms and physical examination. Ophthalmologic monitoring for glaucoma and cataracts is appropriate.

How Prednisone Might Be Benefitting s-IBM. The main benefit may be by suppression of the cytotoxic lymphocytes (mainly CD8 + T-lymphocytes [39,40]) that are considered to be attacking the muscle fibers, and perhaps by suppressing cytotoxic macrophages. Prednisone is also known to stabilize lysosomes; this action would be beneficial if the accumulated membranous whorls in some of the muscle-fiber vacuoles reflect an aggravating pathogenic role of lysosomal instability and intracellular leakage of their lytic enzymes. Whether prednisone can beneficially cause the following is speculative: decrease leukocyte cytokine production and effect; decrease muscle-protein catabolism in proteosomes; and decrease peroxinitrite production and its formation of nitrotyrosine on proteins.

In s-IBM, and potentially in h-IBM, a possible non-anti-dysimmune benefit of prednisone could be related to the following findings. (a) In aneurally cultured human muscle, hydrocortisone decreases βAPP mRNA (41) and prion mRNA (V. Askanas et al., unpublished). (b) In co-cultures of human-muscle plus fetal-rat spinal cord, hydrocortisone enhances neuromuscular-junction formation and maintenance, including junctional-fold formation (42–46). (c) In cultures of fetal-rat ventral spinal cord, hydrocortisone has a trophic influence on acetylcholinesterase-positive neurons, presumably motor neurons (47,48). The foregoing observations are potentially relevant because we have previously observed in both s-IBM and h-IBM: (a) in the non-junctional regions of the vacuolated muscle fibers, up-regulated mRNA and protein of both βAPP and prion (4–6); (b) junctional morphologic abnormalities (VA, unpublished); and (c) loss of normal complete junctionalization (normal junctionalization of a muscle fiber confines transcription of several junctional proteins, such as βAPP and prion, strictly to the post-synaptic junctional region [Fig. 24.04], whereas in s-IBM and h-IBM such transcriptions, indicated by accumulations of mRNAs and proteins, occur ectopically throughout the length of the vacuolated muscle fiber [4–6]).

Despite these theoretical possibilities, the benefit of prednisone treatment in s-IBM is limited, perhaps because it may be ameliorating mainly a dysimmune mechanism without having a major impact on other more severe and progressive mechanisms that produce weakness of muscle fibers. The following observations also suggest that the dysimmune aspect of s-IBM, although very important, is not the major pathogenic mechanism: the benefit resulting from prednisone or IVIG treatment in s-IBM is not as rapidly dramatic, nor of the magnitude initially seen, for example, with prednisone in myasthenia gravis (49–51), or more recently with IVIG in some dysimmune progressive muscular atrophies (52,53), nor as seen with interferon-alpha 2A in fever-responsive neuropathy (54,55).

Could prednisone be benefitting non-muscle aspects of the patient, e.g., arthralgias? In our opinion arthralgias are not a typical aspect of s-IBM, even in the older patients; and the patients usually do not have significant unrelated arthralgias. The s-IBM patients do not have significantly elevated erythrocyte sedimentation rates, rheumatoid-factor titers, or anti-nuclear-antibody titers. We consider that the prednisone-induced increased endurance and decreased fatigue does not have a significant arthralgia-ameliorating component, nor a non-specific feeling of well-being.

High-Dose Intravenous-Pulse Methylprednisolone. This is a technique we employed many years ago for refractory dysimmune neuromuscular diseases, but have not used routinely. Recently, long-term use of this method has been emphasized as an excellent treatment for dermatomyositis (750–1,000 mg methylprednisolone 2–3 times/week for many months, along with azathioprine), and found especially beneficial for the associated pulmonary fibrosis (56). Because this treatment has not been reported in s-IBM, we do not know whether it may be beneficial.

2. Intravenous Immunoglobulin G (IVIG). Using a dose of approximately 0.4 gms/kg body-weight (= 0.18 gm/pound) per day, we initially give, usually as an out-patient, two (or sometimes three) 5-day courses, each course separated by a 2-week interval. If there is benefit of increased endurance and/or strength, typically it is evident within the week following a 5-day course. Because the IVIG-induced benefit usually begins to wain after 2–3 weeks (sometimes after one week) and is gone at 3–4 weeks, IVIG maintenance therapy must be given. We continue the same 5-day courses as necessary, interspersed by no-treatment intervals of 2–3 weeks (infrequently up to 4 weeks). Note that three recent studies (57,58,58a) claiming no statistical benefit of IVIG in s-IBM we consider not only valueless but, in fact, misleading because of faulty design – the IVIG was given on two consecutive days, three times (57,58a) or two times (58) at one-month intervals, but the muscle strength was not measured for efficacy until one month after the last dose. At one month, an IVIG-induced benefit would have dissipated, as noted above, and thus would be missed by that study design. Our own experience is that we see definite benefit for 2–3 weeks after 5-day IVIG courses in the majority of the s-IBM patients treated.

We use a 7.5% solution of the IVIG, administered not faster than 100 ml/hr, the infusion extending at least 4 hours. The slow rate of infusion is especially important for the older s-IBM patients, who often are being treated concurrently for hypertension and/or cardiac insufficiency and/or renal disease (the last necessitating a lower IVIG dosage). We usually pretreat with ibuprophen 400 mg or naproxen 250–500 mg 15 minutes before IVIG and repeat this after 3 hours. To help prevent a possible allergic reaction, we often use 25 mg diphenhydramine at the first or both time points. If actual improvement is not evident after the two (or sometimes three) 5-day courses of IVIG, we do not continue them.

Drawbacks of IVIG treatment include inconvenience to the patient and cost of the drug. Side effects are usually minor, but can include an annoying pruritic rash, increased blood pressure, fluid overload, headache, and, rarely, sterile meningitis (which can be very discomfiting but not dangerous, and recurrence often can be prevented by concurrent i.v. glucocorticoid); the rash, headache, and sterile meningitis often do not recur when the same patient receives further IVIG treatments. If fluid overload occurs, or seems likely to occur, the patient can be given 20–40 mg furosemide 30 minutes before the IVIG and possibly repeated after 3 hours. It can also be given stat slowly intravenously if hypertension, or edema of lungs or ankles, is occurring. A pruritic rash can be treated with topical fluocinonide cream. If IVIG is used long-term, an indwelling catheter is often required. However, a catheter engenders other possible complications, such as septicemia, or thrombosis of a peripheral or central vein. It is preferable to surgically produce an arterio-venous fistula or, second choice, install an artificial A-V shunt.

The mechanism(s) by which IVIG benefits various dysimmune diseases is not established despite various speculations, and how it benefits s-IBM is also not known. (We know that IVIG does not turn off B-lymphocyte production of a monoclonal antibody because during careful monitoring we have seen net increase of IgM and new detectability of an IgM monoclonal antibody developing 2–3 months after each patient had a cumulatively-marked improvement of dysimmune motor neuropathy [36; WKE, unpublished]. IVIG does, though, transiently somewhat decrease total quantitative IgG, IgA and IgM (WKE, unpublished). In s-IBM, IVIG might beneficially interfer with cytokine release or cytokine-receptor recognition by CD8+ lymphocytes, macrophages, or muscle fibers [see Fig. 24.3].)

3. L-Carnitine and Co-Enzyme Q-10 (CoQ, also called Ubiquinone). Both molecules are required for transporting (or shuttling) essentials for energy production by the mitochondrion. Carnitine is necessary to shuttle long-chain fatty-acyl groups (e.g., palmitoyl) across the inner mitochondrial membrane so that within the mitochondrial matrix they can, as fatty-acyl CoAs, be beta-oxidized to provide energy (ATP). CoQ provides, within the mitochondrion, a conduit for transport of electrons from NADH and succinate to cytochromes b, c_1, and c, and thence to cytochrome c oxidase and O_2 for coupling with, and driving, ATP synthesis (oxidative phosphorylation).

In s-IBM, mitochondria can have mitochondrial-DNA deletions that produce segments of muscle fibers which are cytochrome-oxidase (COX) negative (59–62). Carnitine and CoQ are used as treatment in an attempt to facilitate function of muscle-fiber mitochondria that are not yet significantly impaired, for example, ones retaining some or all of their COX enzyme molecules. But carnitine and CoQ would not benefit mitochondria completely lacking COX activity because such mitochondria cannot carry out that last step of electron transport, from cytochrome c to O_2. Some s-IBM patients benefit from carnitine and CoQ.

Possibly relevant is that in muscle carnitine deficiency, which involves defective mitochondrial function, prednisone can be remarkably beneficial (63,64), for unknown reasons. Possibly the ability of prednisone to increase transport of carnitine into muscle fibers plays a role. Perhaps this is an aspect of the prednisone benefit in s-IBM, and possibly prednisone would be more efficacious with concurrent carnitine ± CoQ treatment.

We are giving carnitine (by prescription or non-prescription) as one gm 4–5 times daily, plus CoQ 100–150 mg 4 times daily (CoQ/ubiquinone is only available as non-prescription), both to be taken with food. They are begun separately, at a one-week interval, to allow any side effect to be attributed to one or the other. When started, each is gradually incremented during a 7-day period to reach the target dose. If no benefit is evident after 2 months, they are discontinued, unless prednisone or IVIG is added. The only significant side-effects of carnitine or CoQ we have seen are occasional diarrhea or nausea, and rarely a fish-like halitotic odor from carnitine.

4. Testosterone. We find that testosterone transiently improves muscle endurance and/or strength of men with various neuromuscular disorders, including some with s-IBM and h-IBM (WKE, unpublished). In normal and diseased states, the cellular sites of androgen-benefited neuromuscular function are probably both the muscle fibers and the lower motor neurons, because both have androgen receptors. A beneficial effect of dihydrotestosterone on long axonal outgrowth of neurons, presumably motor neurons, in cultured fetal rat ventral spinal cord has been described (48, 65, 66).

Depo-testosterone enanthate is given to men as 100–200 mg intramuscularly, as tolerated, once weekly (oral androgen is avoided to obviate liver toxicity). If benefit occurs, it typically begins on day 2 and lasts through day 5 or 6. One must monitor the side effects, such as irritability/anger and elevation of prostate-specific antigen (PSA), which can occur at the level of 150–200 mg i.m./week. (We are skeptical of the report of no alteration of mood or behavior during 10 weeks of testosterone 600 mg i.m./week [67], unless at that high dose the androgen-receptor was actually desensitized or downregulated, thereby negating the toxic and beneficial effects of that extremely high dose.) Testosterone can aggravate a diabetic tendency, and if given during prednisone treatment can raise the glucose to very high levels, e.g. > 400 (WKE, unpublished; and 1997 *Physician's Desk Reference*). In our testosterone-treated men, a high level of estradiol (a normal metabolite of testosterone) is produced, of uncertain therapeutic relevance.

The recently introduced androgen patch method of daily drug delivery can be considered for its convenience. Because our men with s-IBM, like other men in the s-IBM age range, can have low-normal or low levels of circulating testosterone, attributed to "normal aging," one might consider an androgen patch as replacement treatment. In women with IBM, one might consider the androgen danazol [used to treat fibrocystic breast disease and endometriosis], after weighing the various possible side-effects, including glucose intolerance.

5. Oral Cyclophosphamide (or Azathioprine). When used, oral cyclophosphamide is given once daily, with food, 2 mg/kg body-weight (or azathioprine 3 mg/kg), to the nearest multiple of 25 (20). The dose is gradually increased to this level during the first 7–10 days. Treatment should be for a minimum of 3 months. *It is obligatory to monitor absolute neutrophil and lymphocyte counts weekly* (or, if rather stable, every 2 weeks). In our method, the objective is to lower the absolute lymphocytes to < 700 and maintain absolute neutrophils (granulocytes) above 2,000 (or above 1,800 if the counts are stable) (37, 68). If neutrophils do go below 2,000 (or 1,800), treatment is interrupted until they reach 2,500, and the cyclophosphamide (or azathioprine) is then resumed at a dose of 25 mg less per day. (Other authors using these drugs to treat s-IBM typically do not give an interruption criterion.)

Note: the "white count" is a useless number reflecting the combination of different cell-types, neutrophils and lymphocytes, that concern opposite therapeutic objectives. The "total white count" concept should be abolished from the medical literature and from medicine in general [37,68]. Likewise, the terms "leucocytes" and "leukopenia" should be expurged from the therapeutic vocabulary (contrary to their recent emphasis [38]). *Obligatory adjunct with oral cyclophosphamide treatment.* We require that the patient drink at least 10 glasses (3 liters) of liquid daily, (albeit inconvenient) to prevent chemotoxic hemorrhagic cystitis and bladder neoplasm (37). Unfortunately, in the 1997 *Physicians' Desk Reference* (69) this high fluid intake daily is not published as a required concomitant of oral cyclophosphamide treatment, and the inappropriate total "white blood cell count" is recommended for safety monitoring! In patients who do not have episodes of hemorrhagic cystitis, late development of neoplasm does not seem to be a problem, in our experience (WKE, unpublished). However, patients who do not take adequate daily fluid and have repeated episodes of hemorrhagic cystitis can later develop bladder neo-plasia, according to the literature (70,71). In one of our cyclophos-phamide-treated, remarkably improved HTLV1 myelopathy patients (34) who, despite our exhortations, had not drunk adequate fluids, bladder can-cer surgery occurred $3\frac{1}{2}$ years after stopping 4 years of oral cyclophos-phamide-plus-prednisone (his treatment-produced restoration of walking remains improved $2\frac{1}{2}$ years after that surgery) (WKE, unpublished).

A second episode of hemorrhagic cystitis indicates that the patient is not taking, and presumably not able to take, adequate fluids; this should prompt consideration of ensuring adequate fluid intake or stopping the cyclophosphamide.

In individual patients with various dysimmune neuromuscular diseases, one can directly compare oral cyclophosphamide and azathioprine. We have had patients who came to us having failed to improve on azathio-prine, but have had an excellent benefit after being switched to oral cyclo-phosphamide (WKE, unpublished); for that reason, we favor oral cyclophosphamide if this type of drug is to be used.

With either cyclophosphamide or azathioprine, a late, post-treatment complication of myelodysplasia can occur; this sometimes can be serious or fatal. Exposure to more than one of these drugs, ± irradiation treat-ment, increases this liklihood.

In reports concerning the use of these drugs for IBM, unfortunately there is usually no mention of close monitoring by frequent absolute neutrophil counts to determine dosage modulation. Also, some of the reported doses of azathioprine are too low compared to our method (for example, a minimum dose of "75 mg/day for 8 weeks" [72] or, concur-rently with methotrexate, "maximum therapy of 150 mg/day or 0.3 mg/kg/day" [73]); these low doses could allow a beneficial effect of azathioprine to be missed.

Intravenous cyclophosphamide can cause very unpleasant acute side effects, and so we do not use it.

6. Methotrexate, Chlorambucil, or Cyclosporin. We do not use these drugs. We previously used chlorambucil successfully in a few dysimmune neuromuscular disease patients (74), but more recent information that it can cause secondary acute leukemia (75) deters us from currently using it.

7. Total-Body Irradiation (TBI). In small dosage, 150 rads total course (15 rads twice weekly for 5 weeks), TBI can produce excellent benefit in some patients with various dysimmune neuromuscular diseases (76, 77).

The remarkable improvement persisted for at least 15 years after one TBI course in our second-treated (76, 77), otherwise-refractory dermatomyositis patient (WKE, unpublished). However, one should be hesitant to use TBI after, or before, cytotoxic-immunosuppression, e.g., with oral cyclophosphamide, azathioprine or similar drugs, because of possible delayed (by several years) myelodysplastic bone-marrow failure or neoplasia. A course of total-nodal irradiation, which involves higher radiation dosages focused on lymph nodes, is more prolonged and thereby more inconvenient and expensive, and is without advantages regarding benefit or side-effects [WKE, unpublished].

8. Pyridostigmine. At doses of 60 mg 3 times daily, one of our otherwise typical autosomal-recessive h-IBM patients has achieved 3 years of modest but useful symptomatic improvement of ptosis (which is not typical of h-IBM or s-IBM), hand function (e.g. writing) and limb strength. In him, the improvement dissipates when treatment is temporarily omitted. Several of our other h-IBM and s-IBM patients have not benefited from pyridostigmine.

9. Various "anti-oxidants". We have not specifically studied these. However, our patients have not reported benefit from using, on their own initiative, vitamin E 400–2,000 U/day, or other non-prescription "antioxidant" formulations. This is despite our findings indicating that "oxidative stress" may play a role in the pathogenesis of the IBM vacuolated muscle fibers (28; 30, 31).

10. Bracing. For drop-foot abnormality, due to peroneal and anterior-tibial muscle weakness, common in both h-IBM and s-IBM, a light-weight drop-foot brace can definitely enhance walking stability and reduce tripping and falling. A different brace is required if there is concurrent weakness of plantar flexion due to gastrocnemius-soleus muscle involvement. Quadriceps muscle weakness impairing normal locking of the knees is the major cause of falling in s-IBM. A simple elastic brace to stabilize the knees can sometimes be beneficial. Use of a walker, often at the insistence of the physician, can be very important for various IBM patients to prevent falling and broken bones.

H. What Should be Measured for Therapeutic Evaluation? The treatments of all of our own neuromuscular-disease patients are evaluated for a 3–6 month period and seek actual improvement, namely increased endurance (decreased fatigue) and/or increased strength, and this is also the goal in s-IBM and h-IBM. Only for amyotrophic lateral sclerosis (ALS) patients are we willing to accept absolute lack of progression during the 3–6 months as a satisfactory treatment result. In none of the neuromuscular diseases are we seeking merely a slowing of disease progression in the 3–6 month therapeutic trials. In general, we believe that if a good treatment is found, the cellular repair and recoverability of muscle fibers (or motor neurons in ALS) will produce at least some increase of muscle endurance and/or strength.

The Medical Research Council scale of grading maximal muscle force from 0–5 is not satisfactory for evaluating modest changes, especially in the grade 4 range. To improve grade 4 evaluation by manual testing, we introduced the "Finger-Force" technique (78).

Over the years, various mechanical systems have been developed for Quantitative Muscle Testing (QMT) to evaluate treatment of neuromuscular diseases, including an original QMT machine designed by one of us (79). Such machines allow measurement of maximal isometric strength; however, increased endurance and decreased fatiguability are not measured, although those parameters seem to be the subtle features of improved muscle function first appreciated by patients. To quantitate endurance, we have previously utilized a moderately heavy weight to evaluate: (a) maximal number of repetitions, or (b) maximal duration of posture maintenance (80). At the onset of testing of a patient (beginning of the therapeutic trial), the weight is chosen separately for each muscle tested to be such that about 5 is the maximal possible (a) number of the full-range repetitions (e.g., biceps flexion with a gripped dumbbell or weighted wrist-cuff), or (b) seconds of maintenance against gravity, e.g., in the sitting position, of (i) biceps maintaining the forearm horizontal with a gripped dumbbell or weighted wrist cuff, or (ii) iliopsoas maintaining hip flexion to keep the foot one inch off the floor with a weighted ankle-cuff. All the tests were video recorded to allow an independent observer to later evaluate the test results.

In our evaluation of IBM treatments, we have not been doing those quantitative measurements of strength and endurance. Instead, we used the more expedient but less precise method of patient self-evaluation and recording of various tasks involving especially endurance/fatiguability during performance of everyday activities, comparing one treatment versus another. Although it is true that psychological factors potentially can influence the self-evaluation method, we conclude that the treatment results summarized below reflect definite practical benefit for some s-IBM patients.

Verification aspects of our patient-self-assessment method include the following: (a) comparing one treatment versus another (and versus a placebo); and (b) return of weakness with reduction of the medication dosage. For example, prednisone benefit is demonstrated if the patient becomes weaker when we decrease the dose, and becomes stronger again when the dose is increased. Likewise, benefit attributable to IVIG is demonstrated if there is an improvement with each course, beginning about day 5–8 of a 5-day IVIG course, maximal about day 8–10, and waning of improvement evident about day 16–23. These IVIG-induced improvements typically summate in the responsive patient. Patients considered to be prednisone or IVIG responders fulfilled these criteria.

I. Inappropriate Surrogate Markers of Benefit in s-IBM. The serum creatine kinase (CK) level typically decreases during prednisone treatment, but because prednisone is well known to decrease serum CK in various muscle diseases when there is no improvement of strength or endurance, a lower serum CK value cannot be considered a surrogate marker of essential muscle benefit (nor of decreased "active inflammation"; we disagree with others [73] on this point). Basically, we treat the patient's weakness and fatiguability, not the CK.

In an individual s-IBM patient, the amount of lymphocytic inflammatory cells in an after-treatment compared with a before-treatment muscle biopsy is not a valid marker of prednisone efficacy on the muscle weakness, for several reasons. (a) The biopsies are small samples of similar, but necessarily different, portions of the body musculature. (b) Different regions of the same muscle at one time-point can have different amounts of lymphocytes; for example, adjacent biopsy samples of s-IBM muscle taken at the same time can differ significantly, one having many lymphocytes and the other few or none. (c) In polymyositis and dermatomyositis, patients taking a glucocorticoid typically have virtually no, or only a few, lymphocytes in their muscle biopsies; thus it would not be surprising that s-IBM patients taking prednisone would have fewer lymphocytes in the muscle biopsy, regardless of prednisone effect on their muscle strength. (d) Early-involved s-IBM muscles have more lymphocytes than later-involved, weaker muscles (which have more vacuolar degeneration) (4–6; unpublished).

J. Study Design. Over the years, our therapeutic approaches have always been to treat each patient as an individual, on a one-by-one basis, because we are looking for actual improvement of the patient with a progressively worsening neuromuscular disease (and, unless the patient had been severely and dangerously weak, we typically incorporate the parameters of withdrawal-of-treatment-causing-slight-worsening and restitution-of-treatment-reinstituting-benefit, as discussed above) (35–37,49–55,81–85). This one-by-one approach has more recently been sanctified by the "n-of-1" designation.

K. Hypothetical curves indicating response of a specific muscle to treatment of s-IBM. In Figure 24.5, Curve E represents an untreated state, or complete unresponsiveness to a treatment attempt. In this example, treatment (Rx) is started when the muscle is weakened down to 60% of normal. With curves A_1 there is a fairly rapid benefit up to 80% of normal function (a 33% increase of the strength existing at time of treatment), resulting from repair of a reversible cellular malfunction. Curve A_2 represents a similar improvement but to only 70% of normal (a 17% increase from pre-Rx status). Both A_1 and A_2 demonstrate maintained improvement.

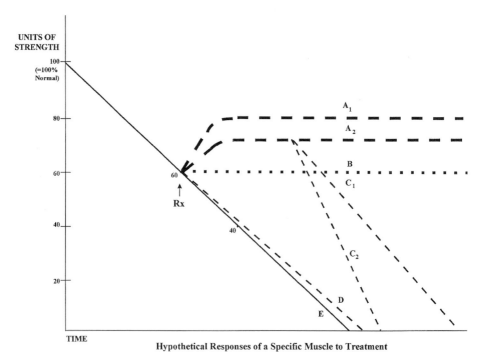

Hypothetical Responses of a Specific Muscle to Treatment

Figure 24.5.

However, the improvement might not be maintained, due to a concurrent cellular disease-process unresponsive to the treatment, resulting in two types of outcome. (i) Curves C_1 demonstrates that benefit from the treatable component (e.g., in s-IBM stopping the presumed cytotoxicity of invading CD8+ lymphocytes) provides the affected muscle fibers an ameliorative legacy of improved function involving a basis to better withstand (but not completely prevent) the insistent deterioration caused by the untreatable-component (e.g., in s-IBM the vacuolar degeneration, mitochondrial abnormality, and abnormal accumulation of proteins), thereby extending the time to reach any given level of further reduced strength. Thus, curve C_1 is set "permanently" at a higher level than the no-treatment curve E and declines approximately parallel to it. Curve C_2 demonstrates a loss of the initial improvement with only minimal residual benefit, such that in time C_2 progressively approaches the no-treatment curve E. Curve B reflects complete stopping of progression, but no improvement (i.e., no cellular repair). Curve D indicates only a minimal slowing of disease progression.

L. Results of Treatment. The literature data on treating s-IBM is reviewed by Griggs and Rose (86), but they did not critique the dosing and testing schedules (*v.s.*). The following results are from patients we have treated. In our patient population we have: (a) 67 s-IBM patients (80% men), including one woman who had had poliomyelitis decades earlier, and one HTLV1 antibody and antigen-positive Persian (Iranian) Muslim man from an HTLV1 endemic region of Iran; (b) 27 patients with autosomal-recessive hereditary IBM, including 25 Persian Jews and two non-Jewish non-Persian Mexican brothers; and (c) 7 patients with autosomal-dominant IBM (non-Jewish non-Persians in four families).

In reference to Fig. 24.5, the later response of an initially responsive s-IBM muscle to a treatment, for example prednisone, seems to follow curve C_1; infrequently it seems to almost follow A_2 for a few years. Nearly normal strength is not restored (as it can be in some dermatomyositis and polymyositis patients). Research must still develop a better treatment, or combination of treatments. It is our general impression that better response to treatment occurs in earlier-involved individual muscles (which usually have more lymphocytic infiltration). Thus a given patient can have some muscles more responsive than others. Younger patients tend to respond better.

Among the s-IBM patients treated with prednisone, 74% (30 of 41) have improvement, including increased limb endurance and strength of limb muscles, and improved swallowing in some. Two men have now been prednisone-responsive, and prednisone-dependent (worsening when the prednisone dosage is transiently reduced), for more than 10 years (response A_2) (unpublished observations); however, one has developed mild diabetes. From IVIG treatment, 75% (6 of 8) have had improvement. The 5-day maintenance courses of IVIG must be repeated every 2–6 weeks. Carnitine and CoQ have produced slight benefit of endurance for 3–12 months, in 75% (9 of 12) of the patients treated. TBI (given 1981–85) benefited 75% (3 of 4) of the treated patients, with improved strength lasting as long as 6–24 months. Oral cyclophosphamide benefited 67% (2 of 3). Oral azathioprine, given by other physicians, benefited none (0 of 4). Weekly intramuscular testosterone, given only to men, provided slight but definite improvement of endurance in 83% (5 of 6).

M. Possible Sequence of Treatments. Virtually all s-IBM patients should be given a trial of treatment. Carnitine plus CoQ can be tried for 1–2 months. Then either prednisone (even if carnitine + CoQ is not beneficial) or IVIG treatment can be added – or treatment can be begun with one of these. Compared with prednisone, benefit from IVIG is evident sooner (within a week after a 5-day course of IVIG) and has many fewer side-effects, but IVIG is more inconvenient and more expensive. IVIG can benefit s-IBM patients who do not respond to prednisone. Side-effects are different between IVIG and prednisone, and each patient's individual potential susceptibility to them will partly determine the choice of treatment. For patients who fail to benefit from prednisone or cannot take it (e.g., hypertensive or diabetic patients), and who cannot be given IVIG, oral cyclophosphamide can be considered.

N. For the Future. Better treatments are certainly needed. We anticipate that additional knowledge of the mechanisms of the cyto- and molecular-pathogenic cascade of both s-IBM and the h-IBMs that is rapidly developing (6) will lead to new treatments directed at key pathogenic steps of: (a) the vacuolar degeneration of muscle fibers in s-IBM, HTLV1-IBM, and the h-IBMs; (b) the dysimmune component of s-IBM and HTLV1-IBM; and (c) the virus, known in HTLV1-IBM and suspected in s-IBM. In s-IBM, eventually treatments may be directed at the first, etiologic step. In the h-IBMs, identification of the different genetic abnormalities and the consequent pathogenic cascades of the several types of h-IBM may direct our treatments toward beneficially affecting those cascades long before "gene-replacement therapy" might ever become achievable. Our own research is oriented toward obtaining more information about the pathogenic cascades of s-IBM, HTLV1-IBM, and the h-IBMs, and seeking commonalities thereof.

References

1. Mendell JR, Sahenk Z, Gales T, Paul L. Amyloid filaments in inclusion body myositis. *Arch Neurol* 48:1229–1234, 1991.
2. Askanas V, Engel WK, Alvarez RB. Enhanced detection of congo-red-positive amyloid deposits in muscle fibers of inclusion-body myositis and brain of Alzheimer disease using fluorescence technique. *Neurology* 43:1265–1267, 1993.
3. Askanas V, Alvarez RB, Mirabella M, Engel WK. Use of anti-neurofilament antibody to identify paired-helical filaments in inclusion-body myositis. *Ann Neurol* 39:389–391, 1996.
4. Askanas V, Engel WK. New advances in the understanding of sporadic inclusion-body myositis and hereditary inclusion-body myopathies. *Curr Opin Rheumatol* 7:486–496, 1995.
5. Askanas V, Engel WK. Sporadic inclusion-body myositis and hereditary inclusion-body myopathies. In: Appel SH (ed), *Current Neurology*, vol. 16, pp. 115–144. Springfield, IL, Mosby-Year Book, 1996.
6. Askanas V, Engel WK. Newest approaches to diagnosis and pathogenesis of sporadic inclusion-body myositis and hereditary inclusion-body myopathies, including molecular-pathologic similarities to Alzheimer disease. Chapter 1, this volume.
7. Engel WK, Cunningham GG. Alkaline phosphatase-positive abnormal muscle fibers of humans. *J Histochem Cytochem* 18:55–57, 1970.
8. Engel WK. Integrative histochemical approach to the defect of Duchenne muscular dystrophy. In: Rowland LP (ed), *Pathogenesis of the Human Muscular Dystrophies*, pp. 277–309. New York, American Elsevier, 1977.
9. Ringel SP, Engel WK, Bender AN. Extrajunctional acetylcholine receptors on myogenously de-innervated muscle fibers. *J Histochem Cytochem* 24:1033–1034, 1976.
10. Askanas V, Engel WK, DiMauro S, Brooks BR, Mehler M. Adult-onset acid maltase deficiency. *N Engl J Med* 294:573–578, 1976.
11. Engel WK, Askanas V. Toxic role of long-chain fatty acids in muscle carnitine deficiency and other LCFA endodissolutions? Dietary LCFA restriction associated with dramatic long-term improvement. *Neurology* 36:94, 1986.
12. Mirabella M, Engel WK, Passinetti G, Finch CE, Askanas V. Denervation of adult human muscle fibers induces apoptosis, evidenced by fragmentation of nuclear DNA, and increased expression of the clusterin (ApoJ) gene. *Neurology* 46:270, 1996.
13. Engel WK. Muscle biopsies in neuromuscular diseases. *Pediatr Clin North Am* 14:963–995, 1967.
14. Engel WK. "Myopathic EMG" – nonesuch animal. *N Engl J Med* 289:485–486, 1973.

15. Engel WK. Brief, small, abundant motor-unit action potentials. *Neurology* 25:173–176, 1975.
16. Luciano CA, Dalakas MC. Inclusion body myositis: no evidence for a neurogenic component. *Neurology* 48:29–33, 1997.
17. Eisen A, Berry K, Gibson S. Inclusion body myositis (IBM): myopathy or neuropathy? *Neurology* 33:1109–1114, 1983.
18. Mitrani-Rosenbaum S, Argov Z, Blumenfeld A, Seidman CE, Seidman JG. Hereditary inclusion body myopathy maps to chromosome 9p1-q1. *Hum Mol Genet* 5:159–163, 1996.
18a. Middleton LT, Christodoulou K, Askanas V, Engel WK et al. *Ann Neurol* 42:414, 1997.
19. Engel WK, Haginoya K, Alvarez RB, Sabetian K, Bajoghli M, Askanas V. Sporadic inclusion-body myositis (s-IBM) in an HTLV1-positive Iranian muslim. *Neurology* 48:A124, 1997.
20. Gilmore TD. Regulation of Rel transcription complexes. In: Goodbourn S (ed), *Eukaryotic Gene Transcription*, pp 102–131. Oxford, IRL Press at Oxford University Press, 1996.
21. Abarbanel JM, Lichtenfeld Y, Zirkin H, Louzon Z, Osimani A, Farkash P, Herishanu Y. Inclusion body myositis in post-poliomyelitis muscular atrophy. *Acta Neurol Scand* 78:81–84, 1988.
22. Dalakas MC, Leon-Monzon M, Illa I, Culper E. Viruses, immunodeficiency and inclusion body myositis. Chapter 18, this volume.
23. Inclusion body myositis in HIV-1 and HTLV-1 infected patients. Cupler EJ, Leon-Monzon M, Miller J, Semino-Mora C, Anderson TL, Dalakas MC. *Brain* 119:1887–1893, 1996.
24. Askanas V, Engel WK. Reovirus-like particles in cultured muscle fibers of a patient with a chronic vacuolar myopathy. *Neurology* 28:386, 1978.
25. Askanas V, McFarland H, Engel WK, Rodman RB. Electronmicroscopic (EM) and immunoperoxidase studies of measles-infected human cultured muscle: possible relevance to nonspecific vacuolar myopathy (NVM). *Neurology* 31:57, 1981.
26. Engel WK, Askanas V. Overlooked avian oncornavirus in cultured muscle – functionally significant? *Science* 192:1252–1253, 1976.
27. Askanas V, Engel WK. Chick muscle in tissue culture: the ubiquity of viral infection. *Acta Neuropathol* (Berl) 32:271–279, 1975.
28. Yang C-C, Alvarez RB, Engel WK, Askanas V. Nitric-oxide induced oxidative stress in muscle fibers of hereditary inclusion-body myopathy (h-IBM) and sporadic inclusion-body myositis (s-IBM). *Neurology* 48:331A–332A, 1997.
29. Haginoya K, Alvarez RB, Engel WK, Askanas V. Light- and electron-microscopic immunolocalization of interleukins 1α, 1β and 6 in vacuolated muscle fibers of sporadic inclusion-body myositis (s-IBM). *Neurology* 48:A126, 1997.
30. Askanas V, Sarkozi E, Alvarez RB, McFerrin J, Engel WK, Siddique T. Superoxide-dismutase-1 (SOD1) gene and protein in vacuolated muscle fibers of sporadic inclusion-body myositis (s-IBM), hereditary inclusion-body myopathy (h-IBM), and cultured human muscle after β-amyloid precursor protein (APP) gene transfer. *Neurology* 46:487, 1996.
31. Yang C-C, Alvarez RB, Engel WK, Askanas V. Increase of nitric oxide synthases and nitrotyrosine in inclusion-body myositis. *NeuroReport* 8:153–158, 1996.

32. McFerrin J, Price SM, Baqué S, Engel WK, Askanas V. Overexpression of çamyloid precursor protein (βAPP) gene in cultured normal human muscle using adenovirus vector prevents formation of neuromuscular junctions (NMJs) and functional innervation: relevance to inclusion-body myositis (s-IBM). *Neurology* 48:A332, 1997.
33. Hohlfeld R, Engel AG. Induction of HLA-DR expression on human myoblasts with interferon-gamma. *Am J Pathol* 136:503–508, 1990.
34. Engel WK, Hanna CJ, Misra AK. HTLV1-associated myelopathy. *N Engl J Med* 323:552, 1990.
35. De Vivo DC, Engel WK. Remarkable recovery of a steroid responsive recurrent polyneuropathy. *J Neurol Neurosurg Psychiatry* 33:62–69, 1970.
36. Engel WK, Borenstein A, DeVivo DC, Schwartzman RI, Warmolts JR. High-single-dose alternate-day prednisone (HSDAD-PRED) in the treatment of dermatomyositis/polymyositis complex. *Trans Am Neurol Assoc* 7:272–275, 1972.
37. Engel WK, Dalakas MC. Treatment of neuromuscular diseases. In: Wiederholt WC (ed), *Therapy for Neurologic Disorders*, pp. 51–101. New York, Wiley, 1982.
38. Griggs RC, Mendell JR, Miller RG. *Evaluation and treatment of myopathies*. Philadelphia, F.A. Davis Company, 1995.
39. Engel AG, Arahata K. Monoclonal antibody analysis of mononuclear cells in myopathies: II. Phenotypes of autoinvasive cells in polymyositis and inclusion-body myositis. *Ann Neurol* 16:209–215, 1984.
40. Hohlfeld R, Bender A, Engel AG. Muscle-fiber T Cells in IBM: antigen-presenting cells or innocent bystanders? Chapter 17, this volume.
41. Sarkozi E, Askanas V, McFerrin J, Johnson SA, Engel WK. Regulation of the β-amyloid precursor protein (βAPP) gene in cultured human muscle fibers. *Neurobiol Aging* 15:S158–159, 1994.
42. Braun S, Askanas V, Engel WK, Ibrahim EM. Long-term treatment with glucocorticoids increases synthesis and stability of junctional acetylcholine receptors on innervated cultured human muscle. *J Neurochem* 60:1929–1935, 1993.
43. Askanas V, McFerrin J, Park-Matsumoto YC, Lee CS, Engel WK. Glucocorticoid increases acetylcholinesterase and organization of the postsynaptic membrane in innervated cultured human muscle. *Exp Neurol* 115:368–375, 1992.
44. Park YC, Askanas V, Engel WK. Influence of hydrocortisone (HC) on the development of neuromuscular junctions (NMJs) in cultured human muscles. *J Neurol Sci* 98:181–182, 1990.
45. Askanas V, McFerrin J, Lee CS, Park YC, Engel WK. Hydrocortisone (HC) influences molecular and morphologic properties of neuromuscular junctions (NMJs) of innervated cultured human muscle. *Neurology* 40:313, 1990.
46. McFerrin J, Askanas V, Engel WK. Hydrocortisone (HC) increases dystrophin immunoreactivity and causes dystrophin aggregation in aneurally cultured human muscle. *Soc Neurosci* 18:229, 1992.
47. Mariotti C, Askanas V, Kanda T, Engel WK. Influence of hydrocortisone (HC) on fetal rat ventral spinal cord neurons in vitro. *J Neurol Sci* 98:170, 1990.
48. Askanas V, Mariotti C, Engel WK. Trophic factors for cultured lower motor neurons. In: Rowland LP (ed), *Amyotrophic Lateral Sclerosis and*

Other Motor Neuron Diseases (Advances in Neurology, vol. 56), pp. 37–56. New York, Raven Press, 1991.

49. Warmolts JR, Engel WK, Whitaker JN. Alternate-day prednisone in a patient with myasthenia gravis. *Lancet* 2:1198–1199, 1970.

50. Engel WK, Warmolts JR. Myasthenia gravis: a new hypothesis of the pathogenesis and a new form of treatment. *Ann NY Acad Sci* 183:72–87, 1971.

51. Warmolts JR, Engel WK. Benefit from alternate-day prednisone in myasthenia gravis. *N Engl J Med* 286:17–20, 1972.

52. Engel WK, Hanna CJ. Intravenous immunoglobulin: excellent benefit in otherwise refractory progressive muscular atrophy with IgM monoclonal gammopathy. *Ann Neurol* 32:279, 1992.

53. Engel WK. Rapid and continued improvement from intravenous immunoglobulin treatment of asymmetrical chronic progressive muscular atrophy after 19 years of disease progression. *Ann Neurol* 38:333–334, 1995.

54. Engel WK, Adornato BT. Long-term interferon alpha-2A (Iα) benefits otherwise intractable chronic fever-responsive schwannian immune neuropathy (FR-SIN). *Neurology* 42:467, 1992.

55. Engel WK, Adornato BT. Fever-responsive neuropathy (FRN) benefitted by long-term interferon alpha-2A (Iα) treatment. *Can J Neurol Sci (Suppl)* 4:S44, 1993.

56. Genge A, Karpati G. Intermittent, high dose, intravenous glucocorticoid (GC) treatment (Rx) is preferred to high dose oral GC administration in adult dermatomyositis (DM). *Neurology* 48:A321, 1997.

57. Dalakas MC, Sonies B, Dambrosia J, Sekul E, Cupler E, Sivakumar K. Treatment of inclusion-body myositis with IVIg: a double-blind, placebo-controlled study. *Neurology* 48:712–716, 1997.

58. Dalakas MC, Sonies B, Koffman B, Spector S, Sivakumar K, Cupler E, Lopez-Devine J. High-dose intravenous immunoglobulin (IVIg) combined with prednisone in the treatment of patients with inclusion-body myositis (IBM): a double blind, randomised controlled trial. *Neurology* 48:A332, 1997.

58a. Amato AA, Barohn RJ, Jackson CE, Papert EJ, Sahenk Z, Kissel JT. Inclusion-body myositis: treatment with intravenous immunoglobulin. *Neurology* 44:1516–1518, 1994.

59. Oldfors A, Moslemi A-R, Fyhr I-M, Holme E, Larsson N-G, Lindberg C. Mitochondrial DNA deletions in muscle fibers in inclusion body myositis. *J Neuropathol Exp Neurol* 54:581–587, 1995.

60. Desnuelle C, Paquis V, Paul R, Engel WK, Saunières A, Alvarez RB, Askanas V. mtDNA analysis in muscle of patients with sporadic inclusion-body myositis and hereditary inclusion-body myopathy. Chapter 22, this volume.

61. Paquis V, Paul R, Askanas V, Engel WK, Desnuelle C. mtDNA deletions in muscle of sporadic inclusion-body myositis (S-IBM) and hereditary inclusion-body myopathy (H-IBM). *Neurology* 45:445, 1995.

62. Santorelli FM, Sciacco M, Tanji K, Shanske S, Vu TH, Golzi V, Griggs RC, Mendell JR, Hays AP, Bertorini TE, Pestronk A, Bonilla E, DiMauro S. Multiple mitochondrial DNA deletions in sporadic inclusion body myositis: a study of 56 patients. *Ann Neurol* 39:789–795, 1996.

63. Engel AG, Angelini C. Carnitine deficiency of human skeletal muscle with associated lipid-storage myopathy: a new syndrome. *Science* 179:899, 1973.

64. Prockop LD, Engel WK, Shug AL. Nearly fatal muscle carnitine deficiency with full recovery after replacement therapy. *Neurology* 33:1629–1631, 1983.
65. Micaglio G, Askanas A, Engel WK. Dihydrotestosterone influences neurite growth of rat ventral spinal cord cultures (VSCC). *Neurology* 35:246, 1985.
66. Micaglio G, Askanas V, Engel WK. Age-related influence of 5-(alpha) dihydrotestosterone (DHT) on rat ventral spinal cord cultures (VSCC). Presented at the XIII World Congress of Neurology, September 1–6, 1985.
67. Bhasin S, Storer TW, Berman N, Callegari C, Clevenger B, Phillips J, Bunnell TJ, Tricker R, Shirazi A, Casaburi R. The effects of supraphysiologic doses of testosterone on muscle size and strength in normal men. *N Engl J Med* 335:1–7, 1996.
68. Engel WK. Oral immunosuppression for multiple sclerosis (letter to the editor). *Lancet* 339:64–65, 1992.
69. Cytoxan (cyclophosphamide). *Physicians' Desk Reference*, 51st ed., pp. 700–701, Montvale, NJ, Medical Economics, 1997.
70. Kinlen LJ. Incidence of cancer in rheumatoid arthritis and other disorders after immunosuppressive treatment. *Am J Med* 78:44–49, 1985.
71. Castor CW, Bull FE. Review of United States data on neoplasms in rheumatoid arthritis. *Am J Med* 78:33–38, 1985.
72. Joffe MM, Love LA, Leff RL, Fraser DD, Targoff IN, Hicks JE, Plotz PH, Miller FW. Drug therapy of the idiopathic inflammatory myopathies: predictors of response to prednisone, azathioprine, and methotrexate and a comparison of their efficacy. *Am J Med* 94:379–387, 1993.
73. Leff RL, Miller FW, Hicks JE, Fraser DD, Plotz PH. The treatment of inclusion body myositis: a retrospective review and a randomized, prospective trial of immunosuppressive therapy. *Medicine* 72:225–235, 1993.
74. Dalakas MC, Flaum M, Engel WK, Gralnick H, Joshi B. Successful treatment of polyneuropathy in Waldenstrom macroglobulinemia (WM): role of dysproteinemia in pathogenesis of the neuropathy. *Neurology* 30:428, 1980.
75. Leukeran (chlorambucil). *Physicians' Desk Reference*, 50th ed., pp. 1133–1135. Montvale, NJ, Medical Economics, 1996.
76. Engel WK, Lichter AS, Galdi AP. Polymyositis: remarkable response to total body irradiation. *Lancet* 1:658, 1981.
77. Engel WK, Lichter AS, Siddique T. Remarkable improvement sustained 1–2 years following total body irradiation (TBI) treatment of otherwise intractable adult polymyositis/dermatomyositis (PM/DM). *Neurology* 32:120, 1982.
78. Engel WK. Finger force (*ff*): a simple, rapid technique for one observer to reproducibly semiquantitate "grade 4" muscle strength during drug testing. *Muscle Nerve* 9:270, 1986.
79. Dorman JD, Engel WK, Fried DM. Therapeutic trial in amyotrophic lateral sclerosis. Lack of benefit with pancreatic extract and dl-alpha tocopherol in 12 patients. *J Am Med Assoc* 209:257–258, 1969.
80. Engel WK. RNA metabolism in relation to amyotrophic lateral sclerosis. In: Rowland LP (ed), *Amyotrophic Lateral Sclerosis and Other Motor Neuron Diseases (Advances in Neurology*, vol. 56), pp. 125–153. New York, Raven Press, 1991.

81. Resnick JS, Engel WK, Griggs RC, Stam A. Acetazolamide prophylaxis in hypokalemic periodic paralysis. *N Engl J Med* 278:582–586, 1968.
82. Dalakas MC, Engel WK. Chronic relapsing (dysimmune) poly-neuropathy: pathogenesis and treatment. *Ann Neurol* 9:134–145, 1981.
83. Engel WK, Hopkins LC, Rosenberg BJ. Fasciculating progressive muscu-lar atrophy (F-PMA) remarkably responsive to anti-dysimmune treat-ment (ADIT) – a possible clue to more ordinary ALS? *Neurology* 35:72, 1985.
84. Engel WK, Cuneo RA, Levy HB. Polyinosinic-polycytidylic acid treat-ment of neuropathy. *Lancet* 2:503–504, 1978.
85. Engel WK, Prentice AF. Some polyneuropathies (PNs) in insulin-requir-ing adult-onset diabetes (IRAOD) can benefit remarkably from anti-dysimmune treatments. *Neurology* 43:A255–A256, 1993.
86. Griggs RC, Rose M. Evaluation of treatment for sporadic inclusion-body myositis. Chapter 23, this volume.

Index

Aβ, *see* β-amyloid protein
abdominal muscles, 196, 198
acid phosphatase
    diagnostic use, 139–140
    tibial muscular dystrophy, 237
activities of daily living, 247–249
adenovirus vector, 54–59, 67–68
Afghan Jews
    chromosome 9p1-q1, 209
    hereditary-IBM diagnosis, 205–206
    history, 202–204
age at diagnosis, 116, 118
age at onset
    asymptomatic leukoencephalopathy, 213
    as diagnostic criterion, 353
    distal myopathy with rimmed vacuoles,
        246–247, 250
    hereditary-IBM, 191–192
    and prognosis, 122
    sporadic-IBM, 87, 108, 116–117, 353
aging
    muscle and brain, 4
    and sporadic-IBM diagnosis, 353
AIDS, *see* HIV infection
alkaline phosphatase reaction, 7–8, 352
α-1-antichymotrypsin, 47, 50
"Alzheimer-characteristic" proteins
    hereditary-IBM, 47–52
    sporadic-IBM, 24–30, 93
Alzheimer's disease
    linkage analysis, hIBM candidate genes,
        207
    paired-helical filaments, 10
    sporadic-IBM phenotypic similarities,
        63–64
ambulatory period, 120
amyloid deposits; *see also* β-amyloid protein
    hereditary-IBM, 46–47
    oculopharyngeal muscular dystrophy,
        158–159

sporadic-IBM, 20–24, 46–47, 93, 110,
    144–147
amyotrophic lateral sclerosis
    electromyography, 353
    treatment response, 343, 372
amyotrophies, inhomogeneous findings, 89
androgen patch method, 369
angular fibers
    as diagnostic criterion, 84, 142–144, 351
    pathology, 142–144
    Welander distal myopathy, 223
animal retroviruses, 277
ankle-foot orthoses, 347
anterior abdominal muscles
    computed tomography, 196
    histology, 198
anterior tibial muscle, *see* tibialis anterior
    muscle
"anti-oxidant" formulations, 371
antisense studies, 54, 56
ApoE, 39–43
    hereditary-IBM accumulation, 47
    neuromuscular junction immunoreactiv-
        ity, 43
    sporadic-IBM accumulation, 40–43
    T lymphocyte activation role, 184–185
    transport of, 40, 42
ApoE-ε4 allele
    βA4 binding affinity, 184
    in sporadic-IBM, 42–43, 184–185
apoptosis
    atrophic fibers, 142–143
    Marinesco-Sjögren syndrome, 304
    muscle degeneration relationship, 304
    TUNEL technique evidence, 352
areflexia, 88
arthralgias, 365
asymmetrical weakness
    at time of diagnosis, 120
    and prognosis, 122–123